AGGRESSION

Clinical Features and Treatment
Across the Diagnostic Spectrum

AGGRESSION

Clinical Features and Treatment Across the Diagnostic Spectrum

Edited by

Emil F. Coccaro, M.D.
Michael S. McCloskey, Ph.D.

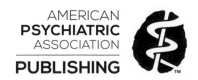

AMERICAN
PSYCHIATRIC
ASSOCIATION
PUBLISHING
TM

Copyright © 2019 American Psychiatric Association Publishing

ALL RIGHTS RESERVED

First Edition

Manufactured in the United States of America on acid-free paper
22   21   20   19   18   5   4   3   2   1

American Psychiatric Association Publishing
800 Maine Avenue SW
Suite 900
Washington, DC 20024-2812
www.appi.org

Library of Congress Cataloging-in-Publication Data
Names: Coccaro, Emil F., Jr. editor. | McCloskey, Michael S., editor.
Title: Aggression : clinical features and treatment across the diagnostic spectrum / edited by Emil F. Coccaro and Michael S. McCloskey. Other titles: Aggression (Coccaro)
Description: First edition. | Washington, D.C. : American Psychiatric Association Publishing, [2019] | Includes bibliographical references and index.
Identifiers: LCCN 2018045843 (print) | LCCN 2018046866 (ebook) | ISBN 9781615372454 (ebook) | ISBN 9781615371532 (pbk. : alk. paper)
Subjects: | MESH: Aggression—psychology | Mental Disorders—psychology Classification: LCC RC569.5.A34 (ebook) | LCC RC569.5.A34 (print) | NLM WM 600 | DDC 616.85/81—dc23
LC record available at https://lccn.loc.gov/2018045843
British Library Cataloguing in Publication Data
A CIP record is available from the British Library.

Contents

Part I
Primary Aggression:
Intermittent Explosive Disorder

Emil F. Coccaro, M.D.
Royce J. Lee, M.D.
Michael S. McCloskey, Ph.D.

Michael S. McCloskey, Ph.D.
Martha K. Fahlgren, M.A.
Emil F. Coccaro, M.D.

Part II
Aggression in Other Psychiatric Disorders

Contributors

Lindsay P. Bodell, Ph.D.
Assistant Professor, Department of Psychology, Western University, London, Ontario, Canada

Samuel R. Chamberlain, M.B./B.Chir., Ph.D., M.R.C.Psych.
Wellcome Trust Clinical Fellow, Department of Psychiatry, University of Cambridge; Honorary Consultant Psychiatrist, Cambridge and Peterborough NHS Foundation Trust, Cambridge, England, United Kingdom

Leslie Citrome, M.D., M.P.H.
Clinical Professor, Department of Psychiatry and Behavioral Sciences, New York Medical College, Valhalla, New York

Emil F. Coccaro, M.D.
E.C. Manning Professor and Director, Clinical Neuroscience and Psychopharmacology Research Unit, Department of Psychiatry and Behavioral Neuroscience, The University of Chicago, Chicago, Illinois

Craig Erickson, M.D.
Professor of Psychiatry, Cincinnati Children's Hospital, Cincinnati, Ohio

Martha K. Fahlgren, M.A.
Doctoral Student, Department of Psychology, Temple University, Philadelphia, Pennsylvania

Jennifer R. Fanning, Ph.D.
Pathways to Independence Instructor, Clinical Neuroscience Research Unit, Department of Psychiatry and Behavioral Neuroscience, The University of Chicago, Pritzker School of Medicine, Chicago, Illinois

Maurizio Fava, M.D.
Professor and Executive Vice-Chair, Department of Psychiatry, Massachusetts General Hospital, Harvard Medical School, Boston, Massachusetts

Sarah E. Fitzpatrick, B.S.
M.D./Ph.D. Student, Yale School of Medicine, New Haven, Connecticut

Daniel J. Fridberg, Ph.D.
Assistant Professor, Department of Psychiatry and Behavioral Neuroscience, The University of Chicago, Illinois

David T. George, M.D.
Senior Investigator, National Institute on Alcohol Abuse and Alcoholism, Bethesda, Maryland

Kyle R. Gerst, M.Sc.
Doctoral Candidate, Department of Psychological and Brain Sciences, Indiana University, Bloomington, Indiana

Caroline W. Grant, B.A.
Intramural Research Training Award recipient, National Institute on Alcohol Abuse and Alcoholism, Bethesda, Maryland

Jon E. Grant, J.D., M.D., M.P.H.
Professor, Department of Psychiatry and Behavioral Neuroscience, The University of Chicago, Illinois

Michael Greenage, D.O.
Assistant Professor and Residency Program Director, Department of Psychiatry and Behavioral Medicine, Virginia Tech/Carilion School of Medicine and Carilion Clinic, Roanoke, Virginia

Rachel L. Gunn, Ph.D.
Postdoctoral Research Fellow, Center for Alcohol and Addiction Studies, Brown University School of Public Health, Providence, Rhode Island

Richard G. Heimberg, Ph.D.
Thaddeus L. Bolton Professor of Psychology, Department of Psychology, Temple University, Philadelphia, Pennsylvania

Iliyan Ivanov, M.D.
Associate Professor, Department of Psychiatry, Icahn School of Medicine at Mount Sinai, New York, New York

Karen M. Jennings, Ph.D., R.N., A.P.R.N.
Assistant Professor, College of Nursing, University of Rhode Island, Kingston, Rhode Island

Paul E. Keck, Jr., M.D.
President and Chief Executive Officer, Lindner Center of HOPE, Mason, Ohio; Frances & Craig Lindner Professor and Executive Vice Chair, Department of Psychiatry and Behavioral Neuroscience, University of Cincinnati College of Medicine, Cincinnati, Ohio

Beth Krone, Ph.D.
Clinical Research Coordinator, Department of Psychiatry, Icahn School of Medicine at Mount Sinai, New York, New York

Royce J. Lee, M.D.
Associate Professor and Medical Director, Clinical Neuroscience and Psychopharmacology Research Unit, Department of Psychiatry and Behavioral Neuroscience, The University of Chicago, Chicago, Illinois

Ellen Leibenluft, M.D.
Director, Section on Bipolar Spectrum Disorders, Emotion and Development Branch, Intramural Research Program, National Institute of Mental Health, Bethesda, Maryland

Brian E. Martens, L.S.W., M.S., C.C.R.C.
Research Coordinator, Lindner Center of HOPE, Mason, Ohio; Research Coordinator, Department of Psychiatry and Behavioral Neuroscience, University of Cincinnati College of Medicine, Cincinnati, Ohio

Michael S. McCloskey, Ph.D.
Associate Professor, Director of Clinical Science Training, and Director of the Mechanisms of Affect Dysregulation Laboratory, Department of Psychology, Temple University, Philadelphia, Pennsylvania

Susan L. McElroy, M.D.
Chief Research Officer, Lindner Center of HOPE, Mason, Ohio; Linda & Harry Fath Professor, Department of Psychiatry and Behavioral Neuroscience, University of Cincinnati College of Medicine, Cincinnati, Ohio

Jeffrey Newcorn, M.D.
Professor, Departments of Psychiatry and Pediatrics, Icahn School of Medicine at Mount Sinai, New York, New York

Emily B. O'Day, B.A.
Doctoral Student in Clinical Psychology, Department of Psychology, Temple University, Philadelphia, Pennsylvania

Laura C. Politte, M.D.
Assistant Professor of Psychiatry and Pediatrics, Carolina Institute for Developmental Disabilities, University of North Carolina Chapel Hill, North Carolina

Robert L. Trestman, Ph.D., M.D.
Professor and Chair, Department of Psychiatry and Behavioral Medicine, Virginia Tech/Carilion School of Medicine and Carilion Clinic, Roanoke, Virginia

Jan Volavka, M.D., Ph.D.
Professor Emeritus, Department of Psychiatry, New York University School of Medicine, New York; Professor, Department of Psychiatry, Charles University School of Medicine, Pilsen, Czech Republic

Jennifer E. Wildes, Ph.D.
Associate Professor and Director of the Eating Disorders Program, Department of Psychiatry & Behavioral Neuroscience, The University of Chicago, Chicago, Illinois

Disclosure of Competing Interests

The following contributors to this book have indicated a financial interest in or other affiliation with a commercial supporter, a manufacturer of a commercial product, a provider of a commercial service, a nongovernmental organization, and/or a government agency, as listed below:

Samuel R. Chamberlain, M.B./B.Chir., Ph.D., M.R.C.Psych.—*Research grant:* Wellcome Trust Clinical Fellowship; *Consultant:* Cambridge Cognition, Shire

Leslie Citrome, M.D., M.P.H.—*Consultant:* Acadia, Alkermes, Allergan, Intra-Cellular Therapies, Janssen, Lundbeck, Merck, Neurocrine, Noven, Otsuka, Pfizer, Shire, Sunovion, Takeda, Teva, Vanda; *Speaker:* Acadia, Alkermes, Allergan, Janssen, Lundbeck, Merck, Neurocrine, Noven, Otsuka, Pfizer, Shire, Sunovion, Takeda, Teva, Vanda; *Shareholder:* Bristol-Myers Squibb, Eli Lilly, J & J Merck, Pfizer; *Royalties:* Wiley (Editor-in-Chief, *International Journal of Clinical Practice*), UpToDate (reviewer), Springer Healthcare (book)

Emil F. Coccaro, M.D.—*Grant:* National Institute of Mental Health; *Consultant and scientific advisory board member:* Avanir Pharmaceuticals, Azevan Pharmaceuticals

Maurizio Fava, M.D.—*See https://mghcme.org/faculty/faculty-detail/ maurizio_fava for listing of lifetime disclosures.*

Jon E. Grant, J.D., M.D., M.P.H.—*Research grants:* American Foundation for Suicide Prevention, Forest Pharmaceuticals, National Center for Responsible Gaming, National Institute on Drug Abuse; Roche; *Editor-in-Chief* (compensation): Springer Publishing (*Journal of Gambling Studies*); *Royalties:* American Psychiatric Association Publishing; Johns Hopkins Press, McGraw-Hill, Oxford University Press, WW Norton

Paul E. Keck, Jr., M.D.—*Consultant:* Lyndra, Otsuka; *Patent:* Dr. Keck is a co-inventor on U.S. Patent No. 6,387,956: Shapira NA, Goldsmith TD, Keck PE Jr (University of Cincinnati): "Methods of Treating Obsessive-Compulsive Spectrum Disorder Comprises the Step of Administering an Effective Amount of Tramadol to an Individual" (filed March 25, 1999; approved May 14, 2002). Dr. Keck has received no financial gain from this patent.

Royce J. Lee, M.D.—*Clinical trial support:* Avanir Pharmaceuticals (for an investigational compound for the treatment of aggression)

Michael S. McCloskey, Ph.D.—*Consultant:* Avanir Pharmaceuticals

Susan L. McElroy, M.D.—*Research support* (as principal investigator or co-investigator): Allergan, Brainsway, Marriott Foundation, Myriad, National Institute of Mental Health, Novo Nordisk, Shire, Sunovion; *Consultant and/or scientific advisory board member:* Bracket, F. Hoffmann–La Roche Ltd., MedAvante, Mitsubishi Tanabe Pharma America, Myriad, Novo Nordisk, Shire, Sunovion; *Patent:* Dr. McElroy is inventor on U.S. Patent No. 6,323,236 B2, "Use of Sulfamate Derivatives for Treating Impulse Control Disorders," and, along with the patent's assignee, University of Cincinnati, OH, has received payments from Johnson & Johnson Pharmaceutical Research and Development, L.L.C., which has exclusive rights under the patent.

Jeffrey Newcorn, M.D.—*Research support:* Enzymotec, Shire, Supernus; *Advisor/Consultant:* Akili Interactive, Alcobra, Arbor, Cingulate Therapeutics, Enzymotec, KemPharm, NFL, NLS Pharma, Rhodes, Shire, Sunovion, Supernus

The following contributors have indicated that they have no financial interests or other affiliations that represent or could appear to represent a competing interest with the contributions to this book:

Lindsay P. Bodell, Ph.D.

Craig Erickson, M.D.

Martha K. Fahlgren, M.A.

Jennifer R. Fanning, Ph.D.

Sarah E. Fitzpatrick, B.S.

Daniel J. Fridberg, Ph.D.

David T. George, M.D.

Kyle R. Gerst, M.Sc.

Caroline W. Grant, B.A.

Michael Greenage, D.O.

Rachel L. Gunn, Ph.D.

Richard G. Heimberg, Ph.D.

Iliyan Ivanov, M.D.

Karen M. Jennings, Ph.D., R.N.

Beth Krone, Ph.D.

Ellen Leibenluft, M.D.

Brian E. Martens, L.S.W., M.S.

Emily B. O'Day, B.A.

Laura C. Politte, M.D.

Robert L. Trestman, Ph.D., M.D.

Jan Volavka, M.D., Ph.D.

Jennifer E. Wildes, Ph.D.

Preface

Aggression is one of our basic drives—a drive that is adaptive in the context that it enables us to secure the resources we need to live and to protect ourselves and our loved ones. However, as human civilization has advanced, aggression has become an increasingly ineffective strategy for productive living in social groups. For the most part, aggressive behavior is not needed to obtain the things we need to live and thrive. Instead, our objectives can usually be achieved through our ability to influence others peacefully (e.g., by reciprocation or through cooperation).

That said, civilizing processes do not negate our basic biological drives, and the instinct to turn to aggressive behavior when we feel threatened remains. Furthermore, the human organism remains saddled with psychobiological systems that may increase the risk of behavioral aggression when selected systems are abnormal in some way. While many consider these systems to involve neurochemistry and neural circuits, influences associated with genetics, epigenetics, and our environmental forces are also extremely important.

For the purposes of this volume, we are defining *human aggression* as behavior by one individual directed at another person or object in which either verbal force or physical force is used to injure, to coerce, or to express anger. Although aggression can occur in the context of a socially sanctioned role (e.g., soldiers or law enforcement) or in the context of a medical condition that affects mental status, we focus mostly on aggression that is impulsive or reactive in nature and aggression that is premeditated or instrumental in nature, though we note that the former is far more prevalent than the latter.

Until recently, aggression was primarily examined as a dimensional construct. The first time that the field of psychiatry considered recurrent and prominent aggressive behavior as a disorder was with the publication of the *Diagnostic and Statistical Manual of Mental Disorders*

(DSM) in 1952 (American Psychiatric Association 1952). This first edition of DSM listed "Passive Aggressive Personality (Aggressive Type)" as a disorder of aggression and described individuals with this disorder as having "a persistent reaction to frustration with irritability, temper tantrums, and destructive behavior" (p. 37). This disorder evolved into "Explosive Personality (Epileptoid Personality Disorder)" for DSM-II in 1968 (American Psychiatric Association 1968). Patients with this disorder were characterized as being aggressive individuals who display intermittently violent behavior and who are "generally considered excitable, aggressive and over-responsive to environmental pressures" with "gross outbursts of rage or of verbal or physical aggressiveness" that are "strikingly different from…[their] usual behavior" (p. 42). This changed, in 1980, with publication of DSM-III (American Psychiatric Association 1980), which included the diagnosis of "Intermittent Explosive Disorder" (IED). IED in DSM-III (and even more so in DSM-IV [American Psychiatric Association 1994]), however, was mostly considered to be a disorder of exclusion and, perhaps, a disorder related in some way to epilepsy, though there has been little evidence for the latter. In fact, the DSM-III and DSM-IV criteria for IED were poorly operationalized in terms of severity and frequency of aggressive behavior and were written in a way that the diagnosis was excluded by the presence of most other disorders. Consequently, little research was done in this area because it appeared that few people could possibly have IED.

This situation changed in the 1990s after the availability of agents acting on the serotonin (5-HT) system became available. A variety of animal and human studies supported the hypothesis that impulsive aggressive rather than premeditated aggression was associated with reduced function of the central 5-HT system. With the then-new availability of fluoxetine in the world market, studies were conducted to see if increasing 5-HT in the brain would reduce aggression in those individuals who were highly aggressive. Findings from initial trials were positive, as were those from the first set of double-blind, placebo-controlled trials. Fluoxetine was not a "magic bullet," but it appeared to reduce impulsive aggression to, at the very least, a moderate degree.

The next question was to determine what kind of diagnosis one could use for further study of impulsive aggressive behavior. The best starting point was with the DSM-III-R criteria for IED (American Psychiatric Association 1987), which investigators, including the editors of this volume, modified to create a set of research diagnostic criteria that could be used for this purpose. Over the next 20 years or more, investigators worked through a few versions of research criteria sets for IED that were later approved for inclusion in DSM-5 (American Psychiatric Association 2013). This work is discussed in Chapter 1 of this volume, on primary aggression. The treatment of IED is then addressed in Chapter 2.

Although IED is the only disorder for which aggression is pathognomonic, several other psychological disorders are associated with aggression, and this complicates their presentation and treatment. The rest of this volume covers aggression that takes place in the context of these other psychiatric disorders. Chapter 3 reviews clinical and treatment aspects of aggression in the context of autism spectrum disorder and other developmental disorders. Chapter 4 reviews the same for disruptive behavioral disorders of childhood, including attention-deficit/hyperactivity disorder, oppositional defiant disorder, and conduct disorder. Chapter 5 focuses on aggression in the context of psychosis, while Chapter 6 focuses on the same in bipolar disorders. Chapter 7 addresses unipolar depressive disorders and reviews aggression in the context of anger attacks in major depression and of disruptive mood dysregulation disorder, a diagnosis that was developed to allow clinicians a clearer picture of chronic irritability in childhood and how it differs from pediatric bipolar disorder. Chapter 8 focuses on aggression in the context of anxiety disorders, while Chapter 9 focuses on aggression in the context of obsessive-compulsive disorder. Chapter 10 focuses on anger and aggression in the context of posttraumatic stress disorder, while the role of aggression in the context of eating disorders is covered in Chapter 11. The role of aggression in alcohol use disorder (including the role of alcohol in aggression) and substance use disorder is discussed in Chapters 12 and 13, respectively. The volume closes with a review of aggression in the context of personality disorders (Chapter 14) followed by an overview of the legal and forensic aspects of aggression (Chapter 15).

This volume is not meant to be comprehensive. For example, we do not include a chapter on aggressive behavior in late life because most of this work has been conducted in the context of agitation in late life and the dementias. While agitation may be confused with aggression, it is not aggression in the way we have defined it. In addition, we have not covered the possible presence of aggression in other psychiatric disorders or medical disorders in this volume.

That said, we hope you find this volume helpful to you in your understanding of aggression, particularly impulsive aggression, in your patients and others in your life.

Emil F. Coccaro, M.D.
Michael S. McCloskey, Ph.D.

References

American Psychiatric Association: Diagnostic and Statistical Manual: Mental Disorders. Washington, DC, American Psychiatric Association, 1952

American Psychiatric Association: Diagnostic and Statistical Manual of Mental Disorders, 2nd Edition. Washington, DC, American Psychiatric Association, 1968

American Psychiatric Association: Diagnostic and Statistical Manual of Mental Disorders, 3rd Edition. Washington, DC, American Psychiatric Association, 1980

American Psychiatric Association: Diagnostic and Statistical Manual of Mental Disorders, 3rd Edition, Revised. Washington, DC, American Psychiatric Association, 1987

American Psychiatric Association: Diagnostic and Statistical Manual of Mental Disorders, 4th Edition. Washington, DC, American Psychiatric Association, 1994

American Psychiatric Association: Diagnostic and Statistical Manual of Mental Disorders, 5th Edition. Arlington, VA, American Psychiatric Association, 2013

PART I

Primary Aggression:
Intermittent Explosive
Disorder

1

Phenomenology and Psychobiology of Aggression and Intermittent Explosive Disorder

Emil F. Coccaro, M.D.
Royce J. Lee, M.D.
Michael S. McCloskey, Ph.D.

Human aggression occurs when an individual assaults or attacks another in the context of defense or in the context of securing access to resources needed for survival. As such, aggression represents a fundamental aspect of human behavior. Over the course of civilization, however, human aggression has become less advantageous, with the use of aggression for reasons other than self-defense generally viewed as unacceptable. In this chapter, we examine the biology of primary aggression both as a continuum and as a clinical diagnosis.

Aggression as a Continuum

Phenomenology

Aggressive behavior can vary in both form and type. With respect to form, aggression can be verbal (e.g., snapping, name-calling, arguments, threats) and/or physical (e.g., throwing things, breaking things, pushing or hitting someone, physically injuring someone). The aggression can also be direct (yelling at or hitting someone) or indirect (gossiping about someone, damaging an object). Indirect aggression aimed at damaging a person's interpersonal relationships is called *relational aggression* (Murray-Close et al. 2010). What all forms of aggression have in common is intent to harm, though the function or "type" of aggression may differ.

Aggression can be *socially sanctioned* (as in, e.g., soldiers and law enforcement) or *medically related*. Neither type of aggression is typically the focus of aggression interventions, because in the former the aggression is not seen as problematic and in the latter there is a clear medical cause for the behavior. Other, more "primary" types of aggression are *premeditated* (i.e., instrumental) aggression and *impulsive* (i.e., affective or reactive) aggression (Barratt et al. 1997; Dodge 1991). The critical difference between these types of aggression is that in premeditated aggression, the harm caused by the aggressive behavior is merely a means to an end (e.g., punching someone to steal his or her wallet), whereas in the case of impulsive aggression the desire to harm another is a primary goal of the aggressive act (e.g., to take revenge). Though aggressive acts can include both instrumental and impulsive facets, most aggression is predominantly impulsive. Furthermore, primary aggression can be viewed both along a continuum (i.e., dimensionally) and as a dichotomy between normative and pathological aggression (i.e., diagnostically).

Psychobiology

Psychobiological studies involving human aggression as a dimension are numerous and involve those related to behavioral genetics and neurobiology (i.e., central and peripheral neurochemistry and dynamic responsiveness to neurotransmitter challenge) and neuroimaging. Impulsive aggressive behavior, in particular, appears to be associated with significant genetic influence and with reduced function in inhibitory neural pathways and/or an imbalance in inhibitory and excitatory influences on behavioral responses to social threat and/or frustration.

Behavioral Genetics

Aggression is under both genetic and environmental influence, with up to 50% of the variability in measures of aggression accounted for by genetic factors (Miles and Carey 1997). Our own twin studies using aggression support these findings, showing that the genetic influence of the aggression increases with the severity of the aggressive acts. Specifically, genetic influence is 28% for verbal aggression, 35% for aggression against objects, and 45% for aggression against others (Coccaro et al. 1997a). In addition, impulsivity is under similar genetic influence in these types of studies, and the genetic correlation of impulsivity and aggression is correspondingly substantial, supporting the conceptualization of aggression as a form of dysregulation (Seroczynski et al. 1999).

Neurobiology

The neurobiological study of human aggression began in the 1970s when Brown and colleagues (1979, 1982) reported a strong inverse relationship between cerebrospinal fluid (CSF) 5-hydroxyindoleacetic acid (5-HIAA) levels, an index of serotonin (5-HT) function, and a lifetime measure of aggressive behavior—a finding consistent with previous animal studies reporting inverse relationships between 5-HT and aggressive responding (Valzelli and Garattini 1968). This relationship has also been reported in other studies of severely aggressive individuals (Linnoila et al. 1983, Virkkunen et al. 1987, 1989) but not in those involving individuals with less intense aggressive behavior (Coccaro et al. 1997b, 1997c; Møller et al. 1996). In addition to this inverse correlation between CSF 5-HIAA and aggression, inverse correlations with aggression have also been reported with the hormonal responsiveness to 5-HT selective agents (Duke et al. 2013), including fenfluramine (an indirect 5-HT agonist: Coccaro et al. 1989, 2010a), ipsapirone (a 5-HT_{1A} agonist: Almeida et al. 2010), and *m*-chlorophenylpiperazine (m-CPP) (a 5-HT_{2C} receptor agonist: Coccaro et al. 1997b; Moss et al. 1990). These latter studies suggest that 5-HT receptors are sub-sensitive to 5-HT activation so that there is a reduction in 5-HT activity and, thus, in 5-HT-mediated behavioral inhibition.

Other neurochemical systems may also be relevant in human aggression. At this time, there are preliminary data supporting positive relationships between aggression and catecholamines (norepinephrine: Coccaro et al. 2003; dopamine: Coccaro and Lee 2010; Limson et al. 1991), other amines (glutamate: Coccaro et al. 2013), peptides (vasopressin: Coccaro et al. 1998; substance P: Coccaro et al. 2012b; neuropeptide Y: Coccaro et al. 2012a), and circulating cytokines (e.g., interleukin-6 [IL-6]: Coccaro et al. 2014; Marsland et al. 2008; Suarez 2003). There are similar data supporting an inverse relationship between aggression and oxytocin (Lee et al. 2009). However, with the exception of studies manipulating 5-HT as a strategy to reduce (Dougherty et al. 1999) or increase (Berman et al. 2009) impulsive aggression, few studies have been conducted to explore how manipulating non-5-HT systems reduces, or has no effect on, impulsive aggressive behavior in humans.

Molecular Genetics

Molecular genetic studies of aggression are far fewer than those for other psychiatric disorders, such as schizophrenia and depressive and bipolar disorders. The first candidate gene study of relevance reported that five individuals, in a Dutch kindred with X-linked borderline intellectual ability, had recurrent impulsive aggressive behavior, low activity for the enzyme monoamine oxidase A (MAO-A), elevated urinary levels of noradrenergic metabolites, and reduced urinary levels of both serotonergic and dopaminergic metabolites (Brunner et al. 1993). Although subsequent studies did not replicate these findings in unaffected males (Rosenberg et al. 2006), a stepwise relationship between low MAO-A activity, early life trauma, and aggression and criminality in young adult males (Caspi et al. 2002), as well as increased aggression in MAO-A knockout mice compared with wild-type mice (Scott et al. 2008), has been reported. A more recent study, involving healthy volunteers, reported an inverse relationship between brain MAO-A activity, assessed with positron emission tomography (PET), and aggression across several cortical and subcortical areas (Alia-Klein et al. 2008).

The next candidate gene study involved polymorphisms of the gene for tryptophan hydroxylase (TPH), an enzyme catalyzing the reaction that serves as the rate-limiting step in the synthesis of 5-HT, with studies involving healthy volunteers reporting a relationship between aggression and the U allele of the TPH polymorphism (Manuck et al. 1999). Another important candidate gene study in this area involves the relationship between polymorphisms of the 5-HT transporter (5-HTT) and antisocial behavior and aggression. Meta-analysis of these studies reveals a moderately strong association between presence of the s allele (with reduced synthesis of the 5-HTT) and aggression across many studies (Ficks and Waldman 2014). A number of other studies report a relationship between polymorphisms for the gene related to catechol O-methyltransferase (COMT), an enzyme that metabolizes norepinephrine and dopamine, and aggression. In one study of patients with schizophrenia, the presence of the Met/Met (low COMT activity) versus the Val/Val (high COMT activity) genotype was associated with aggression (Tosato et al. 2011), a finding confirmed in two meta-analytic studies (Bhakta et al. 2012; Singh et al. 2012). Selected haplotypes of the COMT gene were also associated with aggression in a separate study of schizophrenia patients (Gu et al. 2009), whereas no association between COMT polymorphisms and aggression was reported in a more recent study involving patients with schizophrenia (Mohamed Saini et al. 2015). Another, modestly sized study of individuals with personality disorders reported that individuals with the G allele for COMT had higher aggression scores compared with individuals with other genotypes (Flory et al. 2007), Lastly, individuals with schizophrenia who have the Val/Met genotype for the gene associated with brain-derived neurotrophic factor (BDNF) were reported to have higher aggression scores compared with those with the Val/Val genotype in one study (Spalletta et al. 2010) but not two other studies (Chung et al. 2010; Guan et al. 2014) involving patients with schizophrenia.

Molecular Epigenetics

Beyond strict genetic influence, environmental factors are critical, and these factors account for more of the variance in measures of aggression than do genetic factors (Coccaro et al. 1997a). Environmental factors in aggression include, among others, history of childhood trauma, witnessing of aggression, modeling of aggressive behavior observed in parents and caretakers, history of head trauma, and aversive social interaction in the "here and now" (Crick and Dodge 1996). These factors operate, at least partially, through epigenetic mechanisms that work to turn genes on and off. For example, greater methylation of the 5-HTT promoter has been reported in young adults with prominent histories of physical aggression in whom PET studies also show reduced synthesis of 5-HT, bilaterally, in the orbitofrontal cortex (OFC) (Wang et al. 2012).

Structural Neuroimaging

Neuroimaging studies have begun to identify sites of neurotransmitter action in the brain, mostly in regard to 5-HT. The first published study in this area reported reduced glucose metabolism on PET in the left OFC and anterior cingulate cortex (ACC) in six impulsively aggressive individuals, compared with five healthy control subjects, after *d,l*-fenfluramine challenge (Siever et al. 1999). A similar finding was reported in a larger subject group using m-CPP challenge (New et al. 2002). In addition, a 12-week course of treatment with fluoxetine normalized OFC function in a similar group of impulsively aggressive subjects, supporting the idea that deficits in OFC function are at least partially accounted for by abnormalities in 5-HT function (New et al. 2004a). Other neuroimaging studies suggest that impulsively aggressive individuals have abnormal 5-HT synthesis and reuptake in medial frontal gyrus, anterior cingulate gyrus, superior temporal gyrus, and corpus striatum compared with healthy control subjects (Leyton et al. 2001).

Functional Neuroimaging

In addition to neuroimaging studies relating to neurochemistry, other studies have reported on structural and functional aspects of the brain as they relate to aggression. The first published studies in this area reported reduced glucose utilization in prefrontal and temporal cortices in individuals with a history of violence (Volkow et al. 1995) and an inverse correlation between glucose utilization in the prefrontal cortex with life history of aggression in subjects with personality disorders (Goyer et al. 1994). Later studies suggested metabolic hypoactivity in frontal brain regions, and hyperactivity in subcortical regions, in impulsive aggressive murderers compared with healthy control subjects (Raine et al. 1998). Subsequent structural magnetic resonance imaging (MRI) studies have reported a significant reduction of prefrontal volume in individuals with antisocial personality disorder compared with a control group (Raine et al. 2000). Functional MRI (fMRI) studies of healthy subjects show that anger-inducing paradigms activate the prefrontal cortex (Blair et al. 1999; Damasio et al. 2000; Dougherty et al. 1999; Kimbrell et al. 1999), while similar studies report reduced activity in this area in typically aggressive individuals with borderline personality disorder (Soloff et al. 2000).

In addition to the prefrontal cortex, the amygdala is also involved in the regulation of aggression, as demonstrated by the fact that electrical stimulation of the amygdala increases aggression and amygdalectomy reduces aggression (see Eichelman 1983). Despite this observation, both epileptic patients with episodic aggressive outbursts (van Elst et al. 2000) and individuals with antisocial personality disorder (Veit et al. 2002) have been shown to have reduced amygdalar volume, a finding that might suggest reduced activation of the amygdala when stimulated.

Summary

Studies of aggression as a continuum suggest significant genetic, epigenetic, and biological influences, most notably 5-HT deficits and dysregulation of the frontolimbic brain circuits. Though it is likely that the biobehavioral relationship between aggression and its neurobiological substrate is primarily dimensional in nature, there is also some support for the possibility that pathological aggression is qualitatively distinct from aggression of lesser severity (Ahmed et al. 2010). Furthermore, interventions designed to reduce impulsive aggression require diagnostic criteria for the identification of who could, or should, be treated for problematic impulsive aggressive behavior. To date, the *Diagnostic and Statistical Manual of Mental Disorders* (DSM) diagnosis that best represents pathological primary aggression is intermittent explosive disorder (IED) (American Psychiatric Association 2013).

Impulsive Aggression as Clinical Diagnosis: Intermittent Explosive Disorder

When sufficiently frequent and severe, impulsive aggression may meet the DSM-5 diagnosis of intermittent explosive disorder (American Psychiatric Association 2013; see also Coccaro 2012). Impulsive aggression is also observed in other diagnostic conditions, but when aggression is not directly due to another psychiatric disorder, a diagnosis of IED may be made. In this way, IED represents a disorder of primary impulsive aggression, while other behavioral disorders in which aggression may occur (e.g., psychosis, mania) can be referred to as disorders of secondary aggression.

Phenomenology

Diagnostic Criteria

The essence of recurrent problematic impulsive aggression has been in the DSM since its first edition. However, criteria for IED did not unequivocally require impulsive aggression as its hallmark characteristic until the fifth edition. IED in DSM-5 is characterized by at least one of the following types of impulsive aggressive outbursts (Coccaro 2011): frequent but low-intensity verbal or physical outbursts occurring twice weekly, on average, for at least 3 months or infrequent but high-intensity behavioral outbursts occurring three times per year. The outbursts are out of proportion to stressors (i.e., provocation), impulsive and anger based (i.e., not premeditated), associated with marked distress and impairment, and not better accounted for by another mental disorder or medical condition (i.e., outbursts do not only occur during the presence of another disorder). Generally, IED has its onset in childhood and peaks in adolescence: Studies of adults report the mean age at onset as the midteens (Coccaro et al. 2005; Kessler et al. 2006); studies of adolescents report the mean age at onset as about 12 years (McLaughlin et al. 2012). The mean duration of IED ranges from more than 10 years to nearly the whole lifetime, which suggests a persistent and chronic course without treatment. A large (2:1) preponderance of males over females has been suggested by small clinical reports, though community survey data suggest this ratio is closer to 1.5:1.0 (Kessler et al. 2006). Other sociodemographic variables (e.g., age, race, education, marital status, occupational status, family income) show only modest correlations with IED, suggesting that the disorder cuts cross racial and sociocultural groups (Kessler et al. 2006).

Epidemiology

Though early versions of DSM characterized IED as a "rare" disorder, subsequent studies suggest that IED may be among the more common psychiatric (DSM-IV; American Psychiatric Association 1994) disorders in the United States (Kessler et al. 2006). The National Comorbidity Survey Replication (NCS-R) reported a lifetime prevalence of DSM-IV IED in the United States of 7.3% by "broad criteria" and 5.4% by "narrow criteria," and a past-year prevalence of 3.9%, and 2.7%, respectively (Kessler et al. 2006). Inspection of the data reveals meaningful differences between the two IED types, with "narrow" IED being far more severe than "broad" IED (Coccaro 2012). "Broad" IED stipulates only three aggressive outbursts during a lifetime, whereas "narrow" IED required at least three aggressive outbursts in a single year.

The prevalence of IED may not be as high in non-U.S. countries, however, where the lifetime estimate of DSM-IV IED may range from only 0.1% (i.e., Nigeria) to 1.2% (i.e., Colombia, South Africa), with an average of 0.6%, compared with 2.7% for the United States (Scott et al. 2016). Reasons for this cross-national difference are not known with any certainty but are likely related to variation in general risk factors, cultural factors that have an impact on willingness to disclose information about one's own psychopathology, and other methodological factors.

The lower rate for the United States in the cross-national study is attributable to the fact that the algorithm used to make the DSM-IV diagnosis of IED required the presence of impairment, on the Sheehan Disability Scale, in addition to three anger attacks in the same year. A separate analysis of the U.S. data using different impairment criteria suggests that the lifetime rate of DSM-IV IED in the United States is 3.6% (Coccaro et al. 2017b), down from the 5.4% in the original report (Kessler et al. 2006). In addition, a survey study of more than 5,300 nondeployed army service members (Army STARRS) reported lifetime pre- and postenlistment rates of DSM-IV IED of 15.5% and 4.8%, respectively (Nock et al. 2014). Despite these data, the community rate of DSM-5 IED is not known, because DSM-5 criteria for IED require either low-intensity but high-frequency impulsive aggressive outbursts (Criterion A1) or high-intensity but low-frequency outbursts (Criterion A2).

Since the data instrument used in the NCS-R (Kessler et al. 2006) and the cross-national study (Scott et al. 2016) only sought information about Criterion A2, not A1 (i.e., type of impulsive aggressive outbursts), the prevalence of IED diagnosed on the basis of only Criterion A1 in the NCS-R sample is unknown. New data from our own studies suggest that more than one-fifth of those with current IED meet Cri-

terion A1 only (had only frequent nondestructive/noninjurious outbursts) and not Criterion A2 (E.F. Coccaro et al., data on file). If so,
one might estimate the lifetime prevalence of DSM-5 IED in the United
States as 3.3% (using data from Scott et al. 2016) to 4.4% (using data
from Coccaro et al. 2017b), at least until another community survey is
done assessing the epidemiology of DSM-5 disorders.

Psychosocial Consequences

Not surprisingly, individuals with IED experience significant psychosocial consequences as a result of recurrent, impulsive aggressive behavior. First, global psychosocial function is reduced in individuals
with IED compared with both healthy and psychiatric control subjects (Kulper et al. 2015), as is quality of life experience, even when
differences in global psychosocial function are accounted for (Rynar
and Coccaro 2018). Examined more closely, individuals with IED report greater dysfunction while at work and with family and friends
(Kulper et al. 2015).

Psychiatric Comorbidity

Because impulsive aggressive behavior appears in patients with many
diagnoses, most clinicians have been reluctant to make a diagnosis of
IED in the absence of other psychiatric diagnoses. In fact, impulsive
aggressive behavior is manifest in all humans early in life and before
the onset of other psychiatric disorders. In the vast majority of people,
impulsive aggressive behaviors diminish over time—frequently well
before adolescence (Tremblay 2013). In the adolescent supplement
to the NCS-R, lifetime prevalence of DSM-IV IED by "narrow" criteria was 5.3% (McLaughlin et al. 2012), a rate similar to that found in
adults (Kessler et al. 2006). Clinical studies suggest significant comorbidity of IED with mood disorders, anxiety disorders, and substance use disorders (see, e.g., Coccaro 2011). IED has been reported to
have an earlier age at onset than any of the comorbid disorders, with
the exception of phobic anxiety disorders. This suggests that IED and
the comorbid disorder may be independent or that IED might be a risk
factor for the comorbid disorder. A similar finding was found in a family history study of IED (Coccaro 2010).

　　Some clinical investigators claim that the diagnosis of IED should
not be made in the presence of borderline personality disorder (BPD)
or antisocial personality disorder (AsPD). When the issue is exam-

ined empirically, however, levels of lifetime aggressive behavior among individuals with BPD or AsPD only are markedly lower than the levels among those whose symptoms also meet criteria for IED, indicating that both diagnoses should be made when the criteria for both are met (Coccaro 2012).

Medical Comorbidity

A reanalysis of a large community data set has demonstrated evidence of a relationship between various medical conditions and DSM-IV IED (McCloskey et al. 2010). Specifically, individuals with IED have an increased risk of coronary heart disease, hypertension, stroke, diabetes, arthritis, back and neck pain, ulcer, headaches, and other chronic pain. Another study reports a significant correlation between IED and diabetes (de Jonge et al. 2014). A factor tying together many of these conditions (e.g., coronary heart disease, stroke, arthritis, ulcer) may be abnormalities of immune function. For example, elevations of plasma inflammatory proteins (C-reactive protein [CRP] and IL-6) have been reported in individuals with IED compared with psychiatric and healthy control subjects (Coccaro et al. 2014). In addition, a history of aggressive behavior was also shown to directly correlate with levels of CRP and IL-6. It is not known if these elevations are causal to aggression as suggested by animal studies or merely associated with aggressive behavior (Zalcman and Siegel 2006). However, recent data suggest that the relationship between aggression and elevated levels of inflammatory cytokines is not likely due to changes in serotonin metabolism (Coccaro et al. 2016c).

Those with IED are also at risk for latent toxoplasmosis, a parasite that infects many worldwide. In a recent study involving more than 300 participants (Coccaro et al. 2016d), those with IED were more likely to be seropositive for IgG antibodies to *Toxoplasma gondii* compared with healthy and psychiatric control subjects; *T. gondii* seropositivity was also associated with higher aggression but was not associated with state depression or anxiety scores. Additional studies are needed to determine if there is a rationale for treating the low-grade inflammation, or latent toxoplasmosis, that may be present in individuals with IED.

The medical and comorbid psychiatric problems associated with IED highlight the importance of examining antecedents and correlates of IED in order to identify potential mechanisms of prevention and intervention.

Developmental Antecedents

A history of trauma in childhood has long been thought to be associated with the development of aggression later in childhood and in adolescence (Dodge 1991). The few studies published on IED support this association. For example, Nickerson and colleagues (2012) found that interpersonal traumas and early life traumas are particularly predictive of IED. We also found that IED was associated with higher scores on the Childhood Trauma Questionnaire (CTQ) and lower scores related to parental care relative to both psychiatric and healthy control subjects (Fanning et al. 2014; Lee et al. 2014). Furthermore, CTQ scores were correlated with hostile attribution bias scores that were significantly greater in individuals with IED (Coccaro et al. 2009; Fanning et al. 2014). These findings are consistent with data that strongly suggest that trauma or maltreatment in childhood is associated with aggression in later childhood and/or adolescence and that this relationship is mediated by hostile attribution bias (Coccaro et al. 2009). Taken as whole, these findings suggest that it may be possible to intervene at the level of attribution bias and to reduce the propensity to be impulsively aggressive at a later time in life.

Social Cognition

Although family studies cannot speak to the role of environmental factors, specific study of some of these factors have been conducted in individuals with IED. For example, individuals with IED are more likely to have a childhood history of perceived physical and emotional trauma (Fanning et al. 2014) and altered social-emotional information processing (SEIP; Coccaro et al. 2009; Coccaro et al. 2016a), which is partially mediated by the former. The finding of altered SEIP is extremely important because it speaks to the intrapersonal factors that lead to an aggressive outburst. For example, individuals with IED are less likely to process relevant information in a social interaction involving potential threat (Coccaro et al. 2017a), more likely to attribute hostile motives to the other person in the interaction, and more likely to get angry in these situations (Coccaro et al. 2009, 2017a). Further, the more an individual with IED thinks the other person is behaving in a hostile fashion (even when they are not), the more angry that individual becomes at the other person. Given that the threshold to engage in an impulsively aggressive outburst is regulated by the neurobiological substrate (e.g., reduced inhibition and enhanced activation by neurotransmitter systems and brain circuitry), deficits in SEIP relate to the proximal stimulus to an impulsive, angry, aggressive outburst.

Other Psychological Correlates

Not surprisingly, individuals with IED demonstrate problems in a number of psychological areas. Compared with control subjects, individuals with IED have elevations of relational aggression aimed at damaging interpersonal relationships (Murray-Close et al. 2010); elevations of affective lability and affective intensity (Fettich et al. 2015); immature defense mechanisms, including acting out, dissociation, projection, and rationalization (Puhalla et al. 2016); and reduced emotional intelligence (Coccaro et al. 2015b)—all of which provide a rationale for psychological interventions, particularly those that focus on SEIP. However, there are also biological deficits as potential foci for pharmacological interventions in individuals with IED.

Psychobiology

Behavioral Genetics

Although there are no twin studies of IED to elucidate the degree of genetic influence underlying IED, family studies of IED have been conducted. The one published, controlled family history study of IED reported a significantly increased morbid risk (MR) of IED in first-degree relatives of probands whose symptoms met research criteria for IED (MR=0.34) compared with the relatives of control probands without IED (MR=0.10) (Coccaro 2010). The increased morbid risk of IED in relatives of IED probands was not due to issues of comorbidity in either the probands or the relatives. These findings, which were replicated in a follow-up direct family study conducted by our group (E.F. Coccaro et al., data on file), is consistent with observations from twin studies that report moderate degrees of genetic influence underlying measures of both aggression and impulsivity (Coccaro et al., manuscript in review; Seroczynski et al. 1999).

Neurobiology

Studies of individuals with IED affirm the expected categorical differences in biological markers as a function of aggression. For example, individuals with IED display reduced 5-HT function as evidenced by a reduction in the prolactin response to both *d,l*-fenfluramine (Coccaro et al. 1989; New et al. 2004b), and *d*-fenfluramine challenge (Coccaro et al. 2010a), platelet 5-HTT binding (Coccaro et al. 2010b), and platelet 5-HT itself (Goveas et al. 2004). In addition, individuals with IED display elevated levels of inflammatory markers compared with both healthy and psychiatric control subjects (Coccaro et al. 2014). PET imaging studies have extended these findings in study participants with personality disorders who are impulsively aggressive, most of whom have symptoms that would meet criteria for IED. For example, Frankle et al. (2005) reported reduced availability of the 5-HTT in several cortical and subcortical regions, with availability significantly lowest in the ACC of impulsively aggressive individuals with personality disorders. Although another study did not replicate this finding (van de Giessen et al. 2014), this more recent study did report a significant, positive correlation with 5-HTT availability in the ACC and trait callousness. Among impulsively aggressive individuals in this study, a trend-level, negative partial correlation (with callousness and age as covariates) was observed between trait aggression and 5-HTT availability in the ACC. Finally, a PET study reported increased binding of 5-HT_{2A} receptors in the OFC of impulsively aggressive individuals with personality disorders (Rosell et al. 2010).

Molecular Genetics

Not surprisingly, few molecular genetic studies have been published in IED. Although our group has found little association between IED and viable candidate genes (see, e.g., Vu et al. 2011) or copy number variants (Kumar et al. 2008), other groups examining impulsive aggressive individuals, including those with symptoms that would likely meet criteria for IED, have reported preliminary findings of note. For example, studies in Finland reported that the presence of an L allele (either LL or UL) for the noncoding region of TPH in impulsively aggressive male offenders, but not in other subjects, was associated with reduced CSF 5-HIAA levels (Nielsen et al. 1994). Other studies have reported higher aggression scores in males with personality disorders (many with prominent histories of impulsive aggression) with the LL, compared with the UL or UU, genotype (New et al. 1998), though the reverse was reported in a larger study involving community-recruited study participants (Manuck et al. 1999) and suicide attempters (Rujescu et al. 2002).

Molecular Epigenetics

A recent report found increased methylation of the MAO-A promoter (which will deactivate the promoter and reduce synthesis of MAO-A) in persons with AsPD (many of whom likely had IED) compared with the methylation observed in control subjects (Checknita et al. 2015). Finally, we have recently reported increased methylation in networks of genes relevant for inflammatory processes in a modest-sized sample of individuals with IED, compared with nonaggressive controls (Montalvo-Ortiz et al. 2018), suggesting that epigenetic factors may play a role in the relationship between aggression and inflammation.

Structural Neuroimaging

Studies of individuals with IED affirm categorical differences in structural and functional imaging studies. Individuals with IED display a reduction in gray matter volume in frontolimbic circuits (Coccaro et al. 2016b) abnormalities in the shape of the amygdala and hippocampus (Coccaro et al. 2015a), and reduced fractional anisotropy in the superior longitudinal fasciculus (Lee et al. 2016), all suggesting important structural deficits in critical emotion regulating areas of the brain.

Functional Neuroimaging

fMRI studies also note hyperactivity of the amygdala to hostile social threat (i.e., anger faces) in IED compared with heathy control subjects, with either unchanged or reduced activation of prefrontal cortical regions (Coccaro et al. 2007; McCloskey et al. 2016). Recently, we found that whereas the amygdala exhibits a hyperactive response to anger faces, amygdalar responses to induced emotion are not different in individuals with IED compared with healthy controls (Coccaro et al., manuscript in review). This suggests that heightened amygdalar activity to hostile social threat may be an endophenotype for IED. Finally, we have found important differences in fMRI BOLD responses to videos displaying socially ambiguous situations in which one individual experiences a potentially aggressive event. In these studies we have found that individuals with IED display multiple deficits in corticolimbic activation as a function of the different steps in SEIP. Specifically, compared with healthy control subjects, individuals with IED display reduced activation of medial prefrontal cortex and ACC when watching aggressive versus nonaggressive videos; reduced activation of dorsolateral prefrontal cortex and at the temporoparietal junction while evaluating if the persons in the video were hostile in their actions; and reduced activation of superior prefrontal cortex and the periaqueductal gray when estimating how angry they would be if the potentially aggressive event were to happen to them.

Clinical Vignette

EW is a 27-year-old white male with an M.P.H. degree, currently working as a staff coordinator in a nonprofit health care organization. He has been in a relationship "on and off" for the past 2 years that is troubled now by his aggressive outbursts. He was raised primarily by his mother, whom he described as a strict disciplinarian who often hit him "hard" when he "misbehaved." He had little contact with his father growing up, and has none now, though he was told that his father had a "bad temper" and that that had led to the demise of his father's marriage to his mother. On interview, EW reported that he has had trouble with this "temper" since he was 9 years old, though it did not result in any serious consequences at school. EW denied history of serious health issues or head injuries, and he denied sleepwalking, stammering/stuttering, or enuresis after age 5 years. As he progressed into his teen years, his temper got worse and he had periods in which he lost control of his temper (e.g., yelling and screaming at people, getting into arguments with others) ranging from twice weekly to once daily. These episodes occurred (and still occur) with family members, male friends, girlfriends, and random strangers. He also reported episodes of road rage ("slamming on the brakes and cussing people out in the car"). In addition, he reports physical attacks on objects and breaking them on occasion but not physical attacks on other people. He explained that he "explodes" when he is frustrated or feels disrespected ("dissed") by others. He stated that his aggressive outbursts are never planned and are rarely done to attain a tangible objective. While EW has a history of alcohol bingeing (in college but not currently), he stated that most outbursts do not occur under the influence of alcohol. In recent years he has begun to see how his aggressive outbursts have caused problems for him in his relationships and interactions with others. His current girlfriend recently told him that she's not sure she can stay with him if he doesn't get help for his aggressive outbursts.

Discussion of Vignette

This case highlights many things that are characteristic of IED. First, EW has a history of high-frequency but low-intensity aggressive outbursts that may include assault on objects and others but that do not damage expensive items (e.g., > $50) and/or that cause no injury or only minor injury—a common presentation of IED. Second, EW's impulsive aggressive outbursts apparently began when he was 9 years old (outbursts in IED begin in childhood or generally by adolescence), and the behavior is causing dysfunction in social, educational, or vocational spheres. Third, EW has a history of impulsive aggressive outbursts in first-degree relatives, specifically his father and, perhaps, his mother. Fourth, there is a history of family discord.

Summary

Aggression comes in several forms, though impulsive aggression is, perhaps, the most relevant for the mental health system and psychiatry. Impulsive aggression is dimensional in nature, begins at an early age, and displays important correlates with genetics, psychobiology, and clinical neuroscience. The DSM-5 diagnosis of intermittent explosive disorder was designed to represent the categorical expression of impulsive aggression. As a clinical entity, IED is relatively common in the United States but, perhaps, less common in other countries, and people with this disorder are less commonly treated for it, if at all. Individuals with IED share most of the psychobiological characteristics of those with high levels of impulsive aggression, and the aggression is not likely due to the presence of other psychiatric conditions.

Focusing on the pathophysiology of impulsive aggression has led to a variety of possible treatments, though the most efficacious appear to be treatments that increase brain serotonin activity and that work to reduce both hostile attribution bias and negative emotional response to socially ambiguous interactions with others (see Chapter 2, "Assessment and Treatment of Intermittent Explosive Disorder" for a detailed discussion).

Key Clinical Points

▌ Impulsive aggression is under substantial genetic influence and is associated with anomalies in central neurotransmitter function, particularly those involving serotonin and other neurotransmitters or modulators that inhibit or facilitate aggressive responding.

▌ Clinical neuroscience studies suggest that impulsive aggression is associated with an imbalance in cortical (inhibitory) and subcortical (facilitatory) pathways.

▌ Intermittent explosive disorder (IED) is the categorical expression of impulsive aggressive behavior in humans.

▌ The lifetime prevalence of IED in the United States is estimated at between 3% and 5%.

▌ Most individuals with IED do not seek treatment.

▌ IED includes impulsive aggressive outbursts that are of high frequency but low intensity or of low frequency but high intensity.

▌ IED is comorbid with several psychiatric disorders, but the onset of IED precedes that of these comorbid disorders in most cases.

▌ Treatment of IED should target the neuronal systems associated with a role in impulsive aggression (e.g., serotonin agents; psychosocial interventions that target deficits in social cognition).

References

Ahmed AO, Green BA, McCloskey MS, et al: Latent structure of intermittent explosive disorder in an epidemiological sample. J Psychiatr Res 44(10):663–672, 2010 20064645

Alia-Klein N, Goldstein RZ, Kriplani A, et al: Brain monoamine oxidase A activity predicts trait aggression. J Neurosci 28(19):5099–5104, 2008 18463263

Almeida M, Lee R, Coccaro EF: Cortisol responses to ipsapirone challenge correlate with aggression, while basal cortisol levels correlate with impulsivity, in personality disorder and healthy volunteer subjects. J Psychiatr Res 44(14):874–880, 2010 20378126

American Psychiatric Association: Diagnostic and Statistical Manual of Mental Disorders, 4th Edition. Washington, DC, American Psychiatric Association, 1994

American Psychiatric Association: Diagnostic and Statistical Manual of Mental Disorders, 5th Edition. Arlington, VA, American Psychiatric Association, 2013

Barratt ES, Stanford MS, Felthous AR, et al: The effects of phenytoin on impulsive and premeditated aggression: a controlled study. J Clin Psychopharmacol 17(5):341–349, 1997 9315984

Berman ME, McCloskey MS, Fanning JR, et al: Serotonin augmentation reduces response to attack in aggressive individuals. Psychol Sci 20(6):714–720, 2009 19422623

Bhakta SG, Zhang JP, Malhotra AK: The COMT Met158 allele and violence in schizophrenia: a meta-analysis. Schizophr Res 140(1–3):192–197, 2012 22784685

Blair RJ, Morris JS, Frith CD, et al: Dissociable neural responses to facial expressions of sadness and anger. Brain 122(Pt 5):883–893, 1999 10355673

Brown GL, Goodwin FK, Ballenger JC, et al: Aggression in humans correlates with cerebrospinal fluid amine metabolites. Psychiatry Res 1:131–139, 1979 95232

Brown GL, Ebert MH, Goyer PF, et al: Aggression, suicide, and serotonin: relationships to CSF amine metabolites. Am J Psychiatry 139(6):741–746, 1982 6177256

Brunner HG, Nelen M, Breakefield XO, et al: Abnormal behavior associated with a point mutation in the structural gene for monoamine oxidase A. Science 262(5133):578–580, 1993 8211186

Caspi A, McClay J, Moffitt TE, et al: Role of genotype in the cycle of violence in maltreated children. Science 297(5582):851–854, 2002 12161658

Checknita D, Maussion G, Labonté B, et al: Monoamine oxidase A gene promoter methylation and transcriptional downregulation in an offender population with antisocial personality disorder. Br J Psychiatry 206(3):216–222, 2015 25497297

Chung S, Chung HY, Jung J, et al: Association among aggressiveness, neurocognitive function, and the Val66Met polymorphism of brain-derived neurotrophic factor gene in male schizophrenic patients. Compr Psychiatry 51(4):367–372, 2010 20579509

Coccaro EF: A family history study of intermittent explosive disorder. J Psychiatr Res 44(15):1101–1105, 2010 20488459

Coccaro EF: Intermittent explosive disorder: development of integrated research criteria for Diagnostic and Statistical Manual of Mental Disorders, Fifth Edition. Compr Psychiatry 52(2): 119–125, 2011 21295216

Coccaro EF: Intermittent explosive disorder as a disorder of impulsive aggression for DSM-5. Am J Psychiatry 169(6):577–588, 2012 22535310

Coccaro EF, Lee R: Cerebrospinal fluid 5-hydroxyindolacetic acid and homovanillic acid: reciprocal relationships with impulsive aggression in human subjects. J Neural Transm (Vienna) 117(2):241–248, 2010 20069438

Coccaro EF, Siever LJ, Klar HM, et al: Serotonergic studies in patients with affective and personality disorders. Correlates with suicidal and impulsive aggressive behavior. Arch Gen Psychiatry 46(7):587–599, 1989 2735812

Coccaro EF, Bergeman CS, Kavoussi RJ, et al: Heritability of aggression and irritability: a twin study of the Buss-Durkee aggression scales in adult male subjects. Biol Psychiatry 41(3):273–284, 1997a 9024950

Coccaro EF, Kavoussi RJ, Cooper TB, et al: Central serotonin activity and aggression: inverse relationship with prolactin response to d-fenfluramine, but not CSF 5-HIAA concentration, in human subjects. Am J Psychiatry 154(10):1430–1435, 1997b 9326827

Coccaro EF, Kavoussi RJ, Trestman RL, et al: Serotonin function in human subjects: intercorrelations among central 5-HT indices and aggressiveness. Psychiatry Res 73(1–2):1–14, 1997c 9463834

Coccaro EF, Kavoussi RJ, Hauger RL, et al: Cerebrospinal fluid vasopressin levels: correlates with aggression and serotonin function in personality-disordered subjects. Arch Gen Psychiatry 55(8):708–714, 1998 9707381

Coccaro EF, Lee R, McCloskey M: Norepinephrine function in personality disorder: plasma free MHPG correlates inversely with life history of aggression. CNS Spectr 8(10):731–736, 2003 14712171

Coccaro EF, Posternak MA, Zimmerman M: Prevalence and features of intermittent explosive disorder in a clinical setting. J Clin Psychiatry 66(10):1221–1227, 2005 16259534

Coccaro EF, McCloskey MS, Fitzgerald DA, et al: Amygdala and orbitofrontal reactivity to social threat in individuals with impulsive aggression. Biol Psychiatry 62(2):168–178, 2007 17210136

Coccaro EF, Noblett KL, McCloskey MS: Attributional and emotional responses to socially ambiguous cues: validation of a new assessment of social/emotional information processing in healthy adults and impulsive aggressive patients. J Psychiatr Res 43(10):915–925, 2009 19345371

Coccaro EF, Lee R, Kavoussi RJ: Aggression, suicidality, and intermittent explosive disorder: serotonergic correlates in personality disorder and healthy control subjects. Neuropsychopharmacology 35(2):435–444, 2010a 19776731

Coccaro EF, Lee R, Kavoussi RJ: Inverse relationship between numbers of 5-HT transporter binding sites and life history of aggression and intermittent explosive disorder. J Psychiatr Res 44(3):137–142, 2010b 19767013

Coccaro EF, Lee R, Liu T, et al: Cerebrospinal fluid neuropeptide Y-like immunoreactivity correlates with impulsive aggression in human subjects. Biol Psychiatry 72(12):997–1003, 2012a 22985695

Coccaro EF, Lee R, Owens MJ, et al: Cerebrospinal fluid substance P-like immunoreactivity correlates with aggression in personality disordered subjects. Biol Psychiatry 72(3):238–243, 2012b 22449753

Coccaro EF, Lee R, Vezina P: Cerebrospinal fluid glutamate concentration correlates with impulsive aggression in human subjects. J Psychiatr Res 47(9):1247–1253, 2013 23791397

Coccaro EF, Lee R, Coussons-Read M: Elevated plasma inflammatory markers in individuals with intermittent explosive disorder and correlation with aggression in humans. JAMA Psychiatry 71(2):158–165, 2014 24352431

Coccaro EF, Lee R, McCloskey M, et al: Morphometric analysis of amygdala and hippocampus shape in impulsively aggressive and healthy control subjects. J Psychiatr Res 69:80–86, 2015a 26343598

Coccaro EF, Solis O, Fanning J, Lee R: Emotional intelligence and impulsive aggression in intermittent explosive disorder. J Psychiatr Res 61:135–140, 2015b 25477263

Coccaro EF, Fanning JR, Keedy SK, et al: Social cognition in intermittent explosive disorder and aggression. J Psychiatr Res 83:140–150, 2016a 27621104

Coccaro EF, Fitzgerald DA, Lee R, et al: Frontolimbic morphometric abnormalities in intermittent explosive disorder and aggression. Biol Psychiatry Cogn Neurosci Neuroimaging 1(1):32–38, 2016b 29560894

Coccaro EF, Lee R, Fanning JR, et al: Tryptophan, kynurenine, and kynurenine metabolites: relationship to lifetime aggression and inflammatory markers in human subjects. Psychoneuroendocrinology 71:189–196, 2016c 27318828

Coccaro EF, Lee R, Groer MW, et al: Toxoplasma gondii infection: relationship with aggression in psychiatric subjects. J Clin Psychiatry 77(3):334–341, 2016d 27046307

Coccaro EF, Fanning JR, Fisher E, et al: Social emotional information processing in adults: development and psychometrics of a computerized video assessment in healthy controls and aggressive individuals. Psychiatry Res 248:40–47, 2017a 28012305

Coccaro EF, Fanning JR, Lee R: Intermittent explosive disorder and substance use disorder: analysis of the National Comorbidity Study Replication sample. J Clin Psychiatry 78(6):697–702, 2017b 28252880

Coccaro EF, Keedy SK, Lee RJ, et al: Neural responses to induced emotion and response to social threat in intermittent explosive disorder. Psychiatry Res Neuroimaging (manuscript in review)

Crick NR, Dodge KA: Social information-processing mechanisms in reactive and proactive aggression. Child Dev 67(3):993–1002, 1996 8706540

Damasio AR, Grabowski TJ, Bechara A, et al: Subcortical and cortical brain activity during the feeling of self-generated emotions. Nat Neurosci 3(10):1049–1056, 2000 11017179

de Jonge P, Alonso J, Stein DJ, et al: Associations between DSM-IV mental disorders and diabetes mellitus: a role for impulse control disorders and depression. Diabetologia 57(4):699–709, 2014 24488082

Dodge K: The structure and function of reactive and proactive aggression, in The Development and Treatment of Childhood Aggression. Edited by Pepler DJ, Rubin KHHillside, NJ, Lawrence Erlbaum, 1991, pp 201–218

Dougherty DD, Shin LM, Alpert NM, et al: Anger in healthy men: a PET study using script-driven imagery. Biol Psychiatry 46(4):466–472, 1999 10459395

Duke AA, Bègue L, Bell R, et al: Revisiting the serotonin-aggression relation in humans: a meta-analysis. Psychol Bull 139(5):1148–1172, 2013 23379963

Eichelman B: The limbic system and aggression in humans. Neurosci Biobehav Rev 7(3):391–394, 1983 6199700

Fanning JR, Meyerhoff JJ, Lee R, et al: History of childhood maltreatment in intermittent explosive disorder and suicidal behavior. J Psychiatr Res 56:10–17, 2014 24935900

Fettich KC, McCloskey MS, Look AE, et al: Emotion regulation deficits in intermittent explosive disorder. Aggress Behav 41(1):25–33, 2015 27539871

Ficks CA, Waldman ID: Candidate genes for aggression and antisocial behavior: a meta-analysis of association studies of the 5HTTLPR and MAOA-uVNTR. Behav Genet 44(5):427–444, 2014 24902785

Flory JD, Xu K, New AS, et al: Irritable assault and variation in the COMT gene. Psychiatr Genet 17(6):344–346, 2007 18075475

Frankle WG, Lombardo I, New AS, et al: Brain serotonin transporter distribution in subjects with impulsive aggressivity: a positron emission study with [11C]McN 5652. Am J Psychiatry 162(5):915–923, 2005 15863793

Goveas JS, Csernansky JG, Coccaro EF: Platelet serotonin content correlates inversely with life history of aggression in personality-disordered subjects. Psychiatry Res 126(1):23–32, 2004 15081624

Goyer PF, Andreason PJ, Semple WE, et al: Positron-emission tomography and personality disorders. Neuropsychopharmacology 10(1):21–28, 1994 8179791

Gu Y, Yun L, Tian Y, et al: Association between COMT gene and Chinese male schizophrenic patients with violent behavior. Med Sci Monit 15(9):CR484–CR489, 2009 19721400

Guan X, Dong ZQ, Tian YY, et al: Lack of association between brain-derived neurotrophic factor Val66Met polymorphism and aggressive behavior in schizophrenia. Psychiatry Res 215(1):244–245, 2014 24289908

Kessler RC, Coccaro EF, Fava M, et al: The prevalence and correlates of DSM-IV intermittent explosive disorder in the National Comorbidity Survey Replication. Arch Gen Psychiatry 63(6):669–678, 2006 16754840

Kimbrell TA, George MS, Parekh PI, et al: Regional brain activity during transient self-induced anxiety and anger in healthy adults. Biol Psychiatry 46(4):454–465, 1999 10459394

Kulper DA, Kleiman EM, McCloskey MS, et al: The experience of aggressive outbursts in intermittent explosive disorder. Psychiatry Res 225(3):710–715, 2015 25541537

Kumar RA, McGhee KA, Leach S, et al: Initial association of NR2E1 with bipolar disorder and identification of candidate mutations in bipolar disorder, schizophrenia, and aggression through resequencing. Am J Med Genet B Neuropsychiatr Genet 147B(6):880–889, 2008 18205168

Lee R, Ferris C, Van de Kar LD, et al: Cerebrospinal fluid oxytocin, life history of aggression, and personality disorder. Psychoneuroendocrinology 34(10):1567–1573, 2009 19577376

Lee R, Meyerhoff J, Coccaro EF: Intermittent explosive disorder and aversive parental care. Psychiatry Res 220(1–2):477–482, 2014 25064384

Lee R, Arfanakis K, Evia AM, et al: White matter integrity reductions in intermittent explosive disorder. Neuropsychopharmacology 41(11):2697–2703, 2016 27206265

Leyton M, Okazawa H, Diksic M, et al: Brain regional alpha-[11C]methyl-L-tryptophan trapping in impulsive subjects with borderline personality disorder. Am J Psychiatry 158(5):775–782, 2001 11329401

Limson R, Goldman D, Roy A, et al: Personality and cerebrospinal fluid monoamine metabolites in alcoholics and controls. Arch Gen Psychiatry 48(5):437–441, 1991 1708656

Linnoila M, Virkkunen M, Scheinin M, et al: Low cerebrospinal fluid 5-hydroxyindoleacetic acid concentration differentiates impulsive from nonimpulsive violent behavior. Life Sci 33(26):2609–2614, 1983 6198573

Manuck SB, Flory JD, Ferrell RE, et al: Aggression and anger-related traits associated with a polymorphism of the tryptophan hydroxylase gene. Biol Psychiatry 45(5):603–614, 1999 10088047

Marsland AL, Prather AA, Petersen KL, et al: Antagonistic characteristics are positively associated with inflammatory markers independently of trait negative emotionality. Brain Behav Immun 22(5):753–761, 2008 18226879

McCloskey MS, Kleabir K, Berman ME, et al: Unhealthy aggression: intermittent explosive disorder and adverse physical health outcomes. Health Psychol 29(3):324–332, 2010 20496987

McCloskey MS, Phan KL, Angstadt M, et al: Amygdala hyperactivation to angry faces in intermittent explosive disorder. J Psychiatr Res 79:34–41, 2016 27145325

McLaughlin KA, Green JG, Hwang I, et al: Intermittent explosive disorder in the National Comorbidity Survey Replication Adolescent Supplement. Arch Gen Psychiatry 69(11):1131–1139, 2012 22752056

Miles DR, Carey G: Genetic and environmental architecture of human aggression. J Pers Soc Psychol 72(1):207–217, 1997 9008382

Mohamed Saini S, Razali R, Ibrahim L, et al: Aggression in Malaysian schizophrenia patients: its clinical determinants and association with COMT Val158Met genotypes. Asian J Psychiatr 17:107–108, 2015 26300284

Møller SE, Mortensen EL, Breum L, et al: Aggression and personality: association with amino acids and monoamine metabolites. Psychol Med 26(2):323–331, 1996 8685288

Montalvo-Ortiz JL, Zhang H, Chen C, et al: Genome-wide DNA methylation changes associated with intermittent explosive disorder: a gene-based functional enrichment analysis. Int J Neuropsychopharmacol 21(1):12–20, 2018 29106553

Moss HB, Yao JK, Panzak GL: Serotonergic responsivity and behavioral dimensions in antisocial personality disorder with substance abuse. Biol Psychiatry 28(4):325–338, 1990 2397249

Murray-Close D, Ostrov JM, Nelson DA, et al: Proactive, reactive, and romantic relational aggression in adulthood: measurement, predictive validity, gender differences, and association with intermittent explosive disorder. J Psychiatr Res 44(6):393–404, 2010 19822329

New AS, Gelernter J, Yovell Y, et al: Tryptophan hydroxylase genotype is associated with impulsive-aggression measures: a preliminary study. Am J Med Genet 81(1):13–17, 1998 9514581

New AS, Hazlett EA, Buchsbaum MS, et al: Blunted prefrontal cortical 18fluorodeoxyglucose positron emission tomography response to meta-chlorophenylpiperazine in impulsive aggression. Arch Gen Psychiatry 59(7):621–629, 2002 12090815

New AS, Buchsbaum MS, Hazlett EA, et al: Fluoxetine increases relative metabolic rate in prefrontal cortex in impulsive aggression. Psychopharmacology (Berl) 176(3–4):451–458, 2004a 15160265

New AS, Trestman RF, Mitropoulou V, et al: Low prolactin response to fenfluramine in impulsive aggression. J Psychiatr Res 38(3):223–230, 2004b 15003426

Nickerson A, Aderka IM, Bryant RA, et al: The relationship between childhood exposure to trauma and intermittent explosive disorder. Psychiatry Res 197(1–2):128–134, 2012 22464047

Nielsen DA, Goldman D, Virkkunen M, et al: Suicidality and 5-hydroxyindoleacetic acid concentration associated with a tryptophan hydroxylase polymorphism. Arch Gen Psychiatry 51(1):34–38, 1994 7506517

Nock MK, Stein MB, Heeringa SG, et al; Army STARRS Collaborators: Prevalence and correlates of suicidal behavior among soldiers: results from the Army Study to Assess Risk and Resilience in Servicemembers (Army STARRS). JAMA Psychiatry 71(5):514–522, 2014 24590178

Puhalla AA, McCloskey MS, Brickman LJ, et al: Defense styles in intermittent explosive disorder. Psychiatry Res 238:137–142, 2016 27086223

Raine A, Meloy JR, Bihrle S, et al: Reduced prefrontal and increased subcortical brain functioning assessed using positron emission tomography in predatory and affective murderers. Behav Sci Law 16(3):319–332, 1998 9768464

Raine A, Lencz T, Bihrle S, et al: Reduced prefrontal gray matter volume and reduced autonomic activity in antisocial personality disorder. Arch Gen Psychiatry 57(2):119–127, discussion 128–129, 2000 10665614

Rosell DR, Thompson JL, Slifstein M, et al: Increased serotonin 2A receptor availability in the orbitofrontal cortex of physically aggressive personality disordered patients. Biol Psychiatry 67(12):1154–1162, 2010 20434136

Rosenberg S, Templeton AR, Feigin PD, et al: The association of DNA sequence variation at the MAOA genetic locus with quantitative behavioural traits in normal males. Hum Genet 120(4):447–459, 2006 16896926

Rujescu D, Giegling I, Bondy B, et al: Association of anger-related traits with SNPs in the TPH gene. Mol Psychiatry 7(9):1023–1029, 2002 12399958

Rynar L, Coccaro EF: Psychosocial impairment in DSM-5 intermittent explosive disorder. Psychiatry Res 264:91–95, 2018 29627702

Scott AL, Bortolato M, Chen K, et al: Novel monoamine oxidase A knock out mice with human-like spontaneous mutation. Neuroreport 19(7):739–743, 2008 18418249

Scott KM, Lim CC, Hwang I, et al: The cross-national epidemiology of DSM-IV intermittent explosive disorder. Psychol Med 46(15):3161–3172, 2016 27572872

Seroczynski AD, Bergeman CS, Coccaro EF: Etiology of the impulsivity/aggression relationship: genes or environment? Psychiatry Res 86(1):41–57, 1999 10359481

Siever LJ, Buchsbaum MS, New AS, et al: d,l-Fenfluramine response in impulsive personality disorder assessed with [18F]fluorodeoxyglucose positron emission tomography. Neuropsychopharmacology 20(5):413–423, 1999 10192822

Singh JP, Volavka J, Czobor P, Van Dorn RA: A meta-analysis of the Val158Met COMT polymorphism and violent behavior in schizophrenia. PLoS One 7(8):e43423, 2012 22905266

Soloff PH, Meltzer CC, Greer PJ, et al: A fenfluramine-activated FDG-PET study of borderline personality disorder. Biol Psychiatry 47(6):540–547, 2000 10715360

Spalletta G, Morris DW, Angelucci F, et al: BDNF Val66Met polymorphism is associated with aggressive behavior in schizophrenia. Eur Psychiatry 25(6):311–313, 2010 20430595

Suarez EC: Joint effect of hostility and severity of depressive symptoms on plasma interleukin-6 concentration. Psychosom Med 65(4):523–527, 2003 12883100

Tosato S, Bonetto C, Di Forti M, et al: Effect of COMT genotype on aggressive behaviour in a community cohort of schizophrenic patients. Neurosci Lett 495(1):17–21, 2011 21402125

Tremblay RE: Early development of physical aggression and early risk factors for chronic physical aggression in humans, in Neuroscience of Aggression: Current Topics in Behavioral Neurosciences, Vol 17. Edited by Miczek K, Meyer-Lindenberg A. Berlin, Springer, 2013, pp 315–328

Valzelli L, Garattini S: Behavioral changes and 5-hydroxytryptamine turnover in animals. Adv Pharmacol 6(Pt B):249–260, 1968 5690585

van de Giessen E, Rosell DR, Thompson JL, et al: Serotonin transporter availability in impulsive aggressive personality disordered patients: a PET study with [11C]DASB. J Psychiatr Res 58:147–154, 2014 25145808

van Elst LT, Woermann FG, Lemieux L, et al: Affective aggression in patients with temporal lobe epilepsy: a quantitative MRI study of the amygdala. Brain 123(Pt 2):234–243, 2000 10648432

Veit R, Flor H, Erb M, et al: Brain circuits involved in emotional learning in antisocial behavior and social phobia in humans. Neurosci Lett 328(3):233–236, 2002 12147314

Volkow ND, Tancredi LR, Grant C, et al: Brain glucose metabolism in violent psychiatric patients: a preliminary study. Psychiatry Res 61(4):243–253, 1995 8748468

Virkkunen M, Nuutila A, Goodwin FK, et al: Cerebrospinal fluid monoamine metabolite levels in male arsonists. Arch Gen Psychiatry 44(3):241–247, 1987 2435256

Virkkunen M, De Jong J, Bartko J, et al: Relationship of psychobiological variables to recidivism in violent offenders and impulsive fire setters. A follow-up study. Arch Gen Psychiatry 46(7):600–603, 1989 2472122

Vu TH, Coccaro EF, Eichler EE, et al: Genomic architecture of aggression: rare copy number variants in intermittent explosive disorder. Am J Med Genet B Neuropsychiatr Genet 156B(7):808–816, 2011 21812102

Wang D, Szyf M, Benkelfat C, et al: Peripheral SLC6A4 DNA methylation is associated with in vivo measures of human brain serotonin synthesis and childhood physical aggression. PLoS One 7(6):e39501, 2012 22745770

Zalcman SS, Siegel A: The neurobiology of aggression and rage: role of cytokines. Brain Behav Immun 20(6):507–514, 2006 16938427

2

Assessment and Treatment of Intermittent Explosive Disorder

Michael S. McCloskey, Ph.D.
Martha K. Fahlgren, M.A.
Emil F. Coccaro, M.D.

Intermittent explosive disorder (IED) is the diagnosis used to classify engagement in repeated acts of affective and/or impulsive aggression that are disproportionate to any provocation and not better accounted for by the effects of a substance, medical condition, or other psychological disorder (American Psychiatric Association 2013). Thus, IED is a disorder of primary affective aggression, the only such disorder in DSM-V. Though initially believed to have a very low prevalence (American Psychiatric Association 2000), IED has since been found to occur in approximately 3%–5% of the U.S. population (Kessler et al. 2006), making it one of the more common psychiatric disorders in the United States. Compounding the public impact associated with its relatively high prevalence, IED also typically has a chronic, waxing and waning course, with onset often in adolescence and extending through middle age (Coccaro 2012).

The aggression in IED can include either 1) frequent minor out-bursts such as verbal tirades or minor physical aggression (at least twice a week, on average, over 3 months or longer) (Criterion A1) or 2) infrequent major outbursts that result in physical harm to others or objects (at least three major outbursts in a year's time) (Criterion A2). Individuals meeting only the minor aggression subcriterion (A1) and those meeting only the major aggression subcriterion (A2) have a quite similar clinical presentation and prognosis (Coccaro et al. 2014; Look et al. 2015). However, most individuals with IED have symp-toms that meet both the minor and the major aggression criteria over their lifetime (Coccaro 2012), a presentation that is associated with a more severe and treatment-refractory course (Coccaro et al. 2014; Look et al. 2015).

When untreated, IED is associated with significant functional im-pairments. Several studies have shown that even relative to individuals with other psychiatric disorders, those with IED have greater psycho-social impairment and a poorer quality of life (McCloskey et al. 2006, 2008a; Rynar and Coccaro 2018). Furthermore, compared with indi-viduals with other psychiatric disorders, those with IED are more likely to endorse that their aggressive behavior leads to problems with family, with friends, and at work (Kulper et al. 2015). Individuals with IED are also more likely to have their aggression lead to legal prob-lems (Kulper et al. 2015). Underscoring the severity of the negative impact of untreated IED, a study based on data from a large epidemi-ological sample found that individuals with IED were more likely to have several negative health outcomes, including coronary heart dis-ease, hypertension, and stroke, even after other risk factors were taken into account (McCloskey et al. 2010). IED is also associated with an increased risk of suicidal behaviors and nonsuicidal self-injury among individuals with a personality disorder (Jenkins et al. 2015). Given the breadth and severity of problems affecting millions of indi-viduals, it is essential to establish and implement effective treatment for IED.

Assessment

Assessment for IED is an integral part of an effective treatment ap-proach with respect to both accurate diagnosis and effective monitor-ing of symptoms. Given that IED is a disorder of primary aggression, but one that is often comorbid with other psychiatric disorders, differential diagnosis is key. There is no gold standard for assessing IED, but for most psychiatric disorders, structured clinical interviews are considered the most reliable means of diagnostic assessment (Ventura et al. 1998). The Structured Clinical Interview for DSM-5–Research Version [SCID-5-RV] now includes an optional module on the diagnosis of current IED, located within the SCID Externalizing Disorders module (First et al. 2015). There is also an unpublished stand-alone IED diagnostic interview, the Intermittent Explosive Disorder Module (IED-M; McCloskey and Coccaro 2003), which was developed prior to SCID-5 to diagnose IED in conjunction with a full diagnostic interview (i.e., to assess for comorbid disorders that may better account for the patient's aggressive behavior). A newly developed IED screening questionnaire (Coccaro et al. 2017) can be used as a "quick and dirty" assessment of IED, but this questionnaire should be followed up with a full diagnostic interview before any formal diagnosis is made.

Whether clinicians are using structured or unstructured clinical interviews, two critical aspects of diagnosing IED are whether 1) the aggression was disproportionate to the provocation and 2) the aggression is best accounted for by IED (as opposed to another disorder or condition.) With regard to proportionality of the aggressive response, a rule of thumb is that the aggression is disproportionate to the provocation if either the aggressive interaction was initiated by the patient or the patient increased the level of aggression. As an example, if a person angrily yells at the patient and the patient angrily yells back, this would not be seen as disproportionate to the provocation. However, if a person angrily yells at the patient and the patient responds by charging and physically attacking the person, this level of aggressive response would be seen as disproportionate to the provocation.

With regard to the question of whether the aggression is primary (IED) or secondary to another condition, the key is to determine if the aggression occurs at a frequency and intensity that meet the criteria for IED independent of the condition. So, if a person is only highly aggressive when criteria for a major depressive episode are met, then IED would not be diagnosed. However, if a person exhibits aggressive behavior that meets the criteria for IED when not experiencing a major depressive episode, but becomes more aggressive when depressed, then the criteria for both IED and major depressive disorder would be met. This distinction is especially difficult for chronic disorders that begin in childhood or early adolescence, as in this case there is not a clear "baseline" for aggressive behavior (e.g., posttraumatic stress disorder from early childhood abuse). In that situation, the extent to which aggression is associated with the disorder in question should be considered. If the comorbid disorder is associated with aggression, then the clinician should assess whether the level of aggression seen in the patient is in excess of what is typically found in patients with this comorbid disorder.

Assessment of IED symptom severity should include tracking of anger and aggression. The primary measure used in intervention studies to assess aggression and irritability (anger) is the Overt Aggression Scale—Modified (OAS-M; Coccaro et al. 1991). The OAS-M is a 10- to 15-minute clinical interview that assesses the frequency of a myriad of aggressive behaviors that occurred over the past week. These aggressive behaviors are divided into categories for verbal assault, assault against objects, assault against others, and assault against self. Additional items assess subjective (patient perspective) and objective (interviewer perspective) irritability as well as suicidal thoughts and behaviors. Because it involves a significant time commitment, the OAS-M is often given every other week. If regular use of the OAS-M is not practical, an alternative is for the patient to keep a journal tracking his or her aggressive behavior that can be reviewed with the clinician each week. This has the added benefit of increasing the patient's monitoring of his or her aggressive behavior, which has been shown to reduce negative behavior (Wang et al. 2012). If this approach is used, it is paramount for the clinician to go over the journal each week to reinforce the importance of completing the journal. It is also helpful to periodically assess general life functioning, by using, for example, the 14-item Quality of Life Enjoyment and Satisfaction Questionnaire—Short Form [Q-LES-Q-SF] (Endicott et al. 1993).

Treatment

There is an extensive literature examining treatment for anger and aggression more generally. In contrast, the research examining IED-specific treatment is quite limited, but with extant studies of pharmacological and psychotherapeutic interventions generally showing aggression reductions in IED.

Psychopharmacological Interventions

As noted in Chapter 1 ("Phenomenology and Psychobiology of Aggression and Intermittent Explosive Disorder"), impulsive aggression in general (Seo et al. 2008), and IED specifically (Coccaro et al. 2010), have been associated with dysfunction or deficits in serotonin. Accordingly, research indicates the utility of selective serotonin reuptake inhibitors (SSRIs) to reduce aggression. SSRIs such as fluoxetine (see Coccaro and Kavoussi 1997; Salzman et al. 1995) have demonstrated greater efficacy, compared with placebo, at reducing impulsive aggression in individuals with personality disorders. Sertraline, another SSRI, has also demonstrated efficacy at reducing aggression in a sample of patients with a personality disorder diagnosis (Kavoussi et al. 1994). These clinical findings have been supported by experimental research. SSRIs have been associated with reduction of aggressive behavior in laboratory paradigms, both when administered chronically (Cherek et al. 2002) and when given acutely (Berman et al. 2009), among those with a history of aggressive behavior. However, these findings are not unanimous, as one randomized controlled trial (RCT) found no difference between fluoxetine and placebo in individuals with personality disorders (Rinne et al. 2002).

Though research on SSRIs for IED specifically is sparse, some promising studies exist. A small case study demonstrated that aggression was reduced for a sample of IED patients taking sertraline (Feder 1999). Further, a more rigorous double-blind RCT demonstrated that nearly half of those with IED had reductions in aggression (significantly better than with placebo) and irritability when treated with fluoxetine, with effects becoming apparent as early as week 2 of treatment and being sustained (Coccaro and Kavoussi 1997; Coccaro et al. 2009a).

In addition to SSRIs, other drug classes have demonstrated efficacy at reducing the type of affective aggression seen in IED. Some early case studies suggested the use of beta-blockers to reduce aggressive behavior in IED. One study investigated metoprolol, which proved effective at reducing aggressive outbursts for two individuals who were diagnosed with IED (Mattes 1985). However, both individuals had organic brain injury, which may have better explained the aggression. Supporting this finding, a separate study found that five of eight patients diagnosed with IED treated with propranolol exhibited significantly decreased aggressive symptoms (Jenkins and Maruta 1987).

There is also some evidence for the utility of mood stabilizers and anticonvulsants for reducing problematic aggressive behavior, though the results for IED specifically are mixed. A randomized, placebo-controlled trial demonstrated that lithium was significantly better than placebo at reducing the frequency of aggressive acts in adolescent and young adults who were incarcerated and had a history of chronic impulsive aggression (Sheard et al. 1976). A later comparative investigation found that the anticonvulsant carbamazepine and the beta-blocker propranolol were effective at reducing "rage outbursts," but it was determined that those with IED improved significantly more while taking carbamazepine (Mattes 1990), suggesting that mood stabilizers may be more effective than beta-blockers in IED. Supporting these findings in a clinically aggressive sample, carbamazepine was shown to decrease aggression in a small sample of women with borderline personality disorder (Gardner and Cowdry 1986). A later study of oxcarbazepine, which is similar in structure and properties to carbamazepine, was shown to significantly reduce clinician-rated aggression and was associated with higher patient-rated improvement compared with placebo for those with IED, lending additional support for this treatment (Mattes 2005). However, all anticonvulsants may not be equally effective for IED. In a follow-up study with IED participants, levetiracetam was not more effective than placebo at reducing aggression (Mattes 2008). Further, although the anticonvulsant divalproex has been shown to decrease aggression and irritability in individuals with a personality disorder (Hollander et al. 2003; Kavoussi and Coccaro 1998), it was no better than placebo at reducing aggression in IED (Hollander et al. 2003). Thus, it may be specific properties of particular anticonvulsants (e.g., the blocking of voltage sensitive sodium channels caused by oxcarbazepine) that account for reductions in aggression in IED, rather than general mechanisms of the class of drugs (Mattes 2008).

Phenytoin has also demonstrated some efficacy at improving impulsive aggression specifically. In a study involving 60 incarcerated participants, treatment with phenytoin reduced impulsive (but not premeditated) aggression (Barratt et al. 1997). Supporting the potential utility of phenytoin for IED specifically, a double-blind, placebo-controlled study was conducted with men whose symptoms met DSM-IV [American Psychiatric Association 1994] A and B criteria for

IED (i.e., several episodes of discrete aggression disproportionate to the precipitating stressor) (Stanford et al. 2001). Individuals treated with daily phenytoin had a significantly decreased number of weekly aggressive outbursts when compared with those receiving placebo (Stanford et al. 2001).

To account for these varying potentially effective psychopharmacological interventions, researchers need to determine which drugs work best for whom. Though more evidence (specifically for those with IED) is needed, some research has suggested tailoring drug treatment for IED on the basis of comorbid diagnoses or affective symptoms. McElroy (1999) suggested administering SSRIs for IED patients with co-occurring unipolar depressive symptoms or compulsive behaviors, and mood stabilizers for those with comorbid mania/bipolar symptoms or with affective instability. An investigation conducted under these conditions with a small sample of patients found a significant improvement for those patients treated with divalproex, and a lesser (but still moderate) improvement with SSRIs (McElroy 1999). Overall, existing evidence is most strongly suggestive of SSRIs as an effective treatment for IED, although some evidence exists for the effectiveness of other psychopharmacological agents as well. Further research is needed to establish these links more clearly.

Clinical Vignette

BW is a 32-year-old, married white male who has been working as an accountant for the past 2 years. He was raised by both parents, who divorced only recently. On interview, he reported no psychiatric issues for his mother but noted that his father had frequently displayed both verbal and physical aggression while BW was growing up. Despite this, he denied having witnessed his parents hit each other. He also stated that his younger sister has the same problems he has with aggressive outbursts, though his older brother does not. BW reported one head injury at age 19 during a rugby game. He denied being unconscious but reported having been momentarily dazed and confused for less than a minute and having had a headache for a few hours that same day.

On interview, BW reported having periods in which he frequently loses control of his temper and yells and screams at people and/or gets into arguments with others. These outbursts began early in his teenage years. This behavior occurs every day and rarely less than twice a week. He also reported having frequent episodes of aggression against objects, sometimes breaking moderately expensive ($50–$100) objects several times in any given year. BW admitted to physically hitting another person, but noted that this had happened only three times *in his life* and never three times in any given year. Situations that set him off included "frustrations over little things, things not being where I put them or out of place." He reported that his reactions are much stronger than they should be given the circumstances and have caused problems in his relationships and interactions with others and have affected his work ("my coworkers are cautious of setting me off"), and that these outbursts typically occur when he is not drinking.

Full evaluation determined that BW's symptoms met DSM-5 criteria for current IED, alcohol use disorder (mild) in full remission, and obsessive-compulsive personality disorder. BW was offered cognitive-behavioral therapy (CBT) as a first option, but he declined this type of treatment because of the time commitment. Thus, BW was prescribed escitalopram 10 mg po qd, and the dosage was increased to 20 mg po qd after 1 week. After 3–4 weeks BW reported that he was feeling less irritable and angry, that things that used to bother him did not bother him as much, and that his aggressive outbursts had diminished but were not "gone," with the outbursts, then, occurring about once or twice a week. After 3 months of treatment BW reported that his anger was under much better control and that his outbursts were occurring only a few times a month. This clinical improvement continued for another year while he was taking escitalopram, at which point BW discovered that his anger was returning. He contacted his psychiatrist and wondered if he was receiving generic "Lexapro." His psychiatrist informed him that generic "Lexapro" was not available (at that time) and asked him to read the label on the medication bottle. BW returned to the phone and spelled out the name on the bottle: "P R I L O S E C." The psychiatrist told him he was on the wrong medication because of a pharmacy error and that he would write another prescription for escitalopram. BW began taking escitalopram again the next day and reported regaining control of his anger within 3–4 weeks.

Psychotherapy

IED is associated with several cognitive-affective deficits, including, but not limited to, poor emotion regulation (Fettich et al. 2015), increased affective impulsivity (Puhalla et al. 2016), and hostile attribution biases (Coccaro et al. 2009b; see Chapter 1 in this volume for a more detailed discussion of cognitive-affective deficits in IED). Thus, behavioral treatments targeting these deficits may be effective for reducing aggression among individuals with IED.

As with pharmacological interventions, there is limited research on psychotherapeutic interventions specifically for IED. However, more extensive research has been conducted on treatment for anger problems. A meta-analysis of nearly 100 interventions demonstrated the general efficacy of therapeutic treatment on both anger and aggressive behaviors, as well as an increase in positive behaviors (DiGiuseppe and Tafrate 2003). Overall, the effect size for target symptoms across studies was moderate, though there was significant heterogeneity of variance across outcomes (DiGiuseppe and Tafrate 2003). Notably, aggression had the largest effect size across studies, reflecting the role of anger in aggressive behavior (e.g., (Spielberger et al. 1988) and suggesting the importance of affective treatment targets for aggression interventions.

Although there were no significant differences across types of treatments, most treatments included in this meta-analysis could be classified as CBT, calling into question the sufficient variance in treatment types examined, and suggesting that CBT is an effective method for reducing aggression (DiGiuseppe and Tafrate 2003). Further, CBT, as well as cognitive therapy alone, has demonstrated moderate to large effects at reducing anger and in maintaining these reductions in anger over time, in prior meta-analyses (Beck and Fernandez 1998; Bowman-Edmondson and Cohen-Conger 1996; Tafrate 1995).

In addition to CBT, prior meta-analyses have found that relaxation treatments have had large effects on anger, as has a treatment that implemented a didactic intervention of social and anger management skills (Bowman-Edmondson and Cohen-Conger 1996; Tafrate 1995). A review of these and related therapies for anger and aggression broadly found positive outcomes for a variety of therapies, including cognitive therapy, CBT, relaxation, social skills training, and combinations of these methods (Glancy and Saini 2005). This review supported the findings of the results of the meta-analyses described above and also advocated for a brief (i.e., eight-session) delivery method of cognitive-based therapies to limit attrition while effectively reducing anger and aggression.

However, the studies included in these meta-analyses and reviews did not specifically examine individuals whose symptoms met criteria for IED, instead focusing primarily on anger as the outcome. To date, two studies have included IED participants specifically. The first was an investigation of a protocol to reduce aggressive driving in those with and without IED (Galovski and Blanchard 2002). This study investigated the effectiveness of a CBT intervention (compared with a symptom-monitoring control condition) for 30 aggressive drivers (over two-thirds of whom were court-referred). Notably, 10 participants in this sample had symptoms that met criteria for IED.

This intervention was a 90-minute, 4-week group therapy protocol that involved relaxation strategies, coping skills training, psychoeducation about the impact of aggressive driving, and cognitive restructuring strategies. The outcome of this study was measured through a daily diary of self-reported aggressive driving behaviors. Results demonstrated that both court- and self-referred participants reported a decrease in aggressive driving, though self-referred participants reported a greater decrease in general anger. Overall, all participants evinced decreased driving anger, state anxiety, and general anger.

Importantly, results also demonstrated that despite these general gains, participants with symptoms that met criteria for IED reported far lower improvements in aggressive driving behavior, a finding that did not achieve significance. The authors concluded that individuals with IED may require "more intensive and prolonged treatment" to reduce aggressive driving behaviors than those without the disorder.

The second psychotherapy treatment study involving participants with IED is a pilot randomized clinical trial of a cognitive-behavioral intervention known as *cognitive restructuring, relaxation, and coping skills training* (CRCST) (McCloskey et al. 2008b). This protocol was based on an anger treatment manual (Deffenbacher and McKay 2000), which combined relaxation techniques with cognitive restructuring to reduce anger both in general and in specific situations. The original protocol utilized an eight-session model that first introduced relaxation training, then introduced cognitive restructuring, and finally combined the two strategies for coping skills training (McCloskey et al. 2008b).

In the IED pilot protocol, 45 participants with symptoms that met integrated research (similar to DSM-5) criteria for IED (McCloskey et al. 2006) were randomly assigned to receive individual or group therapy or a wait-list control group. The sessions for each treatment condition emphasized CRCST. The differences in this manual from Deffenbacher and McKay's (2000) treatment protocol included an increase to 12 sessions from 8, to account for previous evidence suggesting that individuals with IED may require longer treatment (Galovski and Blanchard 2002), as well as evidence suggesting that individuals with IED have more difficulty with executive functioning (Best et al. 2002). Additionally, given previous evidence supporting the efficacy of both group (Galovski and Blanchard 2002) and individual therapy (DiGiuseppe and Tafrate 2003) for reducing anger and aggression, both modalities were included. Control participants were directed to focus on self-monitoring of aggression and anger and completed the same assessments as did the CRCST participants.

Results of this study indicated that both group and individual CRCST had large effects overall. Participants in both active treatment conditions reported significantly less anger and aggression after treatment than wait-list control participants. In addition, both CRCST groups had reduced depression scores after treatment. For individual CRCST only, participants reported significantly decreased hostile thoughts and increased quality of life as compared with the wait-list group. Additionally, nearly half the individual therapy participants evinced remission status (e.g., no aggressive acts in the past 2 weeks) at posttreatment.

Notably, though some of these gains (i.e., reduction of aggression and increase of anger control strategies) were evident at midtreatment, others (i.e., anger tendency and response to anger-provoking situations) did not show significant decrease until posttreatment, supporting research that CBT for IED is more effective for broader improvements over a longer period of delivery. Furthermore, these gains were maintained at a 3-month follow-up. Additional pilot data by the authors suggest that IED is superior to a supportive psychotherapy control and that the effects of CBT in treating IED are not affected by most demographic variables or psychiatric comorbidities. (See the clinical vignette below for an example of CBT for IED.) Despite this strong preliminary evidence, clinical trials by independent research groups, as well as additional treatment modalities, are still needed to further investigate effective and evidence-based psychotherapy for IED.

Clinical Vignette and Discussion

RJ is a 40-year-old, white married male who came in for treatment after an incident in which his yelling resulted in his 6-year-old daughter crying and hiding from him in fear. RJ reported a lifelong pattern of dysfunctional aggression beginning in preadolescence, which he attributed to being "passionate." RJ's aggressive outbursts had been predominantly verbal and/or acts of minor property harm (e.g., punching a steering wheel, slamming a door). However, there had also been several acts of major property harm (e.g., breaking his cell phone) and occasional acts of physical aggression, including a fistfight with another customer at the grocery store who "antagonized" RJ after their shopping carts clipped each other. The police were called, but no charges were filed. At the time of the evaluation, RJ reported engaging in minor acts of aggression approximately two or three times per week and more serious acts of property damage about once every 3 months. His aggressive outbursts occurred most often at home and when in the car, though he acknowledged he can also be "a bit prickly" with subordinates at work. RJ stated that his aggressive outbursts have caused problems in several of his social relationships, including being a precipitating factor in his divorce to his first wife (to which he added "so there is one good thing about my aggression,") and have led to his often feeling angry and frustrated, as well as sometimes remorseful and upset at himself. Common aggression antecedents included "unfair situations" and individuals being "disrespectful, stupid, or not following through on what they agreed to." RJ's wife described him as a "kind and very loving husband and father...but he can't let things go." She added that he was "devastated" that his daughter was afraid of him.

A clinical interview revealed that RJ had a past mild alcohol use disorder when he was in college and a past major depressive episode following his divorce 10 years ago. Neither disorder seemed to have a bearing on his current IED symptoms. RJ also reported some turmoil in his childhood, as his father had alcohol problems and was emotionally and occasionally physically abusive toward RJ (which in part led to RJ's strong reaction to seeing his daughter fearful of him).

Treatment started with psychoeducation about IED and a discussion of goals and expectations of treatment. RJ was able to identify several goals of treatment, and after weighing both the costs (e.g., significant time commitment, discussing things that make him angry, perceived change in who he "is") and the benefits (e.g., better relationship with his daughter and wife, less anger at self for losing control) of successful treatment, RJ agreed to begin a 12-session treatment regimen of CBT. Baseline anger and aggression symptoms were obtained using the OAS-M, and RJ was scheduled to begin treatment the following week.

Early treatment sessions focused on increasing RJ's awareness of his anger and aggression cues. This process was facilitated by having

RJ keep an anger log of whenever he became angry. He was asked to identify the situation that preceded his anger, his physiological reaction, and any aggressive or coping behavior. Through this RJ was able to realize that his anger was not "0 to 100" as he originally believed and that his outbursts often were preceded by minor irritations that increased his "baseline anger." RJ also worked on learning relaxation techniques, which was initially difficult for him, as he wanted to "relax faster." This reaction was normalized, but it was also highlighted that trying to force himself to relax faster would lead to the opposite effect. RJ was eventually able to effectively use multiple relaxation techniques (e.g., breathing, visual imagery, progressive muscle relaxation) to reduce the anger from minor irritants. At the same time, he was taught the "time out" technique for highly angering situations so that his anger "cannot get the best of [him]."

As RJ became more comfortable with the relaxation techniques and started to see some benefit from using them, we began to transition into cognitive restructuring. RJ's hostile cognitive biases were framed as a strategy that, though adaptive at one time, was no longer needed. The relationship between thoughts (distortions), feelings (e.g., anger), and behavior (e.g., aggression) was introduced and elaborated on until understanding was demonstrated, which in RJ's case was quite quickly. RJ was introduced to general coping thoughts to use across angering situations ("they are not worth it."), followed by specific types of anger distortions (e.g., "blaming," "catastrophizing," "shoulds") and how to "talk back" to those anger distortions via cognitive restructuring. RJ had a great deal of difficulty with the concepts of "shoulds" being a distortion. What helped it "click" for RJ was when he was asked if he did everything people thought he should. After responding "no" and being asked why, he explained, "Because I decide what is best for me, no matter what other people think." He then sighed and smirked, adding "And other people have the same right… damn it." As RJ continued to work on his anger distortions, he added identifying anger thought to his anger log. After 7 weeks, RJ had reduced the frequency of his aggression by almost 50%.

The later sessions focused on utilizing his relaxation and cognitive restructuring skills in increasingly provocative imaginal exposures (all based on real-life incidents that had led to RJ acting out aggressively). Toward the end of therapy, RJ and the therapist focused on the importance of continuing to use the skills he developed, likening it to exercise in that he did the hardest part by getting into mental shape, but stressing that if he stopped "exercising" altogether he would lose all his gains. They also collaborated on a relapse prevention plan in case he had a major aggressive outburst. This plan included identifying the factors that led to the outburst, coming up with a strategy to deal with it more effectively next time, and making an appointment for a check-in visit with the therapist. By the end of treatment, RJ had reduced his aggression to minor verbal outbursts (yelling, cursing) about twice a month with no property damage or physical aggression of any sort in the past month. RJ's self-reported quality of life also improved by over 50%. Most important to RJ, his daughter was back to "always wanting to be with her daddy."

Summary

Research into effective treatments for IED is still in its infancy. Extant studies support the use of SSRIs and CBT as effective treatments for IED. There is evidence for other pharmacological interventions, particularly when comorbid symptoms are present (McElroy 1999). However, no treatment meets the criteria for an empirically supported treatment (Chambless and Hollon 1998), suggesting the need for more randomized clinical trials on CBT and other interventions.

Key Clinical Points

▌ To date there are no data to suggest the superiority of behavioral or pharmacological treatments for intermittent explosive disorder (IED), so the clinician should consider the patient's preference when deciding which treatment to attempt first. If the aggression problems are severe, a combined approach may be beneficial.

▌ Prior to aggression treatment, individuals should receive a thorough diagnostic interview and medical examination to help the clinician assess for potential conditions other than IED that may better explain the aggression, or that, when the aggression is IED, identify any comorbidities that may impact treatment.

▌ Those with IED are at increased risk for self-harm and suicidal behavior (Jenkins et al. 2015) and thus should be monitored regularly for these thoughts and behaviors.

▌ When treatment is being initiated, it is important to assess the patient's motivation for treatment. This includes addressing the potential negative consequences of engaging in treatment (e.g., time lost, aggravation) and even the potential consequences of successfully treating IED (e.g., people no longer intimidated, loss of identity, realizing it could have been treated years ago). One approach to this is going through the pros and cons of both having IED and being treated for IED.

▪ Medications can meaningfully reduce impulsive aggressive behavior but do not typically eliminate it.

▪ When medications reduce impulsive aggressive behavior, they do not do so by permanently correcting a psychobiological deficit but instead by suppressing the expression of an impulsive aggressive response to frustration and/or social threat.

▪ When cognitive-behavioral therapy (CBT) is decided on to treat IED, consider starting with relaxation training to give the patient a success experience before moving on to cognitive restructuring, which is often more difficult for the patient to master.

▪ As with most disorders, collaboration is a key to successful CBT treatment for IED. Encourage patients to make minor modifications to the treatment to make it more relevant to them. For example, if they prefer a different muscle sequence for progressive muscle relaxation or they have a different term they like to use for an anger distortion, use that to give the patient more of a feeling of investment in and "ownership" of the treatment.

References

American Psychiatric Association: Diagnostic and Statistical Manual of Mental Disorders, 4th Edition. Washington, DC, American Psychiatric Association, 1994

American Psychiatric Association: Diagnostic and Statistical Manual of Mental Disorders, 4th Edition, Text Revision. Washington, DC, American Psychiatric Association, 2000

American Psychiatric Association: Diagnostic and Statistical Manual of Mental Disorders, 5th Edition. Arlington, VA, American Psychiatric Association, 2013

Barratt ES, Stanford MS, Felthous AR, et al: The effects of phenytoin on impulsive and premeditated aggression: a controlled study. J Clin Psychopharmacol 17(5):341–349, 1997 9315984

Beck R, Fernandez E: Cogntive-behavioral therapy in the treatment of anger: a meta-analysis. Cognit Ther Res 22:62–75, 1998

Berman ME, McCloskey MS, Fanning JR, et al: Serotonin augmentation reduces response to attack in aggressive individuals. Psychol Sci 20(6):714–720, 2009 19422623

Best M, Williams JM, Coccaro EF: Evidence for a dysfunctional prefrontal circuit in patients with an impulsive aggressive disorder. Proc Natl Acad Sci USA 99(12):8448–8453, 2002 12034876

Bowman-Edmondson C, Cohen-Conger J: A review of treatment efficacy for individuals with anger problems: conceptual, assessment and methodological issues. Clin Psychol Rev 16:251–275, 1996

Chambless DL, Hollon SD: Defining empirically supported therapies. J Consult Clin Psychol 66(1):7–18, 1998 9489259

Cherek DR, Lane SD, Pietras CJ, et al: Effects of chronic paroxetine administration on measures of aggressive and impulsive responses of adult males with a history of conduct disorder. Psychopharmacology (Berl) 159(3):266–274, 2002 11862359

Coccaro EF: Intermittent explosive disorder as a disorder of impulsive aggression for DSM-5. Am J Psychiatry 169(6):577–588, 2012 22535310

Coccaro EF, Kavoussi RJ: Fluoxetine and impulsive aggressive behavior in personality-disordered subjects. Arch Gen Psychiatry 54(12):1081–1088, 1997 9400343

Coccaro EF, Harvey PD, Kupsaw-Lawrence E, et al: Development of neuropharmacologically based behavioral assessments of impulsive aggressive behavior. J Neuropsychiatry Clin Neurosci 3(2):S44–S51, 1991 1821222

Coccaro EF, Lee RJ, Kavoussi RJ: A double-blind, randomized, placebo-controlled trial of fluoxetine in patients with intermittent explosive disorder. J Clin Psychiatry 70(5):653–662, 2009a 19389333

Coccaro EF, Noblett KL, McCloskey MS: Attributional and emotional responses to socially ambiguous cues: validation of a new assessment of social/emotional information processing in healthy adults and impulsive aggressive patients. J Psychiatr Res 43(10):915–925, 2009b 19345371

Coccaro EF, Lee R, Kavoussi RJ: Aggression, suicidality, and intermittent explosive disorder: serotonergic correlates in personality disorder and healthy control subjects. Neuropsychopharmacology 35(2):435–444, 2010 19776731

Coccaro EF, Lee R, McCloskey MS: Validity of the new A1 and A2 criteria for DSM-5 intermittent explosive disorder. Compr Psychiatry 55(2):260–267, 2014 24321204

Coccaro EF, Berman ME, McCloskey MS: Development of a screening questionnaire for DSM-5 intermittent explosive disorder (IED-SQ). Compr Psychiatry 74:21–26, 2017 28088746

Deffenbacher JL, McKay M: Overcoming Situational and General Anger: A Protocol for the Treatment of Anger Based on Relaxation, Cognitive Restructuring, and Coping Skills Training. Oakland, CA, New Harbinger Publications, 2000

DiGiuseppe R, Tafrate RC: Anger treatment for adults: a meta-analytic review. Clin Psychol Sci Pract 10:70–84, 2003

Endicott J, Nee J, Harrison W, et al: Quality of Life Enjoyment and Satisfaction Questionnaire: a new measure. Psychopharmacol Bull 29(2):321–326, 1993 8290681

Feder R: Treatment of intermittent explosive disorder with sertraline in 3 patients. J Clin Psychiatry 60(3):195–196, 1999 10192598

Fettich KC, McCloskey MS, Look AE, et al: Emotion regulation deficits in intermittent explosive disorder. Aggress Behav 41(1):25–33, 2015 27539871

First MB, Williams JBW, Karg RS, et al: Structured Clinical Interview for DSM-5 (SCID-5)—Research Version. Arlington, VA, American Psychiatric Association, 2015

Galovski TE, Blanchard EB: The effectiveness of a brief psychological intervention on court-referred and self-referred aggressive drivers. Behav Res Ther 40(12):1385–1402, 2002 12457634

Gardner DL, Cowdry RW: Positive effects of carbamazepine on behavioral dyscontrol in borderline personality disorder. Am J Psychiatry 143(4):519–522, 1986 3513634

Glancy G, Saini MA: An evidenced-based review of psychological treatments of anger and aggression. Brief Treatment Crisis Intervention 5(2):229–248, 2005

Hollander E, Tracy KA, Swann AC, et al: Divalproex in the treatment of impulsive aggression: efficacy in cluster B personality disorders. Neuropsychopharmacology 28(6):1186–1197, 2003 12700713

Jenkins AL, McCloskey MS, Kulper D, et al: Self-harm behavior among individuals with intermittent explosive disorder and personality disorders. J Psychiatr Res 60:125–131, 2015 25300440

Jenkins SC, Maruta T: Therapeutic use of propranolol for intermittent explosive disorder. Mayo Clin Proc 62(3):204–214, 1987 3546964

Kavoussi RJ, Coccaro EF: Divalproex sodium for impulsive aggressive behavior in patients with personality disorder. J Clin Psychiatry 59(12):676–680, 1998 9921702

Kavoussi RJ, Liu J, Coccaro EF: An open trial of sertraline in personality disordered patients with impulsive aggression. J Clin Psychiatry 55(4):137–141, 1994 8071257

Kessler RC, Coccaro EF, Fava M, et al: The prevalence and correlates of DSM-IV intermittent explosive disorder in the National Comorbidity Survey Replication. Arch Gen Psychiatry 63(6):669–678, 2006 16754840

Kulper DA, Kleiman EM, McCloskey MS, et al: The experience of aggressive outbursts in intermittent explosive disorder. Psychiatry Res 225(3):710–715, 2015 25541537

Look AE, McCloskey MS, Coccaro EF: Verbal versus physical aggression in intermittent explosive disorder. Psychiatry Res 225(3):531–539, 2015 25534757

Mattes JA: Metoprolol for intermittent explosive disorder. Am J Psychiatry 142(9):1108–1109, 1985 4025634

Mattes JA: Comparative effectiveness of carbamazepine and propranolol for rage outbursts. J Neuropsychiatry Clin Neurosci 2(2):159–164, 1990 2136070

Mattes JA: Oxcarbazepine in patients with impulsive aggression: a double-blind, placebo-controlled trial. J Clin Psychopharmacol 25(6):575–579, 2005 16282841

Mattes JA: Levetiracetam in patients with impulsive aggression: a double-blind, placebo-controlled trial. J Clin Psychiatry 69(2):310–315, 2008 18232724

McCloskey MS, Coccaro EF: Questionnaire and interview measures of aggression in adults, in Aggression: Psychiatric Assessment and Treatment. Edited by Coccaro EF. New York, Marcel Dekker, 2003, pp 195–214

McCloskey MS, Berman ME, Noblett KL, et al: Intermittent explosive disorder–integrated research diagnostic criteria: convergent and discriminant validity. J Psychiatr Res 40(3):231–242, 2006 16153657

McCloskey MS, Lee R, Berman ME, et al: The relationship between impulsive verbal aggression and intermittent explosive disorder. Aggress Behav 34(1):51–60, 2008a 17654692

McCloskey MS, Noblett KL, Deffenbacher JL, et al: Cognitive-behavioral therapy for intermittent explosive disorder: a pilot randomized clinical trial. J Consult Clin Psychol 76(5):876–886, 2008b 18837604

McCloskey MS, Kleabir K, Berman ME, et al: Unhealthy aggression: intermittent explosive disorder and adverse physical health outcomes. Health Psychol 29(3):324–332, 2010 20496987

McElroy SL: Recognition and treatment of DSM-IV intermittent explosive disorder. J Clin Psychiatry 60 (suppl 15):12–16, 1999 10418808

Puhalla AA, Ammerman BA, Uyeji LL, et al: Negative urgency and reward/punishment sensitivity in intermittent explosive disorder. J Affect Disord 201:8–14, 2016 27155024

Rinne T, van den Brink W, Wouters L, et al: SSRI treatment of borderline personality disorder: a randomized, placebo-controlled clinical trial for female patients with borderline personality disorder. Am J Psychiatry 159(12):2048–2054, 2002 12450955

Rynar L, Coccaro EF: Psychosocial impairment in DSM-5 intermittent explosive disorder. Psychiatry Res 264:91–95, 2018 29627702

Salzman C, Wolfson AN, Schatzberg A, et al: Effect of fluoxetine on anger in symptomatic volunteers with borderline personality disorder. J Clin Psychopharmacol 15(1):23–29, 1995 7714224

Seo D, Patrick CJ, Kennealy PJ: Role of serotonin and dopamine system interactions in the neurobiology of impulsive aggression and its comorbidity with other clinical disorders. Aggress Violent Behav 13(5):383–395, 2008 19802333

Sheard MH, Marini JL, Bridges CI, et al: The effect of lithium on impulsive aggressive behavior in man. Am J Psychiatry 133(12):1409–1413, 1976 984241

Spielberger CD, Krasner SS, Solomon EP: The experience, expression, and control of anger, in Health Psychology: Individual Differences and Stress. Edited by Janisse MP. New York, Springer, 1988, pp 89–108

Stanford MS, Houston RJ, Mathias CW, et al: A double-blind placebo-controlled crossover study of phenytoin in individuals with impulsive aggression. Psychiatry Res 103(2–3):193–203, 2001 11549407

Tafrate RC: Evaluation of strategies for adult anger disorders, in Anger Disorders: Definition, Diagnosis, and Treatment. Edited by Kassinove H. Washington, DC, Taylor & Francis, 1995, pp 109–129

Ventura J, Liberman RP, Green MF, et al: Training and quality assurance with the Structured Clinical Interview for DSM-IV (SCID-I/P). Psychiatry Res 79(2):163–173, 1998 9705054

Wang CJ, Fetzer SJ, Yang YC, et al: The efficacy of using self-monitoring diaries in a weight loss program for chronically ill obese adults in a rural area. J Nurs Res 20(3):181–188, 2012 22902977

Aggression in Other Psychiatric Disorders

3

Aggression in Autism Spectrum Disorder and Other Neurodevelopmental Disorders

Laura C. Politte, M.D.
Sarah E. Fitzpatrick, B.S.
Craig Erickson, M.D.

Neurodevelopmental disorders (NDDs) are a diverse category of syndromes sharing several features: onset in early childhood, delay in one or more areas of development, functional impairment, and persistence of symptoms across the lifespan (American Psychiatric Association 2013). Impairment may be specific to one area (as in a specific learning disorder) or more general (as in intellectual disability), and NDDs frequently co-occur. Autism spectrum disorder (ASD) is a specific NDD characterized by impairment in social communication, coupled with restricted, repetitive patterns of behavior. Individuals with ASD and other NDDs may exhibit additional maladaptive behaviors, including aggression and self-injury, which often cause greater stress and disability than the core features of the NDD (Lecavalier et al. 2006).

Phenomenology

Aggression is behavior that is threatening or likely to cause harm and may be verbal, physical, or destructive of property. Physical aggression in NDD may also be self-directed (e.g., biting, slapping, scratching oneself) and is termed *self-injurious behavior*. Aggression can be proactive or reactive in nature. Proactive aggression is planful, goal-oriented, and frequently motivated by an external reward, whereas reactive aggression occurs in reaction to a perceived threat or intentional harm from others (Fite et al. 2009). Children with ASD are more likely to exhibit reactive than proactive aggression (Farmer et al. 2015), which can stem from deficits in emotion regulation, impulse control, and accurate interpretation of social intent.

Clinical rating scales can be useful in systematically assessing aggressive behavior in individuals with NDD and are summarized in Table 3–1. Aggression can also be directly observed and recorded by a behavior analyst conducting a functional behavior assessment (FBA), as described in the section "Clinical Approach and Treatment."

Epidemiology

Some studies indicate a higher prevalence of aggressive behavior in individuals with ASD compared with typically developing peers and those peers with other NDDs, though reports are inconsistent. ASD-specific research has yielded variable prevalence estimates for aggressive behavior, ranging from 15% (Matson and Rivet 2008) to 56% (Kanne and Mazurek 2011). In some studies, individuals with intellectual disability and comorbid ASD more frequently demonstrated aggression than individuals with intellectual disability alone (McClintock et al. 2003; Tsakanikos et al. 2007). Common predictors of aggression in normative populations, such as male sex, parental education attainment, and parental marital status, do not consistently predict aggression in children with ASD (Farmer et al. 2015; Hartley et al. 2008; Kanne and Mazurek 2011). Greater impairment in language, cognition, and adaptive functioning may contribute to aggressive behavior in children with ASD (Dominick et al. 2007; Hartley et al. 2008).

TABLE 3–1. Rating scales for assessment of aggressive behavior in neurodevelopmental disorders

Rating scale	Description	Rater	Target population
Aberrant Behavior Checklist (ABC) Irritability subscale (Aman et al. 1985)	15 items, rated from 0 (not a problem) to 3 (severe problem) Items focused on irritability, agitation, and mood swings	Parent or caregiver	Children and adults with intellectual disability
Child Behavior Checklist (CBCL) Aggressive Behavior subdomain (Achenbach 2001)	Frequency of behaviors rated on 4-point Likert scale (0–4)	Parent	Children (preschool and school-age forms available)
Overt Aggression Scale (Yudofsky et al. 1986); Overt Aggression Scale–Modified (OAS-M; Sorgi et al. 1991)	Track frequency and severity of behavior in four areas: verbal aggression, physical aggression against objects, physical aggression against self, physical aggression against others	Inpatient clinician	Children and adults on inpatient units
Children's Scale of Hostility and Aggression: Reactive/ Proactive (C-SHARP; Farmer and Aman 2009)	Five factors: verbal aggression, bullying, covert aggression, hostility, physical aggression Differentiates proactive and reactive forms of aggression using Provocation Scale (ranging from –2 [reactive] to +2 [proactive])	Parent	Children with neurodevelopmental disorders
Adult Scale of Hostility and Aggression: Reactive/ Proactive (A-SHARP; Matlock and Aman 2011)	Uses same factor structure for Problem Scale and Provocation Scale as C-SHARP	Caregiver	Adults with neurodevelopmental disorders

Aggression is clearly associated with negative outcomes for children with ASD, including impaired social relationships (Luiselli 2009), placement in restrictive school or residential settings (Dryden-Edwards and Combrinck-Graham 2010), use of physical intervention (Dagnan and Weston 2006), and increased risk of maltreatment (Stith et al. 2009). Aggressive behavior in students also contributes to teacher burnout (Otero-López et al. 2009), which may have a negative impact on the quality of education. Caregivers of youth with ASD and aggression report increased stress levels (Neece et al. 2012), financial problems, lack of support services, and negative impact on day-to-day family life and well-being (Hodgetts et al. 2013).

Psychobiology

Neuroimaging

Several brain regions and neural networks have been implicated in aggressive behavior in humans (Rosell and Siever 2015), though few studies have specifically investigated the neurobiological correlates of aggressive behavior in ASD and other NDDs. A recent structural magnetic resonance imaging (MRI) study examined various brain region volumes in subjects with ASD with and without behavioral dysregulation, defined as a sum of the T-scores of the Attention Problems, Aggressive Behavior, and Anxiety/Depression subscales of the CBCL greater than 180 (Ni et al. 2018). In this study, boys with ASD (ages 7–17) and behavioral dysregulation ($n=53$) demonstrated larger regional gray matter volumes in the right fusiform gyrus than boys with ASD without dysregulation ($n=28$), and smaller gray matter volumes in the anterior prefrontal cortex and left lateral occipital/superior parietal cortex than typically developing control subjects ($n=61$). Dysregulation was associated with smaller gray matter volumes in the orbitofrontal cortex independent of ASD diagnosis. Statistical differences in regional brain volumes between ASD and control subjects no longer existed after adjustment for the presence of dysregulation, suggesting that this behavioral construct ("behavioral dysregulation") may be associated with specific morphological differences across diagnostic categories.

In a separate brain volume region of interest study, smaller brain stem volume was also a predictor of aggressive behavior in children with

ASD, a finding consistent with the literature on aggression in other psychiatric conditions (Lundwall et al. 2017). Observational data suggest that children with aggressive behavior are more likely to have epileptiform discharges on electroencephalogram (EEG) (Mulligan and Trauner 2014), though this relationship is likely mediated by severity of autism.

Further neuroimaging research is needed to characterize the brain regions, functional networks, and molecular activity associated with aggressive behavior in the context of ASD and other NDDs, as identification of specific endophenotypes could lead to more targeted treatment options.

Molecular Genetics

Though the body of literature pertaining to genetic correlates of behavior is still relatively small, recent advances have been made in linking specific genotypes to aggression in ASD and other NDDs. Approaches to understanding this relationship include characterization of behavioral phenotypes in animal models with specific genotypes, and large-scale genotyping in humans with specific disorders, with and without a behavior of interest.

The serotonin transporter gene (*SLC6A4*) is an autism candidate gene because of its association with anxiety, aggression, and attention (Brune et al. 2006). In a sample of 73 subjects with autistic disorder (DSM-IV criteria), having two copies of the L (long) allele (L/L genotype) at the serotonin transporter gene promoter polymorphism (5-HTTLPR) was associated with higher ratings of aggression and stereotyped/repetitive behavior on the Autism Diagnostic Interview—Revised (Brune et al. 2006). In 50 males (ages 8–24 years) with fragile X syndrome (FXS), the L/L 5-HTTLPR genotype was also associated with more severe aggression, destructive behavior, and stereotypy, indicating the influence of genetic polymorphisms across NDDs (Hessl et al. 2008). Replication in larger samples is needed.

The upstream variable number tandem repeat (uVNTR) polymorphism within the X-linked monoamine oxidase A gene (*MAOA*) promoter region is also associated with neurophysiological, neuroanatomical, and behavioral changes in humans (Cohen et al. 2011). A sample of boys with ASD (*N*=119) and their unaffected parents genotyped for the *MAOA*-uVNTR polymorphism found an association between the low-activity three-repeat *MAOA* allele, more severe social communication impairment, and aggression (Cohen et al. 2011). Interestingly, boys with the high-activity four-repeat *MAOA* allele demonstrated greater irritability and aggression when their mothers were homozygous for the four-repeat *MAOA* allele compared with children of heterozygous mothers. It is possible that during gestation, maternal serotonin levels, which vary in association with *MAOA* polymorphism status, may affect areas of brain development governing emotional reactivity and response to environment (Cohen et al. 2011). By contrast, *MAOA* genotype did not correlate with aggressive behavior in males with FXS ($N=50$), though individuals with FXS with the four-repeat allele were more likely to take selective serotonin reuptake inhibitor (SSRI) or serotonin-norepinephrine reuptake inhibitor (SNRI) medication, possibly reflecting a higher propensity for mood and anxiety disorders in this group (Hessl et al. 2008).

A large-scale analysis of copy number variants (CNVs) in children with developmental delay, intellectual disability, and/or autism ($N=$ 29,085) identified an association between a truncating mutation in the gene *ZMYND11* (at locus 10p15.3) and aggressive behavior, tantrums, and rage episodes in three of five affected individuals (Coe et al. 2014). No case-control subjects carried the mutation in *ZMYND11*, which is purported to play an inhibitory role in transcription regulation and neuronal differentiation early in development (Coe et al. 2014).

The gene *STXBP1* encodes a protein (syntaxin-binding protein 1) that plays a role in synaptic vesicle docking and fusion (Stamberger et al. 2016). Mutations in *STXBP1* in humans almost uniformly cause intellectual disability and epilepsy, with some individuals also exhibiting autism or aggressive behavior (Stamberger et al. 2016). Heterozygous *Stxbp1* knockout mice demonstrate a high level of aggression that is mitigated by treatment with the ampakine CX516, which potentiates excitatory (glutamatergic) transmission (Miyamoto et al. 2017). This finding suggests that aggressive behavior associated with *STXBP1* mutation may be mediated by an imbalance in excitatory/inhibitory neurotransmission.

Clinical Approach and Treatment

Assessment of the individual with an NDD and aggression should begin with a thorough characterization of the aggressive behavior, its purported causes, and any consequences of the behavior. It is important to determine the type(s) of aggression present, including verbal aggression, physical aggression toward others, property destruction, and self-injury. Discerning the frequency, duration, and intensity of the behavior helps determine the overall risk and recommended treatment. Safety concerns should always be elicited, including escalation from verbal threats to physical violence, the severity of physical harm inflicted, use of weapons, and risk of accidental injury (e.g., running away toward a busy road during a rage episode). For individuals with severe, persistent aggression or self-injury presenting serious risk of harm, psychiatric hospitalization or residential treatment may be necessary. Standardized ratings scales can be helpful for characterizing aggressive behavior (see Table 3–1).

A careful history includes an assessment of factors, or antecedents, that may contribute to the aggressive behavior. For example, severe functional communication impairment can lead to frustration and use of aggression as a means to express displeasure or discomfort. Establishing when and where the aggression occurs provides clues about possible triggers, such as social problems, learning difficulties, fatigue, hunger, and parent-child conflict. Importantly, medical problems should always be considered first and, if present, treated, particularly in children with limited means of communication. Relatively common sources of discomfort that may drive aggression include gastrointestinal issues (e.g., constipation, gastric reflux), ear infections, abscesses, dental problems, headaches, and urinary tract infections. Sleep disturbance is also common in children with ASD and other NDDs and can have a negative impact on daytime behavior (Hirata et al. 2016; Mazurek and Sohl 2016). Comorbid psychiatric disorders, such as depression and anxiety, can lead to aggressive behavior and should be systematically screened for and treated.

An FBA conducted by a trained behavioral professional (such as a board-certified behavior analyst, or BCBA) is a valuable tool for developing a hypothesis about the antecedents, function(s), and consequences that may be maintaining a maladaptive behavior. Common "functions" for aggressive behavior in individuals with NDDs can include 1) attention from others, 2) avoidance or escape from demands or unpleasant stimuli, 3) access to preferred items or activities, and 4) automatic reinforcement (e.g., seeking tactile sensory input, in service of a compulsive ritual) (Iwata et al. 1994). Understanding the antecedents and function(s) of the aggressive behavior allows for a well-designed behavior intervention plan (BIP) that includes environmental modification and teaching of adaptive replacement behaviors. An FBA further includes analysis of the consequences of the behavior, which may serve to reinforce (strengthen) or reduce the behavior. For example, if a child with limited language shrieks and bites his wrist when asked to do a counting activity and his teacher removes the activity, escape from the nonpreferred activity (the consequence) is likely to reinforce the shrieking and biting, making it more likely to occur again in the future.

Nonpharmacological Treatment of Aggression in NDDs

Learning theory and operant behavior principles form the basis for current behavioral treatments of aggression in ASD (Powers et al. 2011). These principles rely on careful observation and definition of behavior, as well as the recognition that behavior serves a function (Soorya et al. 2011). *Applied behavior analysis* (ABA), a systematic approach to defining and shaping specific behaviors (Cooper et al. 2007), is a preferred, evidence-based method for teaching new skills and reducing maladaptive behaviors in ASD (Campbell 2003; Roth et al. 2014; Wong et al. 2015). An FBA should form the foundation of the behavioral treatment (Powers et al. 2011).

After the antecedents, function(s), and consequences of an individual's aggressive behavior are determined, a behavior plan based on reinforcement principles can be developed. In recent years, differential reinforcement of other behavior has emerged as one of the most frequently used treatments for aggression in ASD (Matson et al. 2005). In differential reinforcement, caregivers provide the individual with positive reinforcement in the absence of the aggressive behavior or when the individual demonstrates an appropriate replacement behavior. For example, if a child with ASD pinches himself when he is frustrated with his schoolwork, he may be taught to use a "break card" to request a break instead. When he appropriately uses the break card, his teacher rewards him with praise for his good choice and 10 minutes to engage in a quiet activity of his choice before returning to the activity. His teacher would purposely ignore any recurrent pinching behavior and remind the child to use his break card.

Functional communication training (FCT) involves teaching a person to appropriately request access to a desirable consequence (e.g., social attention, preferred items/activities) to reduce inappropriate behaviors. For example, a child may be taught to touch a picture of his mother, rather than hitting her, to gain her attention. FCT is an effective and commonly used approach to reducing aggressive behavior in children with communication impairment (Braithwaite and Richdale 2000; Carr and Durand 1985), particularly when used in conjunction with extinction strategies (Kurtz et al. 2011).

Pharmacological Treatment of Aggression in NDDs

Aggressive behavior is a common and often devastating problem for individuals with ASD and their families, and the treatment of ASD-associated irritability, including aggression, tantrums, and self-injury, has been a major focus of pharmacological research. Considerably less research has focused on treating aggression in other NDDs, though results from ASD trials are often used to guide treatment in these populations. Second-generation antipsychotics (SGAs) are considered first-line pharmacotherapy for the treatment of aggression in ASD. Following several large randomized controlled trials (RCTs) that demonstrated robust reduction in aggressive behavior in youth with ASD, the U.S. Food and Drug Administration (FDA) approved risperidone and aripiprazole for the treatment of irritability in this population (Marcus et al. 2009; McCracken et al. 2002; Owen et al. 2009; Shea et al. 2004). First-generation antipsychotics, antiepileptic drugs (AEDs), other mood stabilizers, and glutamatergic modulators are sometimes used to treat ASD-associated irritability, though with less robust evidence supporting their use (see Table 3–2 for a brief review of selected controlled pharmacological trials in ASD).

Second-Generation Antipsychotics

SGAs include risperidone, aripiprazole, olanzapine, quetiapine, ziprasidone, paliperidone, lurasidone, and clozapine.

Risperidone is a robust dopamine D_2 receptor antagonist with additional antagonist activity at $\alpha_{1/2}$-adrenergic and histaminergic receptors. Numerous case reports, open-label studies, and double-blind, placebo-controlled trials of risperidone have demonstrated its efficacy as a treatment for ASD-associated aggression, self-injury, and se-

TABLE 3–2. Pharmacological management of aggression in autism spectrum disorder (selected controlled trials)

Medication	Study	Study design	N	Age (years)	Details	Adverse events
Risperidone	McCracken et al. 2002	8-week RPCT	101	5–17	Risperidone > placebo on ABC-I and CGI-I	Weight gain, increased appetite, fatigue
	Shea et al. 2004	8-week RPCT	79	5–12	Risperidone superior to placebo on ABC-I	Somnolence, weight gain
	RUPP Autism Network 2005	Part 1: 16-week open-label extension	63	5–17	Sustained improvement on ABC-I	Weight gain
		Part 2: 8-week double-blind placebo-substitution	32	5–17	62.5% relapse rate in placebo group	Increased aggression in placebo group
	Aman et al. 2015	Naturalistic 21-month follow-up	84	5–17	Sustained improvement on ABC-I; significant rate of continued use	Weight gain, excessive appetite, enuresis

TABLE 3–2. Pharmacological management of aggression in autism spectrum disorder (selected controlled trials) *(continued)*

Medication	Study	Study design	N	Age (years)	Details	Adverse events
Aripiprazole	Marcus et al. 2009	8-week RPCT (fixed dose)	218	6–17	Aripiprazole>placebo on ABC-I	Weight gain, sedation, EPS
	Owen et al. 2009	8-week RPCT (flexible dose)	98	6–17	Aripiprazole>placebo on ABC-I, CGI-I	Weight gain
	Marcus et al. 2011	52-week, open-label extension of 2009 trial	330	6–17	Aripiprazole>placebo on ABC-I, CGI-I	Weight gain, increased appetite, vomiting, insomnia
Olanzapine	Hollander et al. 2006	8-week RPCT	11	6–14	Olanzapine>placebo on CGI-I, but not on OAS-M	Weight gain, sedation
N-acetylcysteine (NAC)	Hardan et al. 2012	12-week RPCT	29	3.2–10.7	NAC>placebo on ABC-I	Mild gastrointestinal symptoms

Note. ABC-I=Aberrant Behavior Checklist—Irritability subscale; CGI-I=Clinical Global Impressions—Improvement scale; EPS = extrapyramidal symptoms; OAS-M=Overt Aggression Scale—Modified; RPCT=randomized, placebo-controlled trial; RUPP=Research Units on Pediatric Psychopharmacology.

vere tantrums, and in 2006, risperidone became the first medication to be approved by the FDA for the treatment of irritability in youth with ASD (CenterWatch 2009). A pivotal RCT of risperidone in 101 children (ages 5–17) with autism and severe behavioral disturbance found that 69% of the children taking risperidone substantially improved after 8 weeks of treatment, compared with 12% in the placebo group (McCracken et al. 2002). Two-thirds of responders maintained this benefit at 6 months, and a similar proportion (62.5%) relapsed with placebo substitution during a blinded discontinuation phase. Additional open-label and controlled trials of risperidone in children with ASD and severe irritability support short-term response rates in the range of 54% to 72% (Malone et al. 2002; McDougle et al. 1998; Nagaraj et al. 2006; Shea et al. 2004; Troost et al. 2005). Notably, the addition of manualized parent training to risperidone resulted in improved outcome scores and lower risperidone doses compared with risperidone alone in one large clinical trial (Aman et al. 2009). Common side effects of risperidone in this population include sedation, increased appetite, weight gain, and elevated prolactin levels (Martin et al. 2004; McCracken et al. 2002; Scahill et al. 2016; Shea et al. 2004). No significant differences in extrapyramidal symptoms (EPS) were found between risperidone and placebo in the largest studies (McCracken et al. 2002; Shea et al. 2004). As in other clinical populations, a minority of children with ASD treated with risperidone may develop hyperglycemia and insulin resistance (Sukasem et al. 2018).

Aripiprazole has a unique mechanism of action as a partial D_2 receptor and serotonin 5-HT_{1A} receptor agonist, and a 5-HT_{2A} receptor antagonist. Aripiprazole appears to differentially act as an agonist or antagonist depending on local dopamine concentrations (Erickson et al. 2010). In 2009, aripiprazole became the second agent approved by the FDA for the treatment of irritability in children ages 6–17 years with autism on the basis of positive results from two large sponsored RCTs (Marcus et al. 2009; Owen et al. 2009). Overall treatment response was similar in both trials (55.8% vs. 52.2%), as measured by the same outcome criteria used in the pivotal risperidone trial (Aberrant Behavior Checklist—Irritability [ABC-I] subscale score reduction of at least 25% and Clinical Global Impressions—Improvement [CGI-I] rating of "much improved" or "very much improved"). The effect size (0.87) was somewhat lower for aripiprazole than for risperidone, and significant residual symptoms presumably persisted for some individuals, as the mean endpoint ABC-I subscale score was only slightly lower than the minimum entrance-criterion score of 18 (indicating irritability of at least moderate severity) (Owen et al. 2009). When aripiprazole was flexibly dosed up to 15 mg/day, the optimal dosing for most participants was 5–10 mg daily (Owen et al. 2009). Sedation and somnolence were the most commonly reported adverse effects, followed by weight gain, EPS, and vomiting (Marcus et al. 2009; Owen et al. 2009). High-density lipoprotein declined in 30% of individuals, though clinically significant elevations of total cholesterol (5.2%), low-density lipoprotein (6.5%), triglycerides (4.6%), and serum glucose (1.9%) were less common. Mean serum prolactin levels declined from baseline to endpoint, consistent with its partial D_2 agonist mechanism of action. When 85 aripiprazole responders with ASD who were enrolled in a 13- to 26-week RCT were re-randomly assigned to receive aripiprazole or placebo for 16 weeks, the time to relapse of severe behavioral challenges did not significantly differ between groups (Findling et al. 2014). However, the hazard ratio (0.57) and number needed to treat (NNT=6) suggested that at least some individuals may benefit from long-term treatment with aripiprazole.

Studies of other SGAs for the treatment of aggressive behavior in individuals with ASD are generally limited and have yielded mixed results. Two open-label trials of olanzapine, a D_2 and 5-HT_{2A} receptor antagonist, reported high response rates (6 of 7 and 5 of 6 participants) (Malone et al. 2001; Potenza et al. 1999), though results from an additional two studies were less robust (3 of 25 and 12 of 40 participants were responders) (Fido and Al-Saad 2008; Kemner et al. 2002). Weight gain was substantial across studies and often treatment-limiting.

Open-label studies of quetiapine in ASD, though limited, have suggested minimal efficacy and poor tolerability due to excessive sedation, weight gain, and increased aggression or agitation (Findling et al. 2004; Martin et al. 1999), although one study suggested that quetiapine may be helpful for sleep disturbance and aggression, the latter possibly because of its sedative effects (Golubchik et al. 2011).

Ziprasidone has shown promise in the treatment of aggression in ASD, though published data are limited to one open-label study (*N*=12; 75% treatment response; Malone et al. 2007), one case series (*N*=12; 50% treatment response; McDougle et al. 2002), and two case reports (Duggal 2007; Goforth and Rao 2003). Ziprasidone may be a weight-neutral treatment option for individuals with ASD in whom weight gain is a significant concern. Initial sedation is common, and electrocardiographic monitoring for QTc prolongation with ziprasidone is recommended (Taylor 2003).

Evidence for the efficacy of paliperidone, the major active metabolite of risperidone, is limited to one open-label study ($N=25$; mean age=15 years; Stigler et al. 2012) and three case reports (Kowalski et al. 2011; Stigler et al. 2010). In the open-label study, 21 of 25 participants (84%) responded favorably to treatment, suggesting paliperidone may have some benefit for aggression in individuals with ASD (Stigler et al. 2012). As with risperidone, the most common adverse effects were weight gain (average of 2.2 kg in 8 weeks), elevated prolactin levels, and mild EPS.

Lurasidone is an SGA with mixed dopamine and serotonin antagonism and lower propensity for causing weight gain. In a multicenter RCT of 150 children ages 6–17 years old with ASD and aggressive behavior, lurasidone was not superior to placebo for improvement on the primary outcome measure, the ABC-I subscale (Loebel et al. 2016).

Finally, limited case reports suggest that clozapine may be beneficial for individuals with ASD accompanied by severe aggression (Beherec et al. 2011; Chen et al. 2001; Gobbi and Pulvirenti 2001; Lambrey et al. 2010), particularly when rapid control is imperative, though no controlled trials have been reported. Clozapine carries the potential for severe adverse effects, including cardiomyopathy, lowered seizure threshold, and agranulocytosis (Maayan and Correll 2011). Standard monitoring procedures for clozapine include frequent white blood cell count (WBC) analysis to monitor for agranulocytosis. Blood draws can be especially difficult in highly irritable or aggressive individuals with ASD, and clozapine is rarely used in this population.

First-Generation Antipsychotics

Haloperidol is the only first-generation antipsychotic that has been systematically studied in individuals with ASD. These studies did not target aggression specifically, but rather described significant improvement in withdrawal, stereotypy, and learning (Anderson et al. 1989; Campbell et al. 1978, 1982). Sedation and acute dystonic reactions were common. In one prospective study, 40 of 118 (33.9%)

children with ASD treated with haloperidol for 6 months developed dyskinesias, most commonly upon withdrawal of medication (Armenteros et al. 1995). Because of the higher risk of movement disorders with haloperidol compared with SGAs, haloperidol is rarely a first-line treatment for aggression in children with ASD and other NDDs.

Antiepileptic Drugs

AEDs are sometimes prescribed off-label in youth with ASD to treat aggressive behavior, though with limited evidence for benefit. A systematic review of seven randomized, placebo-controlled trials of AEDs in ASD ($N=171$), including four studies of valproic acid, one of lamotrigine, one of topiramate, and one of levetiracetam, revealed no significant change in irritability symptoms (Hirota et al. 2014). Valproic acid has been most extensively studied, though small sample sizes, heterogeneity within samples, and, in one study, a large placebo response limit the ability to draw definitive conclusions about the efficacy of valproic acid for aggression in NDDs. Current evidence does not support the use of valproic acid for the treatment of aggression in NDDs, though it may be a consideration for select patients requiring treatment for both seizures and aggressive behavior.

Lithium

There is little evidence to support the use of lithium for treating aggressive behavior in individuals with ASD and other NDDs. In a retrospective review of 30 hospitalized children with ASD and mood disorders, 43% were rated as "much improved" or "very much improved" on the CGI-I scale; however, significant adverse effects included vomiting, tremor, fatigue, irritability, and enuresis (Siegel et al. 2014). Presently, there is no clear evidence to support the use of lithium for aggression behavior in the absence of significant mood symptoms.

N-acetylcysteine

N-acetylcysteine (NAC), a prodrug of cysteine, modulates glutamate transmission and has antioxidant properties, and this has led to interest in NAC as a treatment for several neuropsychiatric disorders. In a small, 12-week RCT of NAC for children with ASD ($N=33$; ages 3–10 years; follow-up data available for 29 of the children), NAC was superior to placebo for reduction of irritability as measured by the

ABC-I subscale (Hardan et al. 2012). NAC was well tolerated, with few side effects reported aside from mild gastrointestinal upset. In two small, subsequent RCTs, NAC added to risperidone treatment for aggressive behavior in children with ASD was superior to risperidone alone (Ghanizadeh and Moghimi-Sarani 2013; Nikoo et al. 2015). By contrast, NAC has not proved beneficial for social communication impairment in children with ASD (Dean et al. 2017; Wink et al. 2016). Further evidence from larger studies, including determination of optimal dosing and formulation, is needed to guide potential use of NAC in NDD populations.

Clinical Vignette

TB, a 14-year-old male with severe ASD, intellectual disability, and minimal expressive language, is referred to a local developmental center for evaluation of aggressive behavior. He has engaged in self-injurious behaviors, including head banging and wrist biting, since he was a toddler, though the intensity and frequency of these behaviors have increased over the past year. TB has a large, nonhealing ulceration on his left wrist from repetitive biting, and he has made several holes in the walls at home by head banging. In the past several months, TB has also begun hitting his parents, teachers, and speech therapist when they try to help him transition from a preferred activity (such as shaking a shoestring or watching YouTube videos) to a nonpreferred activity (such as a sorting task). His aggression toward others sometimes appears impulsive and unprovoked, particularly when people approach him too quickly. Because of a recent growth spurt, he now has an intimidating physical presence and can hit forcefully; as a result, his parents and teachers tend to back off from demands when he adopts a threatening posture or hits. TB is no longer allowed to attend a vocational training site off school grounds because of his aggressive and unpredictable behavior, and his parents are beginning to consider residential living options. Upon interview, his parents also express concerns about his erratic sleep patterns (often awake until 2 or 3 A.M., engaging in stereotyped jumping and pacing), short attention span, rigid adherence to routines and rituals, and minimal social interest.

On exam, TB presents as a tall, overweight young man with a large head circumference, wide-set eyes, broad nasal bridge, and a large, cracked callous on the dorsal surface of his left wrist. He spends much of the appointment pacing around the room, occasionally vocalizing loudly while jumping up and down. He appears to grow impatient with the appointment and attempts to leave the room; when his mother blocks the door with her hand, he shrieks and bites his wrist but responds to verbal redirection to use his electronic tablet. He is also observed to bite his wrist while calmly using the tablet, but with less intensity. His physical exam is unremarkable for any evidence of infection or other skin lesions. He pulls the physician's hair when she attempts to look in his ears, calming when his mother holds his hands down. A point-of-care urinalysis is unremarkable.

TB is referred to a local ABA agency, and he is placed on a 6-month waiting list for services. The behavioral specialist designs a BIP for school that identifies the target behaviors, antecedents, and proposed functions of the behaviors (e.g., to escape from unpleasant stimuli; to access things he wants; automatic reinforcement). The BIP provides intervention guidelines for teachers, including planned ignoring of low-intensity aggression and self-injury, teaching of nonverbal strategies for requesting breaks (e.g., picture cards, sign language), praise and "free choice time" for appropriately requesting breaks, and redirection back to the academic activity once he is calm again.

Though his behavior at school improves substantially with implementation of the BIP, he still exhibits intermittent severe outbursts both at home and at school that are difficult to manage. He is prescribed risperidone at a dosage of 0.5 mg daily, and the dosage is increased over the course of several weeks up to 1.5 mg daily. His parents and teachers agree that he is noticeably calmer, less aggressive, and more easily redirected back to nonpreferred tasks since he started taking risperidone. His sleep patterns also improve. TB exhibits less repetitive movement (e.g., jumping, pacing) when taking risperidone, but also less willingness to engage in physical activity in general. His appetite and food intake increase noticeably as well, and he gains 15 pounds over the first 3 months of treatment with risperidone. He is referred to a respite care agency to provide additional caregiver support, allowing him to remain safely in his family's home. As his behavior improves, he is also able to leave campus with his class to participate in vocational training.

Discussion of Vignette

This case illustrates a common presentation of aggressive behavior and self-injury in a young adult with a severe developmental disability. Several factors may be contributing to TB's recent escalation in behavior, including hormonal changes related to puberty, sleep disturbance, inadvertent reinforcement (i.e., removal of demands), and sensory processing differences. A thorough physical exam and urinalysis helped to rule out a medical explanation for his behavioral change, and in the absence of focal findings, further laboratory workup was not pursued. The BIP was helpful in identifying a variety of probable functions for his behavior, including: 1) escape/avoidance of unpleasant stimuli (unexpected physical proximity) and nonpreferred activities (academic tasks and chores); 2) access to preferred activities (computer time); and 3) tactile sensory stimulation (biting his hand and pulling his hair while otherwise relaxed). The BIP was designed to address each of these functions differentially and to avoid reinforcing the aggression through attention (positive reinforcement) and removal of demands (negative reinforcement). TB needed additional instruction in functional communication to use nonverbal strategies (i.e., break cards) to make appropriate requests when feeling overwhelmed.

In this case, TB's aggressive behavior was best treated with a combination of behavioral therapy, functional communication training, and medication management. While risperidone was quite helpful for reducing the severity of his behaviors, adverse effects included weight gain and physical fatigue. The risk-benefit balance of using atypical antipsychotics for aggressive behavior should be reassessed on an ongoing basis to ensure that the therapeutic effects of the medication continue to outweigh any negative effects on physical health. This vignette highlights the intensity of services often required to best care for patients with severe NDDs, requiring considerable effort and collaboration on the part of the parents, school staff, therapists, and patient.

Summary

Aggression is a common behavioral challenge in individuals with NDDs, particularly in those with the most severe phenotypes. Its impact is often devastating to families, leading to caregiver burnout, increased financial burden, and loss of educational opportunities. Considerable research effort has been devoted to the treatment of aggressive behavior, with ABA-based therapy and atypical antipsychotics, particularly risperidone and aripiprazole, emerging as the nonpharmacological and pharmacological treatments of choice, respectively. Careful consideration of the factors and functions maintaining the aggressive behavior is critical to developing a successful treatment plan. Often, the chronicity and severity of aggressive behavior require a team approach to treatment, with close communication and coordination among parents, teachers, allied health professionals, behavioral specialists, physicians, and patients. As our knowledge about the neurobiological underpinnings of various NDDs continues to grow, more targeted treatment options are greatly needed.

Key Clinical Points

▌ When evaluating individuals with neurodevelopmental disorders (NDDs) and aggressive behavior, the clinician should first consider possible sources of physical discomfort, particularly in those with severe communication impairment and sudden change in behavior. Comprehensive physical examination and laboratory workup, when indicated by physical findings, constitute a first-line assessment.

▌ Functional behavior assessment is a useful tool for identifying the antecedents, functions, and consequences that may be maintaining aggressive behavior and is the foundation for an individualized behavior intervention plan.

▌ Behavioral therapy based on the principles of applied behavior analysis (ABA) is an evidence-based intervention for both core symptoms of autism spectrum disorder (ASD) and associated maladaptive behaviors. Though few studies have evaluated ABA therapy for individuals with NDDs other than ASD, this approach is likely beneficial for behavioral problems in these other disorders as well.

▌ Two second-generation antipsychotics, risperidone and aripiprazole, have U.S. Food and Drug Administration approval for the treatment of irritability, including aggressive behavior and self-injury, in children with ASD. These medications are considered first-line treatment for aggression that is severe or does not improve with an appropriate course of behavioral therapy, though the metabolic risks must be balanced against its therapeutic benefits.

▌ Optimal treatment of aggressive behavior in individuals with NDDs requires considerable effort and collaboration among team members, including patients, parents, clinicians, teachers, therapists, and community support agencies.

References

Achenbach TM: Manual for the ASEBA School-Age Forms and Profiles. Burlington, University of Vermont, Research Center for Children, Youth, and Families, 2001

Aman M, Rettiganti M, Nagaraja HN, et al: Tolerability, safety, and benefits of risperidone in children and adolescents with autism: 21-month follow-up after 8-week placebo-controlled trial. J Child Adolesc Psychopharmacol 25(6):482–493, 2015 26262903

Aman MG, Singh NN, Stewart AW, et al: The Aberrant Behavior Checklist: a behavior rating scale for the assessment of treatment effects. Am J Ment Defic 89(5):485–491, 1985 3993694

Aman MG, McDougle CJ, Scahill L, et al; Research Units on Pediatric Psychopharmacology Autism Network: Medication and parent training in children with pervasive developmental disorders and serious behavior problems: results from a randomized clinical trial. J Am Acad Child Adolesc Psychiatry 48(12):1143–1154, 2009 19858761

Anderson LT, Campbell M, Adams P, et al: The effects of haloperidol on discrimination learning and behavioral symptoms in autistic children. J Autism Dev Disord 19(2):227–239, 1989 2663834

Armenteros JL, Adams PB, Campbell M, et al: Haloperidol-related dyskinesias and pre- and perinatal complications in autistic children. Psychopharmacol Bull 31(2):363–369, 1995 7491393

American Psychiatric Association: Diagnostic and Statistical Manual of Mental Disorders, 5th Edition. Arlington, VA, American Psychiatric Association, 2013

Beherec L, Lambrey S, Quilici G, et al: Retrospective review of clozapine in the treatment of patients with autism spectrum disorder and severe disruptive behaviors. J Clin Psychopharmacol 31(3):341–344, 2011 21508854

Braithwaite KL, Richdale AL: Functional communication training to replace challenging behaviors across two behavioral outcomes. Behav Interv 15(1):21–36, 2000

Brune CW, Kim SJ, Salt J, et al: 5-HTTLPR genotype-specific phenotype in children and adolescents with autism. Am J Psychiatry 163(12):2148–2156, 2006 17151167

Campbell JM: Efficacy of behavioral interventions for reducing problem behavior in persons with autism: a quantitative synthesis of single-subject research. Res Dev Disabil 24(2):120–138, 2003 12623082

Campbell M, Anderson LT, Meier M, et al: A comparison of haloperidol and behavior therapy and their interaction in autistic children. J Am Acad Child Psychiatry 17(4):640–655, 1978 370186

Campbell M, Anderson LT, Small AM, et al: The effects of haloperidol on learning and behavior in autistic children. J Autism Dev Disord 12(2):167–175, 1982 7174605

Carr EG, Durand VM: Reducing behavior problems through functional communication training. J Appl Behav Anal 18(2):111–126, 1985 2410400

CenterWatch: Drug information: FDA-approved drugs. 2009. Available at: http://www.centerwatch.com/ drug-information/fda-approved-drugs/ year/2009. Accessed April 10, 2018.

Chen NC, Bedair HS, McKay B, et al: Clozapine in the treatment of aggression in an adolescent with autistic disorder. J Clin Psychiatry 62(6):479–480, 2001 11465533

Coe BP, Witherspoon K, Rosenfeld JA, et al: Refining analyses of copy number variation identifies specific genes associated with developmental delay. Nat Genet 46(10):1063–1071, 2014 25217958

Cohen IL, Liu X, Lewis ME, et al: Autism severity is associated with child and maternal MAOA genotypes. Clin Genet 79(4):355–362, 2011 20573161

Cooper JO, Heron TE, Heward WL: Applied Behavior Analysis, 2nd Edition. New York, Pearson, 2007

Dagnan D, Weston C: Physical intervention with people with intellectual disabilities: the influence of cognitive and emotional variables. J Appl Res Intellect Disabil 19(2):219–222, 2006

Dean OM, Gray KM, Villagonzalo KA, et al: A randomised, double blind, placebo-controlled trial of a fixed dose of N-acetyl cysteine in children with autistic disorder. Aust N Z J Psychiatry 51(3):241–249, 2017 27316706

Dominick KC, Davis NO, Lainhart J, et al: Atypical behaviors in children with autism and children with a history of language impairment. Res Dev Disabil 28(2):145–162, 2007 16581226

Dryden-Edwards RC, Combrinck-Graham L: Developmental Disabilities From Childhood to Adulthood: What Works for Psychiatrists in Community and Institutional Settings. Baltimore, MD, Johns Hopkins University Press, 2010

Duggal HS: Ziprasidone for maladaptive behavior and attention-deficit/hyperactivity disorder symptoms in autistic disorder. J Child Adolesc Psychopharmacol 17(2):261–263, 2007 17489724

Erickson CA, Stigler KA, Posey DJ, et al: Aripiprazole in autism spectrum disorders and fragile X syndrome. Neurotherapeutics 7(3):258–263, 2010 20643378

Farmer CA, Aman MG: Development of the Children's Scale of Hostility and Aggression: Reactive/Proactive (C-SHARP). Res Dev Disabil 30(6):1155–1167, 2009 19375274

Farmer C, Butter E, Mazurek MO, et al: Aggression in children with autism spectrum disorders and a clinic-referred comparison group. Autism 19(3):281–291, 2015 24497627

Fido A, Al-Saad S: Olanzapine in the treatment of behavioral problems associated with autism: an open-label trial in Kuwait. Med Princ Pract 17(5):415–418, 2008 18685284

Findling RL, McNamara NK, Gracious BL, et al: Quetiapine in nine youths with autistic disorder. J Child Adolesc Psychopharmacol 14(2):287–294, 2004 15319025

Findling RL, Mankoski R, Timko K, et al: A randomized controlled trial investigating the safety and efficacy of aripiprazole in the long-term maintenance treatment of pediatric patients with irritability associated with autistic disorder. J Clin Psychiatry 75(1):22–30, 2014 24502859

Fite PJ, Stoppelbein L, Greening L: Proactive and reactive aggression in a child psychiatric inpatient population. J Clin Child Adolesc Psychiatry38(2):199–205, 2009 19283598

Ghanizadeh A, Moghimi-Sarani E: A randomized double blind placebo controlled clinical trial of N-acetylcysteine added to risperidone for treating autistic disorders. BMC Psychiatry 13:196, 2013 23886027

Gobbi G, Pulvirenti L: Long-term treatment with clozapine in an adult with autistic disorder accompanied by aggressive behaviour. J Psychiatry Neurosci 26(4):340–341, 2001 11590976

Goforth HW, Rao MS: Improvement in behaviour and attention in an autistic patient treated with ziprasidone. Aust N Z J Psychiatry 37(6):775–776, 2003 14636398

Golubchik P, Sever J, Weizman A: Low-dose quetiapine for adolescents with autistic spectrum disorder and aggressive behavior: open-label trial. Clin Neuropharmacol 34(6):216–219, 2011 21996644

Hardan AY, Fung LK, Libove RA, et al: A randomized controlled pilot trial of oral N-acetylcysteine in children with autism. Biol Psychiatry 71(11):956–961, 2012 22342106

Hartley SL, Sikora DM, McCoy R: Prevalence and risk factors of maladaptive behaviour in young children with autistic disorder. J Intellect Disabil Res 52(10):819–829, 2008 18444989

Hessl D, Tassone F, Cordeiro L, et al: Brief report: aggression and stereotypic behavior in males with fragile X syndrome—moderating secondary genes in a "single gene" disorder. J Autism Dev Disord 38(1):184–189, 2008 17340199

Hirata I, Mohri I, Kato-Nishimura K, et al: Sleep problems are more frequent and associated with problematic behaviors in preschoolers with autism spectrum disorder. Res Dev Disabil 49–50:86–99, 2016 26672680

Hirota T, Veenstra-Vanderweele J, Hollander E, et al: Antiepileptic medications in autism spectrum disorder: a systematic review and meta-analysis. J Autism Dev Disord 44(4):948–957, 2014 24077782

Hodgetts S, Nicholas D, Zwaigenbaum L: Home sweet home? Families' experiences with aggression in children with autism spectrum disorders. Focus Autism Other Dev Disabl 28(3):166–174, 2013

Hollander E, Wasserman S, Swanson EN, et al: A double-blind placebo-controlled pilot study of olanzapine in childhood/adolescent pervasive developmental disorder. J Child Adolesc Psychopharmacol 16(5):541–548, 2006 17069543

Iwata BA, Dorsey MF, Slifer KJ, et al: Toward a functional analysis of self-injury. J Appl Behav Anal 27(2):197–209, 1994 8063622

Kanne SM, Mazurek MO: Aggression in children and adolescents with ASD: prevalence and risk factors. J Autism Dev Disord 41(7):926–937, 2011 20960041

Kemner C, Willemsen-Swinkels SH, de Jonge M, et al: Open-label study of olanzapine in children with pervasive developmental disorder. J Clin Psychopharmacol 22(5):455–460, 2002 12352267

Kowalski JL, Wink LK, Blankenship K, et al: Paliperidone palmitate in a child with autistic disorder. J Child Adolesc Psychopharmacol 21(5):491–493, 2011 22040196

Kurtz PF, Boelter EW, Jarmolowicz DP, et al: An analysis of functional communication training as an empirically supported treatment for problem behavior displayed by individuals with intellectual disabilities. Res Dev Disabil 32(6):2935–2942, 2011 21696917

Lambrey S, Falissard B, Martin-Barrero M, et al: Effectiveness of clozapine for the treatment of aggression in an adolescent with autistic disorder. J Child Adolesc Psychopharmacol 20(1):79–80, 2010 20166802

Lecavalier L, Leone S, Wiltz J: The impact of behaviour problems on caregiver stress in young people with autism spectrum disorders. J Intellect Disabil Res 50(Pt 3):172–183, 2006 16430729

Loebel A, Brams M, Goldman RS, et al: Lurasidone for the treatment of irritability associated with autistic disorder. J Autism Dev Disord 46(4):1153–1163, 2016 26659550

Luiselli J: Aggression and noncompliance, in Applied Behavior Analysis for Children With Autism Spectrum Disorders. Edited by Matson JL. New York, Springer, 2009, pp 175–187

Lundwall RA, Stephenson KG, Neeley-Tass ES, et al: Relationship between brain stem volume and aggression in children diagnosed with autism spectrum disorder. Res Autism Spectr Disord 34:44–51, 2017 28966659

Maayan L, Correll CU: Weight gain and metabolic risks associated with antipsychotic medications in children and adolescents. J Child Adolesc Psychopharmacol 21(6):517–535, 2011 22166172

Malone RP, Cater J, Sheikh RM, et al: Olanzapine versus haloperidol in children with autistic disorder: an open pilot study. J Am Acad Child Adolesc Psychiatry 40(8):887–894, 2001 11501687

Malone RP, Maislin G, Choudhury MS, et al: Risperidone treatment in children and adolescents with autism: short- and long-term safety and effectiveness. J Am Acad Child Adolesc Psychiatry 41(2):140–147, 2002 11837403

Malone RP, Delaney MA, Hyman SB, et al: Ziprasidone in adolescents with autism: an open-label pilot study. J Child Adolesc Psychopharm 17(6):779–790, 2007 18315450

Marcus RN, Owen R, Kamen L, et al: A placebo-controlled, fixed-dose study of aripiprazole in children and adolescents with irritability associated with autistic disorder. J Am Acad Child Adolesc Psychiatry 48(11):1110–1119, 2009 19797985

Marcus RN, Owen R, Manos G, et al: Aripiprazole in the treatment of irritability in pediatric patients (aged 6–17 years) with autistic disorder: results from a 52-week, open-label study. J Child Adolesc Psychopharmacol 21(3):229–236, 2011 21663425

Martin A, Koenig K, Scahill L, et al: Open-label quetiapine in the treatment of children and adolescents with autistic disorder. J Child Adolesc Psychopharmacol 9(2):99–107, 1999 10461820

Martin A, Scahill L, Anderson GM, et al: Weight and leptin changes among risperidone-treated youths with autism: 6-month prospective data. Am J Psychiatry 161(6):1125–1127, 2004 15169706

Matlock ST, Aman MG: Development of the Adult Scale of Hostility and Aggression: Reactive-Proactive (A-SHARP). Am J Intellect Dev Disabil 116(2):130–141, 2011 21381948

Matson JL, Dixon DR, Matson ML: Assessing and treating aggression in children and adolescents with developmental disabilities: a 20-year overview. Educ Psychol 25(2–3):151–181, 2005

Matson JL, Rivet TT: The effects of severity of autism and PDD-NOS symptoms on challenging behaviors in adults with intellectual disabilities. J Dev Phys Disabil 20(1):41–51, 2008

Mazurek MO, Sohl K: Sleep and behavioral problems in children with autism spectrum disorder. J Autism Dev Disord 46(6):1906–1915, 2016 26823076

McClintock K, Hall S, Oliver C: Risk markers associated with challenging behaviours in people with intellectual disabilities: a meta-analytic study. J Intellect Disabil Res 47(Pt 6):405–416, 2003 12919191

McCracken JT, McGough J, Shah B, et al; Research Units on Pediatric Psychopharmacology Autism Network: Risperidone in children with autism and serious behavioral problems. N Engl J Med 347(5):314–321, 2002 12151468

McDougle CJ, Holmes JP, Carlson DC, et al: A double-blind, placebo-controlled study of risperidone in adults with autistic disorder and other pervasive developmental disorders. Arch Gen Psychiatry 55(7):633–641, 1998 9672054

McDougle CJ, Kem DL, Posey DJ: Case series: use of ziprasidone for maladaptive symptoms in youths with autism. J Am Acad Child Adolesc Psychiatry 41(8):921–927, 2002 12164181

Miyamoto H, Shimohata A, Abe M, et al: Potentiation of excitatory synaptic transmission ameliorates aggression in mice with Stxbp1 haploinsufficiency. Hum Mol Genet 26(24):4961–4974, 2017 29040524

Mulligan CK, Trauner DA: Incidence and behavioral correlates of epileptiform abnormalities in autism spectrum disorders. J Autism Dev Disord 44(2):452–458, 2014 23872941

Nagaraj R, Singhi P, Malhi P: Risperidone in children with autism: randomized, placebo-controlled, double-blind study. J Child Neurol 21(6):450–455, 2006 16948927

Neece CL, Green SA, Baker BL: Parenting stress and child behavior problems: a transactional relationship across time. Am J Intellect Dev Disabil 117(1):48–66, 2012 22264112

Ni HC, Lin HY, Tseng WI, et al: Neural correlates of impaired self-regulation in male youths with autism spectrum disorder: A voxel-based morphometry study. Prog Neuropsychopharmacol Biol Psychiatry 82:233–241, 2018 29129723

Nikoo M, Radnia H, Farokhnia M, et al: N-acetylcysteine as an adjunctive therapy to risperidone for treatment of irritability in autism: a randomized, double-blind, placebo-controlled clinical trial of efficacy and safety. Clin Neuropharmacol 38(1):11–17, 2015 25580916

Otero-López JM, Castro C, Villardefrancos E, et al: Job dissatisfaction and burnout in secondary school teachers: student's disruptive behaviour and conflict management examined. Eur J Education Psychol 2(2):99–111, 2009

Owen R, Sikich L, Marcus RN, et al: Aripiprazole in the treatment of irritability in children and adolescents with autistic disorder. Pediatrics 124(6):1533–1540, 2009

Potenza MN, Holmes JP, Kanes SJ, et al: Olanzapine treatment of children, adolescents, and adults with pervasive developmental disorders: an open-label pilot study. J Clin Psychopharmacol 19(1):37–44, 1999 9934941

Powers MD, Palmieri MJ, D'Eramo KS, et al: Evidence-based treatment of behavioral excesses and deficits for individuals with autism spectrum disorders, in Evidence-Based Practices and Treatments for Children With Autism. Edited by Reichow B, Doehring P, Cicchetti DV, et al. New York, Springer, 2011, pp 55–92

Research Units on Pediatric Psychopharmacology Autism Network: Risperidone treatment of autistic disorder: longer-term benefits and blinded discontinuation after 6 months. Am J Psychiatry 162(7):1361–1369, 2005 15994720

Rosell DR, Siever LJ: The neurobiology of aggression and violence. CNS Spectr 20(3):254–279, 2015 25936249

Roth ME, Gillis JM, Reed FDD: A meta-analysis of behavioral interventions for adolescents and adults with autism spectrum disorders. J Behav Ed 23(2):258–286, 2014

Scahill L, Jeon S, Boorin SJ, et al: Weight gain and metabolic consequences of risperidone in young children with autism spectrum disorder. J Am Acad Child Adolesc Psychiatry 55(5):415–423, 2016 27126856

Shea S, Turgay A, Carroll A, et al: Risperidone in the treatment of disruptive behavioral symptoms in children with autistic and other pervasive developmental disorders. Pediatrics 114(5):e634–e641, 2004 15492353

Siegel M, Beresford CA, Bunker M, et al: Preliminary investigation of lithium for mood disorder symptoms in children and adolescents with autism spectrum disorder. J Child Adolesc Psychopharmacol 24(7):399–402, 2014 25093602

Soorya L, Carpenter L, Romanczyk R: Applied behavior analysis, in Textbook of Autism Spectrum Disorders. Edited by Hollander E, Kolevzon A, Coyle JT. Washington, DC, American Psychiatric Publishing, 2011, pp 525–536

Sorgi P, Ratey J, Knoedler DW, et al: Rating aggression in the clinical setting. A retrospective adaptation of the Overt Aggression Scale: preliminary results. J Neuropsychiatry Clin Neurosci 3(2):S52–S56, 1991 1687961

Stamberger H, Nikanorova M, Willemsen MH, et al: STXBP1 encephalopathy: a neurodevelopmental disorder including epilepsy. Neurology 86(10):954–962, 2016 26865513

Stigler KA, Erickson CA, Mullett JE, et al: Paliperidone for irritability in autistic disorder. J Child Adolesc Psychopharmacol 20(1):75–78, 2010 20166801

Stigler KA, Mullett JE, Erickson CA, et al: Paliperidone for irritability in adolescents and young adults with autistic disorder. Psychopharmacology (Berl) 223(2):237–245, 2012 22549762

Stith SM, Liu T, Davies LC, et al: Risk factors in child maltreatment: a meta-analytic review of the literature. Aggress Violent Behav 14(1):13–29, 2009

Sukasem C, Vanwong N, Srisawasdi P, et al: Pharmacogenetics of risperidone-induced insulin resistance in children and adolescents with autism spectrum disorder. Basic Clin Pharmacol Toxicol January 25, 2018 [Epub ahead of print] 29369497

Taylor D: Ziprasidone in the management of schizophrenia: the QT interval issue in context. CNS Drugs 17(6):423–430, 2003 12697001

Troost PW, Lahuis BE, Steenhuis MP, et al: Long-term effects of risperidone in children with autism spectrum disorders: a placebo discontinuation study. J Am Acad Child Adolesc Psychiatry 44(11):1137–1144, 2005 16239862

Tsakanikos E, Costello H, Holt G, et al: Behaviour management problems as predictors of psychotropic medication and use of psychiatric services in adults with autism. J Autism Dev Disord 37(6):1080–1085, 2007 17053989

Wink LK, Adams R, Wang Z, et al: A randomized placebo-controlled pilot study of N-acetylcysteine in youth with autism spectrum disorder. Mol Autism 7:26, 2016 27103982

Wong C, Odom SL, Hume KA, et al: Evidence-based practices for children, youth, and young adults with autism spectrum disorder: a comprehensive review. J Autism Devel Disord 45(7):1951–1966, 2015 25578338

Yudofsky SC, Silver JM, Jackson W, et al: The Overt Aggression Scale for the objective rating of verbal and physical aggression. Am J Psychiatry 143(1):35–39, 1986 3942284

4

Aggression in Disruptive Behavioral Disorders Beginning in Childhood

Beth Krone, Ph.D.
Iliyan Ivanov, M.D.
Jeffrey Newcorn, M.D.

Aggression is a well-studied, multidimensional phenomenon that may be parsed by cognition, affect, and behavior, and represents the most common reason for referral to psychiatric care in youth. In children and adolescents, it frequently occurs in context of attention-deficit/hyperactivity disorder (ADHD) and the disruptive behavioral disorders (DBDs). Although this chapter will focus on aggression in the context of those diagnoses, it is important to remember that aggression can also occur in a variety of other conditions and that for a large subgroup of youth with aggressive behavior, criteria for any specific psychiatric diagnosis may not be met.

ADHD is a neurodevelopmental disorder not characterized by aggression per se; but symptoms characteristic of some ADHD presentations, such as impulsivity, low frustration tolerance, and impatience, may predispose or exacerbate aggressive behaviors. ADHD often occurs with DBDs. In recognition of commonalities across DBDs, DSM-5 saw the reclustering of several disorders into a supraordinate category named "Disruptive, Impulse-Control, and Conduct Disorders" (American Psychiatric Association 2013). This category includes oppositional defiant disorder (ODD), intermittent explosive disorder, conduct disorder (CD), pyromania, kleptomania, and other and unspecified disruptive, impulse-control, and conduct disorder.

Current theoretical models of aggression are interactionist and bridge the historical divide between views of aggression as a primary biological or temperamental characteristic and sociobehavioral views of aggression as a learned behavior, or as a deficit of cognitive control. Anderson and Bushman's (2002) General Aggression Model (GAM) is a social learning theory that views aggression as a learned process with correlates in biological priming and plasticity, but without temperament or biologically based factors of mental illness as predisposing factors to aggression (Ferguson and Dyck 2012). Ferguson and colleagues' (2008) Catalyst Model is a diathesis-stress model of biological vulnerabilities and social cognition that provides an epigenetic framework for aggressive processes among youth with DBDs. This has led to a wealth of research indicating genetic or biological predispositions to aggressive cognitions or affect, environments teaching maladaptive aggressive cognitions or behavioral expression, and impaired cognitive control capacities conferring risk for inappropriately expressing aggression.

Aggression as a research construct and treatment target is often conceptualized along continuums of effortful control, intent, or affect, and these conceptualizations aid in characterizing DBDs. The terms *proactive aggression* and *reactive aggression* delineate the continuum of effortful control. "Proactive" indicates planned use of aggression for goal attainment, requiring effortful control. Consequences of proactive aggression vary by intent. Among individuals with the ability or desire to self-monitor and regulate their aggressive tendencies in prosocial ways, proactive aggression is often considered "healthy" and sometimes associated with leadership abilities and social popularity. Proactive aggression may also be channeled into socially sanctioned behaviors with ill intent or consequence (e.g., military-led genocide) or unsanctioned behaviors with ill intent (e.g., premeditated murder) without necessarily meeting cultural criteria for a DBD diagnosis; however, deliberate acts of aggression with ill intent are required for meeting 3 of 8 criteria for ODD, and at least 8 of 15 criteria for CD.

"Reactive" indicates impulsive, spontaneous, unplanned aggression in response to a stimulus and is characterized by an inability to exert effortful control. About 50% of youth with DBDs with ADHD express this sort of aggression, because this comorbidity is characterized by less developmental ability to exert effortful control and regulate affect (González-Peña et al. 2013).

The terms *predatory* or *instrumental* and *affective* or *hostile* sometimes delineate a continuum of affect. "Predatory/instrumental" describes a state of controlled, deliberate, purposeful aggression for personal gain. This state is associated with DBDs involving predation and callousness, such as the specifiers associated with CD (or the DSM-5 equivalent term "limited prosocial emotions," "lack of remorse or guilt," or "callous/lack of empathy"), or antisocial personality disorder (AsPD), or the experimental construct known as "callous and unemotional traits" (CU). "Affective/hostile" describes spontaneous, emotionally driven aggression whether used for personal gain or not. Affective/hostile aggression is a characteristic feature of ODD and is frequently expressed as symptoms of irritability and vindictiveness. It is important to note that reactive aggression and hostile aggression can and often do exist in the same individuals, with or without CU traits.

Phenomenology

Disruptive Behavioral Disorders

Attention-Deficit/Hyperactivity Disorder

ADHD is characterized by overactivity, poor attentional control, and impulsivity that lead to impairment in multiple functional domains. ADHD is not in and of itself characteristic of pathological aggression, but the symptoms of ADHD are considered by some to represent the extremes in a range of temperamental characteristics that have long been associated with aggression among youth without ADHD (González-Peña et al. 2013). Not all youth with ADHD experience overactivity or impulsivity, or are aggressive, but overall, an ADHD diagnosis is a predictor of aggression, particularly among youth with

ADHD characterized by more severe symptoms of overactivity and impulsivity (Arron et al. 2011). Up to 60% of youth with ADHD are also diagnosed with DBDs because of these associated risks.

Oppositional Defiant Disorder

ODD is characterized by three symptom dimensions: angry, irritable mood; argumentative, defiant behavior; and vindictiveness. Generally the first DBD diagnosis assigned to a youth's behaviors, ODD symptoms may progress to those of CD (sometimes quickly), and eventually to AsPD in adulthood. With proper treatment, and in some cases without treatment, ODD usually resolves within 3 years of first diagnosis in approximately 60%–70% of youth. However, approximately 30% of youth with ODD go on to develop CD, and youth with earlier-onset ODD, usually in the context of a variety of other social or biological risk factors, are three times more likely to do so.

Conduct Disorder

CD occurs along a continuum, with mild, moderate, and severe forms describing escalating levels of aggression and interpersonal violence. CD is also subtyped by age at onset in youth or adolescence (i.e., childhood [before age 10 years], adolescent [age 10 years or older], or unspecified onset) and by interpersonal and emotional functioning, with earlier onset and less prosocial emotion generally associated with greater severity. DSM-5 introduced the specifier "with limited prosocial emotions" to describe youth previously referred to as having CU traits. This group encompasses at least two of the following characteristics: a) lack of remorse or guilt; b) callous/lack of empathy; c) unconcern about performance (at school or in other important activities); and d) shallow or deficient affect (including manipulative use of emotions). Pathological aggression persisting into late adolescence, age 18 years or older, presents the highest risk for the most severe academic, occupational, peer, and family problems, and the greatest risk for substance abuse and incarceration.

Epidemiology

The national prevalence rate for ADHD is approximately 8%, with some states reporting a prevalence of 10%–15%. Projected lifetime risk for being diagnosed with a DBD is approximately 24% (Kessler et al. 2005), with childhood prevalence at 3.5% for CD and 2.8% for ODD among youth collecting Social Security Income (SSI) benefits for severe disability (Boat et al. 2015), and 6.8% and 12.6%, respectively, for all ranges of severity within diagnosis in other national samples (Merikangas et al. 2010). Across cultures, male-to-female prevalence ratio of ADHD is 2:1 (Arnett et al. 2015), but aggression and DBDs are more highly gender dependent (acquired behavior) than sex specific (Demmer et al. 2017).

Stereotypes of aggression and DBDs as sex specific, with males more often committing acts of physical violence and females more often committing acts of covert (hidden) relational aggression, are fueled by statistics showing that girls are less likely than boys to get into physical fights (e.g., 16.5% vs. 28.4%; Centers for Disease Control and Prevention and Youth Risk Behavior Survey 2016) in Western societies. Yet large meta-analyses find that males are only moderately (1.59:1) more likely to have ODD than females worldwide, because DBD prevalence does not differ by sex in non-Western cultures (Demmer et al. 2017), such as in India (Mishra et al. 2014) or South Korea (Park et al. 2015), or in more socially egalitarian Western cultures, such as in Spain (López-Villalobos et al. 2014). Even within the United States, communities that value gender equality produce fewer males with DBDs (Lei et al. 2014).

Aggression toward people or animals and destruction of property encompass 9 of the 15 criteria for diagnosing CD in DSM-5. Since the 1990s, youth violence has been the third leading cause of death among youth ages 10–24 years in the United States, and many of the youth committing these crimes will have a diagnosis of CD. Each year, approximately half a million youth receive emergency health care for violence-related injuries, averaging 1,642 emergency room visits and 13 murders each day (Centers for Disease Control and Prevention, National Center for Injury Prevention and Control 2014). In 2015, 605 children were arrested for murder, 2,745 were arrested for forcible rape, and 21,993 were arrested for aggravated assault, while 14.3% of property crime arrests and 10% of all violent crime arrests involved children under the age of 18 (Federal Bureau of Investigation 2015). In 2015, 16.2% of youth carried a weapon (5.3% carried a gun) for their own protection in the month prior to being surveyed, while 20% reported being aggressively bullied at school (with bullying also being a criterion for CD) (Kann et al. 2016).

Psychobiology

Behavioral Genetics

Twin studies consistently report higher concordance rates for aggression among monozygotic compared with dizygotic twins (Button et al. 2004), with heritability estimates ranging from 0.28 to 0.72. Among adopted-away children whose biological parents were diagnosed with AsPD, children who had both biological vulnerability (family history of AsPD) and environmental risk (i.e., adverse adoptive environment) were found to have higher levels of aggression than children with either biological or environmental vulnerability alone. Familial risk factors such as having a parent with mood disorder, substance abuse, AsPD, CD, or a serious mental health issue (or having a sibling with a DBD or presence of comorbid neurobiological disorder, such as autism spectrum disorder) suggest a possible mechanism for genetic inheritance of biological diatheses (i.e., traits) or disorders that prime individuals toward aggression and contribute to DBD diagnoses (Powis and Oliver 2014).

Neurobiological Studies

Impulsive aggression has often been related to dysfunction in serotonergic neurocircuitry, although a large number of other neurotransmitters are involved. Reduced serotonin (5-HT) synthesis, depletion of 5-HT stores, or destruction of 5-HT neurons, and reduced cerebrospinal fluid levels of the 5-HT metabolite 5-hydroxyindoleacetic acid (5-HIAA), have all been correlated with measures of aggressive behavior. However, these effects are receptor and region specific, and this specificity may be responsible for some of the contradictory findings in human trials. Activation 5-HT_{1A} and 5-HT_{1B} receptors in mesolimbic areas is related to decreased trait aggression, for example, whereas activation of 5-HT_{1A} and 5-HT_{1B} receptors in the medial prefrontal cortex or septal area is related to increased number of aggressive acts (Takahashi et al. 2012). Further, psychopathology may be moderated as much by the timing of neurotransmission and reuptake as by the quantity of available neurotransmitter. The phasic and tonic flow of catecholamines is regulated by a complex interplay of molecules that directly and indirectly affect 5-HT neurotransmission.

The role of norepinepherine and dopamine in pathological aggression is due to central and autonomic nervous system innervations that regulate physiological arousal. While higher levels of arousal are part of the normal autonomic response to stress, preparing individuals for potentially necessary aggressive behavior, hyperarousal is associated with impulsive aggression (and also with aggression in the context of anxiety). Hypoarousal may be of greater clinical significance in DBDs, as behavioral research has shown that persistently low heart rate, an indicator of low autonomic activity, is associated with both DBDs and CU traits and is associated with aggressive and criminal behavior in adults, adolescents, and school-age children (Portnoy and Farrington 2015). Similarly, low skin conductance, another measure of reduced autonomic reactivity, has also been associated with aggressive behaviors in childhood and may indicate an aggressive phenotype that is specific to DBDs in humans.

Reactive aggression is more often associated with peripheral cortisol, which is a primary corticosteroid produced in response to psychological or physical stressors. Associations are nonlinear and complex; aggression correlates to high cortisol among neurobiologically healthy, stressed people, but low cortisol levels correlate to early onset and persistence of aggression among people with DBDs (Murakami et al. 2006).

Stress hormones interact with testosterone and estrogen and influence estrogen conversion among adults, priming stimulatory neurons, sensitizing them and making aggressive responses more (or less) likely among adults. These effects have not been found among prepubertal youth. Current research on prenatal androgen exposure may reveal insights into childhood behavioral priming, though it is unlikely to account for large differences in DBD prevalence.

Molecular Genetics and Epigenetics

Candidate genes most consistently linked to aggression are the 5-HT serotonin transporter (5-HTT) gene and the genes for three enzymes that have an important role in the homeostasis, inactivation, and clearance of dopamine and norepinephrine: monoamine oxidase (MAO), catechol O-methyltransferase (COMT), and dopamine beta-hydroxylase (DBH). Human studies have demonstrated that a rare mutation in the MAO-A gene is associated with impulsively violent behavior expressed over multiple generations. Risk for physical aggression during adulthood may be increased by the interaction of low MAO-A activity in the context of early trauma exposure (Verhoeven et al. 2012). Similarly, youth with early exposure to parental antisocial behaviors who were homozygous for the long variant of 5-HTT expressed higher levels of antisocial behavior than those with other genetic markers (Cicchetti et al. 2012). Other 5-HTT gene alleles are also indicators of aggression, anxiety, and depression in the context of alcohol abuse, stress vulnerability, and reactive aggression.

MAO-A deficiency, which leads to higher levels of 5-HT metabolites but lower levels of norepinephrine and dopamine, has also been linked to impulsive aggression and criminal behavior among humans. Effects of MAO-A variants are highly dependent on environmental exposures to epigenetic triggers and appear to moderate stress reactivity versus resilience. These interactions highlight the interdependence of multiple neurotransmitters in homeostatic regulation of aggression. More evidence of this complexity comes from the dorsal raphe nucleus (DRN), which is the largest serotogenic focal point in the central nervous system and is richly innervated with corticotropin-releasing factor (CRF) neuropeptide receptors. CRF activity in the DRN is strongly associated with marked impulsive aggression, particularly in the context of early life stress, and CRF receptors are involved in the regulation of serotonin along projections from the DRN into the limbic system, striatum, and prefrontal cortex, allowing regulation of homeostasis in these dopamine-rich areas.

Epigenetics is critical as well since it is thought that environmental risk factors work through epigenetic mechanisms governing gene expression. Such environmental risk factors include maternal smoking; drug or alcohol use during pregnancy; harsh or inconsistent parenting style; neglect; physical, emotional, or sexual abuse of the child; and disrupted family environment (including, but not restricted to, domestic violence, poverty, and parental contact with the criminal justice system). Exposure to environmental violence can contribute to both behaviorally acquired (learned) or epigenetic pathways (as in the context of the 5-HT regulator MAO-A) to DBDs (Caspi et al. 2002). For example, tryptophan hydroxylase 2 is also known to moderate the development of aggression in stress-affected young mice (Takahashi et al. 2012). In addition, the 5-HT genotype for the 5-HT$_{2B}$ receptor acts as an epigenetic diathesis for increased emotionally driven impulsive aggression and suicidality that may occur with depression in the context of alcohol consumption (Bevilacqua et al. 2010).

Neuroimaging

Findings from neuroimaging studies implicate the orbital prefrontal cortex (which inhibits limbic and other subcortical regions), anterior cingulate cortex (which manages incoming affective stimuli), and ventromedial prefrontal cortex (which regulates emotion processing) in DBDs. Studies in youth with CD have shown deactivation of the anterior cingulate cortex and reduced activation in the left amygdala in response to negative stimuli (Marsh et al. 2013), as well as reduced gray matter volume in both cortical and subcortical regions (Rogers and De Brito 2016) reflecting possible impairments in the recognition and cognitive control of emotional stimuli.

Clinical Approach and Treatment

In the context of DBDs, trajectories of disorder are identifiable as early as the preschool years. Events such as child abuse or domestic violence exposure exacerbate predispositions through social learning. Poor peer relationships may result from unregulated aggression as the child acts out against gentler friends, or such relationships may act as an added stressor as the child is bullied. Inadequate problem-solving patterns or presence of a neurodevelopmental disorder also contributes to the diathesis and predicts development of impulsive aggression. These factors also contribute to the development of planned aggression, which generally starts later in childhood or adolescence and is fueled by aggressive role models, biological maturation, and a sense of reward from aggressive behaviors.

Childhood aggression is not a stable trait, and psychopathology may resolve with intervention. Among youth with DBDs, aggression resolves in about 50% of cases, usually following three distinct developmental trajectories of resolution or maintenance. Without intervention, childhood aggression may continue or escalate over time, leading to AsPD and continued violence, contributing to poverty cycles through domestic abuse and/or incarceration.

Clinical Assessment

Clinical assessment may include structured, semistructured, or open interviews, questionnaires, and/or specific objective testing, and requires comprehensive understanding of psychological, behavioral, cognitive, and diagnostic considerations related to the nature, context, and severity of aggression. Assessment begins with an interview of the patient and relevant others to understand the nature of the aggressive behaviors (e.g., proactive-reactive, instrumental/predatory-hostile/impulsive) and the context of the behaviors (e.g., where and when the behaviors occur, precipitating or triggering events, rewards or consequences that maintain behaviors). Underlying medical or neurological predispositions (e.g., seizure activity, lead poisoning, head trauma, substance use) are assessed during this interview and through specialized medical testing, when appropriate. A mental status exam is part of this process as well and includes evaluation of ideation or plan to harm self or others and assessment of the potential for carrying out these plans (e.g., access to weapons). Imminent risk to any individual carries a legal obligation to warn the potential target and possibly other authorities, although laws vary. Comorbidities should also be explored as factors that require additional treatment or may impede treatment.

Treatment

Psychosocial interventions can target either impulsive or planned aggression. While medication is generally reserved for treatment of impulsive aggression, improvement is often relative, and multimodal intervention is optimal.

Pharmacological Treatments

Medication treatment of ADHD is an effective initial strategy for treating youth with ADHD and comorbid aggression. Psychostimulants are first-line medication treatments for ADHD, with effect sizes that are superior to those of nonstimulant medications. Numerous studies have shown that youth whose aggression occurs primarily in the context of ADHD often benefit from treatment with stimulants alone, with efficacy demonstrated for both overt and covert aggression. One meta-analysis found overall weighted mean effect sizes of 0.84 for overt aggression and 0.69 for covert aggression (Connor et al. 2002). Moreover, there is evidence that stimulants are effective in treating behavioral symptoms in children with ADHD and comorbid ODD/CD (Gadow et al. 2008). For instance, one placebo-controlled study of 84 youth with CD, two thirds of whom also had symptoms that met criteria for ADHD, found that methylphenidate (MPH) reduced behaviors specific to CD, independent of severity of ADHD symptoms (Klein et al. 1997). Nevertheless, a substantial proportion of children with ADHD that is well treated with stimulants (approximately 60%; Blader et al. 2009) do not achieve sufficient reduction in aggressive behavior with stimulant treatment alone (Jensen et al. 2007) and require pharmacological augmentation.

Though effective, stimulant treatment of aggression is limited by the relatively short duration of action (even in the case of long-acting stimulants). Because aggression can be present at any time of the day, treatments that last all day are highly desirable. Nonstimulant medications such as atomoxetine (ATX) and the extended-release α_2-adrenergic agonists, both of which are evidence-based treatments for ADHD, generally have a longer duration of action than stimulants and can be used for treating aggression in ADHD. Furthermore, ATX was found to be modestly effective in treating ODD symptoms in youth with ADHD (Newcorn et al. 2005), pointing to the possible value of ATX for aggressive children with ADHD—but probably not as a first-choice recommendation. One report from an open–label study showed that the combination of ATX and olanzapine appeared promising for treating aggression in ADHD and comorbid DBD (Holzer et al. 2013).

There are several reports on the possible beneficial effects of clonidine and guanfacine for the treatment of aggression in the context of ADHD (Wilens et al. 2012). Several other studies have shown that guanfacine can increase frustration tolerance and decrease irritability (Connor et al. 2010); this is relevant because these symptoms are frequently present in youth with impulsive aggression. Clonidine has been shown to be effective in reducing aggression in adolescents with ADHD (Hazell and Stuart 2003), though the latter study used clonidine to augment stimulant response and did not study clonidine as monotherapy. Of note, both long-acting clonidine and guanfacine are approved by the U.S. Food and Drug Administration (FDA) for combination treatment with stimulants for ADHD, meaning that there are safety data to support combined therapy in patients with ADHD and aggression.

Stimulants have also been used in combination with anticonvulsants and antipsychotics for control of aggressive symptoms, and there is a growing literature to support this practice. For instance, combined use of stimulants and antipsychotics has been found to be beneficial in controlling physical aggression in children with ADHD (Aman et al. 2014) as well as in youth with comorbid ADHD and CD (Blair et al. 2015). Divalproex has been shown to be effective in treating impulsive aggression, as evidenced by results of an open trial by Blader et al. (2009) in children 6–13 years of age with ADHD plus ODD/CD and aggression thought to be refractory to stimulants. A separate report from the same group (Blader et al. 2013), based on a study with a placebo-controlled design, further documented the beneficial effects of combined treatment with divalproex and stimulant in youth with ADHD and aggression not adequately controlled with optimized stimulant monotherapy. Divalproex has also been shown to reduce the explosive aggression associated with comorbid bipolar disorder and CD, possibly because of its mood-stabilizing properties.

Divalproex may therefore potentially have a dual role in the treatment of aggression: as an intervention for a primary underlying disorder (e.g., bipolar disorder) and as a symptom-target treatment of aggression. In one review, Munshi et al. (2010) examined the utility of 10 anticonvulsant agents in childhood aggression in the context of mood disorders, concluding that there is some evidence to support the use of anticonvulsant agents in pediatric aggression, with the major caveat that controlled trials in pediatric bipolar disorder have not produced promising outcomes. The authors further concluded that valproate is the best-supported agent for aggression and should be considered as a first-line treatment for aggressive youth with mood disorders.

Antipsychotics are not specifically approved by the FDA for treating aggressive behaviors in youth with DBDs (though risperidone is approved for the treatment of aggression in youth with autism). The combination of stimulants with risperidone was evaluated by the Treatment of Severe Childhood Aggression (TOSCA) study in children ages 6–12 years with ADHD and ODD or CD and severe physical aggression. In this double-blind, randomized controlled trial, the participants received stimulant medication for 3 weeks, titrated for optimal effect, while parents received parent training for behavioral management. After 3 weeks, the treatment was augmented with risperidone or placebo for the subjects either who failed to show sufficient clinical response or whose behavior deteriorated. The risperidone group showed moderate improvement in aggression ratings at the end of 9 weeks (Aman et al. 2014), mostly for participants with unplanned aggression and disruptive behavior, rather than callous, planned aggression. A reanalysis of these data indicated that risperidone augmentation was beneficial for a select group of youth with greater clinical impairment (Barterian et al. 2017).

Blair et al. (2015) suggest that the use of stimulants and atypical antipsychotics in combination may be helpful for youth with CD with CU traits, which is more difficult to treat and generally thought to have a poorer prognosis. Several open-label trials (e.g., Kronenberger et al. 2007) have been conducted with quetiapine, suggesting that this medication can be used successfully with MPH in patients with ADHD and aggression, with comorbid ODD or CD. As the prescribing rates of antipsychotic medications have increased substantially in recent years because of their use for the treatment of aggression (Burcu et al. 2014), it should be noted that the combination of stimulants and antipsychotic medication has only sometimes and not always convincingly been found to be useful in controlling physical aggression in children with ADHD (Aman et al. 2014; Linton et al. 2013). A recent randomized clinical trial that included an acute phase and a 52-week follow-up treatment study examined the efficacy of behavioral parent training (BPT)+stimulant treatment versus BPT+stimulant treatment augmented with risperidone for youth with very severe forms of aggression (Gadow et al. 2016). The authors did not find any difference in aggression between the two drug arms, and twice as many families in the risperidone group (23% vs. 11%) discontinued medication entirely. Another review of the overall use of second-generation antipsychotics (SGAs) reported cautiously optimistic effects of risperidone in reducing aggression in the short term in children ages 5–18 with DBDs (Loy et al. 2012), but found no evidence supporting the use of quetiapine for DBDs in children and adolescents. Another review reported that four placebo-controlled studies support the short-term efficacy of low-dose risperidone in youth with a subaverage IQ (Pringsheim and Gorman 2012).

Concerns about the utility of antipsychotics in the treatment of aggression are evident from a recent survey of child psychiatrists, which found that 75% would not prescribe SGAs for children with ADHD and aggression. Further, 61% felt that adjustment of their primary ADHD treatment would be sufficient to manage aggression (Mann et al. 2017). Additional concerns are related to long-term safety, primarily because of metabolic side effects of SGAs. It is documented that concomitant use of stimulants and antipsychotics does not adequately combat the metabolic effects of antipsychotics, contrary to speculation (Linton et al. 2013). Despite these reservations, existing data do not suggest significantly worse adverse effects for stimulant and antipsychotic medications used in combination for aggression compared with monotherapy. Moreover, reports from recent studies using the oral hypoglycemic agent metformin for weight control in youth who receive antipsychotics are promising. Finally, the decision to add an antipsychotic agent is often considered only after failed trials of stimulant and/or nonstimulant monotherapy and combination of stimulant medication with behavioral interventions. In the context of severe impairment and prior treatment failures, addition of a medication with potential benefit can be justified even if there are risks to be managed.

Other agents have also been studied in the pharmacological treatment of childhood aggression. Both lithium and haloperidol were superior to placebo in reducing behavioral symptoms among children with treatment-resistant conditions, but haloperidol was more sedating. Subsequent studies of lithium have supported this finding, though the effect sizes favoring lithium have been lower. Beta-blockers such as propranolol (often given in higher doses) have been used to treat aggression in patients with organic brain dysfunction and DBDs (often in combination with stimulants), but data are limited. Recent clinical trials with fish oil in impulsive aggression indicate that long-term preventive treatment of aggression may be feasible, even among youth with DBDs (Meyer et al. 2016). Others (e.g., Raine et al. 2016) have reported positive results using omega-3 fatty acids as an adjunctive therapy to cognitive-behavioral interventions for reducing aggression in high-risk youth.

Overall, several different classes of medications have shown predominantly short-term benefits in the treatment of aggressive behaviors in the context of ADHD alone or ADHD comorbid with CD. However, treatment with any single agent is often not effective, and frequently combined regimens are used. Combinations of stimulants with antipsychotic or anticonvulsants have shown the most robust clinical effects among certain populations with DBDs, but there are concerns about safety and tolerability. Nonstimulants may be used to avoid side effects related to stimulants, and metformin may help manage the weight gain that frequently accompanies antipsychotic treatment.

Psychotherapeutic Treatments

Psychotherapeutic interventions are empirically supported for the treatment of impulsive and planned aggression and factors that serve to maintain aggression (e.g., affect and behavioral dysregulation, social information processing deficits, or coercive or abusive parenting behaviors).

Behavioral parent training is a first-line treatment for preschoolers with ODD and has utility throughout childhood. It works to reduce aggression by increasing positive parent-child interactions, emotional communication skills, parenting consistency, and the use of effective behavioral rewards systems (Kaminski et al. 2008), and by teaching parents to reinforce appropriate behaviors and skills in their children (Waller et al. 2013).

Cognitive-behavioral therapy (CBT) is an empirically supported treatment for addressing social cognitive deficits associated with aggression: addressing hostile attribution biases, interpreting social cues, processing emotions, and predicting consequences. CBT and BPT are generally more effective when offered together. While BPT appears to be most effective for younger youth, CBT is more effective for older youth. Modular approaches that allow treatment of comorbid psychopathology and other facets of family dysfunction tend to improve outcomes above those of single evidence-based treatments (Weisz et al. 2012).

Multimodal Psychosocial Approaches

Multisystemic treatment (MST) and *multidimensional treatment foster care* (MTFC) are empirically supported for high-risk youth with aggressive, antisocial behaviors that have resulted in out-of-home placement and involvement with the juvenile justice system. MST and MTFC use well-established, developmentally appropriate strategies in highly intensive, tailored treatments to reduce rates of recidivism, arrest, criminal offenses, substance-related offenses, and out-of home placement in the highest-risk youth.

Community Prevention Programs

Early intervention is a collection of long-term services initiated in or before preschool to build resilience and prevent aggression and conduct problems.

School-Based Violence Prevention Programs

School-based violence prevention programs are at least moderately successful when focused on developing positive school climate and reducing bullying and peer rejection (Hong and Espelage 2012; Multisite Violence Prevention Project 2009). Antibullying programs share many features with other school-based violence prevention programs and have been found to decrease bullying at school by 23% and victimization by 20% (Ttofi and Farrington 2012).

Clinical Vignette

MM is a 9-year-old male who lives with both biological parents. He has two siblings. His parents have had a loving but difficult relationship with all of their children, with the children having frequent behavioral outbursts and excessively demanding parents' and teachers' attention. MM's mother was a full-time parent who was hospitalized for treatment of anorexia just prior to her pregnancy with MM. MM's father worked long hours.

MM's parents and teachers became aware of his rigid, inattentive, and disruptive behaviors and a restricted range of emotions when he was 4 years old. He began receiving treatment from his public school counselor at that time. School intervention targeted social skills, anger management, and anxiety. Despite displaying adequate social skills when playing with his next-door neighbor (who was diagnosed and treated for ADHD and disruptive behavior), MM had no friends in school and deliberately started fights by antagonizing other children.

By age 7 years, MM had begun to display a persistent pattern of work refusal, rule violations, and attention seeking, despite being highly intelligent. He had a short fuse and was verbally abusive to both teachers and peers, and his outbursts frightened his classmates. School personnel pressed for professional intervention. After initial resistance, the parents consulted a play therapist. They ended therapy after three sessions because the therapist requested a medication evaluation. By age 8 years, MM's mother expressed concerns over escalating aggression in the home and reported fearing she was "raising a serial killer." MM's father dismissed these concerns and attributed his wife's distress to her own mental illness, saying she was overreacting to "normal boy, rough-and-tumble behaviors." School personnel supported MM's mother's concerns and expressed relief that she was finally acknowledging the severity of MM's behavior problems. MM was evaluated and rated in the very severe ranges for Callous/Unemotional traits, Narcissism, and Impulsivity on both the teacher- and parent (mother's)–report Antisocial Process Screening Device scales. Conners' Teacher Rating Scale (CTRS) Oppositional behaviors were > 4.5 standard deviations (SD), and ADHD behaviors > 2 SD, above the norm. Scores on the Conners' Parent Rating Scale were equally high. Upon interview, both parents endorsed seven symptoms of inattention and five symptoms of hyperactivity, ongoing since age 4, meeting criteria for ADHD. They endorsed seven symptoms of ODD and two symptoms of CD. They endorsed four symptoms of generalized anxiety disorder (not reported by MM). MM received a diagnosis of ADHD and ODD, with features of CD and DSM-IV anxiety not otherwise specified.

BPT was initiated but discontinued after three sessions, with MM's father stating that he did not need to improve his parenting techniques. The family started a 6-week trial of ATX, beginning at 0.5 mg/kg and increasing to 1.4 mg/kg. Symptoms of ADHD and ODD improved but did not resolve. On a follow-up CTRS, Oppositional score fell to > 3 SD above the norm, and ADHD score was in the normal range. MM's mother reported exacerbated aggression at home.

After a washout period, OROS-MPH was started at 18 mg and titrated to a dose of 72 mg over 3 weeks. While MM was taking the OROS-MPH at a dose of 72 mg, MM's teacher placed his behavior in the lowest 10% as compared with his peers and rated his CTRS Oppositional behaviors as being > 3.5 SD above the norm. Ratings of ADHD behaviors on both the CTRS and CPRS were in the normal range. CPRS Oppositional behaviors were > 2.5 SD above the norm. Reduced appetite, weight loss, and difficulty sleeping with relative lack of improvement in aggression prompted OROS-MPH discontinuation.

Given the relative failure of stimulant and nonstimulant medications for the aggression when given in monotherapy, the relatively better tolerability of ATX than OROS-MPH, and the relatively positive response of ADHD symptoms to ATX, it was decided to pursue a combined treatment regimen with a medication. The ATX was restarted and titrated to a dose of 1.2 mg/kg to control the ADHD, and a low dose of risperidone (0.5 mg bid) was added to better control the aggression that was present at school and at home.

Discussion of Vignette

Particularly in the context of ADHD and DBDs, as seen in the case of MM, pathological aggression transcends socioeconomic status and can manifest in enriched environments with traditional nuclear families and external structural supports. Behavioral genetics research points to the multiple biological vulnerabilities experienced by MM, beginning with heritability of ADHD and genetic vulnerability to other mental health problems, compounded by epigenetic diatheses in the perinatal environment as maternal health status and well-being begin to influence development. Social-cognitive processes impacting MM's development and contributing to more severe symptoms of ADHD and DBDs include the following:

▪ A family context of stressful and aggressive relationships between parents and siblings, compounding use of ineffective parenting practices

▪ The family's cultural perceptions and biases resulting in the family being slow to recognize and address emerging (then ongoing) behavioral problems

▪ Social stigma resulting in the family being resistant to acknowledging relational problems and remediating their parenting practices—which is the first-line, evidence-based behavioral therapy for ODD and aggression among youth younger than 10 years

▪ Broader relational problems extending beyond the home environment, hindering integration of a therapeutic approach across home and school settings and leading to functional impairment (e.g., peer relational problems and social isolation, reinforcing the maladaptive social-cognitive schemas developed in the home environment, and/or child relationship problems with teachers contributing to problems acquiring scaffolded socioemotional development curricula, and further impairing MM's educational attainment as the child refused to complete work or attend lessons)

In addition to peer and care-provider negative attributions impacting MM's sense of self, biases among his adult care providers led to distortions of behavioral ratings (e.g., through inattention misrated as deliberate ignoring, and affective "lashing out" being reported as vindictiveness or dislike of others). This is not to say that all cases of more severe and earlier-onset aggression are dismissible as bias and misattribution, but misattributions for behaviors are common in context of ADHD and more so in context of ADHD + DBDs. Features of ADHD hyperactive-impulsive type, including low frustration tolerance and impatience, contributed to MM's lashing out at small provocations and his work refusal at school, although these were underreported as ADHD symptoms. These features of ADHD often contribute to reports of ODD as hostility and irritability, or defiant behavior. In MM's case, these also contributed to development of maladaptive sociocognitive loops and were identified as key problems that fueled growing academic underachievement and social impairment. Features of ODD as vindictiveness can contribute to reports of CD as callous lack of empathy for the people who are recipients of the vindictive behavior, or a lack of remorse or guilt for the vindictive behaviors. However, empathy and guilt require perspective taking that is short-circuited by maladaptive social cognitions that often develop as a feature of ADHD. As such, treatment of ADHD can improve the overall clinical picture, as it did with MM. In MM's case, long-term medication treatment, psychological and behavioral interventions implemented at school, and socioeconomic resources provided by his parents shifted his development toward improved symptomatic, behavioral, and academic functioning and placed him with the 50% of youth for whom DBDs resolve or mainly resolve, leaving traits of callousness and aggression in a small subset of these.

Summary

Several evidence-based psychosocial and pharmacological interventions exist to treat acute presentations, and perhaps alter lifespan trajectories, of aggression in the context of DBDs; however, there is little meaningful evidence of amelioration and treatment efficacy for monotherapy in approximately 60% of cases over the long term. Combined therapies are not much more effective in the long term, although they may provide greatly needed respite and hope for families in crisis situations. There is an urgent need to identify effective, accessible, and tolerable interventions that are both developmentally appropriate and suitable for youth from diverse backgrounds, and those who present with heterogeneous symptom profiles. In light of promising epigenetic findings and elucidation of multiple biological pathways involved in the development and maintenance of both aggression and DBD-related aggression, there is promise for the development of safer, more effective, and more specific interventions.

Key Clinical Points

▮ Aggression is not a psychiatric diagnosis itself, but it can accompany many psychiatric diagnoses. Within the disruptive behavioral disorders (DBDs), intent and ability to control aggressive behaviors help to define and differentiate presentations: overt physical aggression is a key factor in diagnosing conduct disorder; relational aggression displayed as oppositionality, vindictiveness, and defiance is a key factor in diagnosing oppositional defiant disorder (ODD); and, while not a key factor in diagnosing attention-deficit/hyperactivity disorder (ADHD), aggression often stems from the impulsivity that makes youth with ADHD easily frustrated and unable to inhibit impulsive responses.

▮ Aggression and DBDs are identifiable in early childhood. Young children exhibiting symptoms of ADHD, ODD, and aggression, and those exposed to trauma, should be evaluated for intervention to ameliorate risk factors leading to compounding psychosocial adversity and long-term trajectory of disorder.

▮ Treatment should focus on building skills in areas of weakness. Typically, this process involves improving self-regulation of emotion, building expressive language for goal achievement and social communication, developing critical thinking and problem-solving skills, and developing empathy and insight among younger children (or some older youth with DBDs). Treatment should also focus on building support systems for the child by improving relationships within the home (e.g., behavioral parent training [BPT]), within the classroom (e.g., communicating with teachers and establishing school supports), and/or within the larger community (e.g., accessing high-quality after-school activities).

▋ Prevention includes minimizing a child's exposure to violence via methods such as BPT or family therapy, peer mediation, and limited or scaffolded use of violent media. When exposure to violence cannot be prevented, treating trauma early may prevent or reduce sequelae.

▋ A variety of structured and semistructured assessment measures are available. Obtaining information from multiple informants in multiple settings is essential for differentiating normal from pathological aggression and for characterizing aggression, its intent, and affective nature.

▋ Various medications are potentially useful. Differential diagnosis is key, and identifying treatable conditions accompanying the presentation of aggression can aid in directing intervention.

References

Aman MG, Bukstein OG, Gadow KD, et al: What does risperidone add to parent training and stimulant for severe aggression in child attention-deficit/hyperactivity disorder? J Am Acad Child Adolesc Psychiatry 53(1):47.e1–60.e1, 2014 24342385

American Psychiatric Association: Diagnostic and Statistical Manual of Mental Disorders, 5th Edition. Arlington, VA, American Psychiatric Association, 2013

Anderson CA, Bushman BJ: Human aggression. Annu Rev Psychol 53:27–51, 2002 11752478

Arnett AB, Pennington BF, Willcutt EG, et al: Sex differences in ADHD symptom severity. J Child Psychol Psychiatry 56(6):632–639, 2015 25283790

Arron K, Oliver C, Moss J, et al: The prevalence and phenomenology of self-injurious and aggressive behaviour in genetic syndromes. J Intellect Disabil Res 55(2):109–120, 2011 20977515

Barterian JA, Arnold LE, Brown NV, et al: Clinical implications from the Treatment of Severe Childhood Aggression (TOSCA) Study: a re-analysis and integration of findings. J Am Acad Child Adolesc Psychiatry 56(12):1026–1033, 2017 29173736

Bevilacqua L, Doly S, Kaprio J, et al: A population-specific HTR2B stop co-
don predisposes to severe impulsivity. Nature 468(7327):1061–1066,
2010 21179162

Blader JC, Schooler NR, Jensen PS, et al: Adjunctive divalproex versus placebo for children with ADHD and aggression refractory to stimulant
monotherapy. Am J Psychiatry 166(12):1392–1401, 2009 19884222

Blader JC, Pliszka SR, Kafantaris V, et al: Callous-unemotional traits, proactive aggression, and treatment outcomes of aggressive children with at-
tention-deficit/hyperactivity disorder. J Am Acad Child Adolesc
Psychiatry 52(12):1281–1293, 2013 24290461

Blair RJ, Leibenluft E, Pine DS: Conduct disorder and callous-unemotional
traits in youth. N Engl J Med 372(8):784, 2015 25693027

Boat T, Wu J; Committee to Evaluate the Supplemental Security Income
Disability Program for Children With Mental Disorders: Mental Disor-
ders and Disabilities Among Low-Income Children. Washington, DC,
National Academies Press, 2015

Burcu M, Zito JM, Ibe A, et al: Atypical antipsychotic use among Medicaid-
insured children and adolescents: duration, safety, and monitoring implications. J Child Adolesc Psychopharmacol 24(3):112–119, 2014 24690011

Button TM, Scourfield J, Martin N, et al: Do aggressive and non-aggressive
antisocial behaviors in adolescents result from the same genetic and environmental effects? Am J Med Genet B Neuropsychiatr Genet
129B(1):59–63, 2004 15274042

Caspi A, McClay J, Moffitt TE, et al: Role of genotype in the cycle of violence
in maltreated children. Science 297(5582):851–854, 2002 12161658

Centers for Disease Control and Prevention, National Center for Injury Prevention and Control: Web-Based Injury Statistics Query and Reporting
System (WISQARS). 2014. Available at: https://www.cdc.gov/injury/
wisqars/index.html. Accessed April 11, 2018.

Centers for Disease Control and Prevention, Youth Risk Behavior Survey:
Trends in the prevalence of behaviors that contribute to violence on
school property national YRBS: 1991–2015. National Center for HIV/
AIDS, Viral Hepatitis, and TB Prevention: Division of Adolescent and
School Health, 2016. Available at: https://www.cdc.gov/healthyyouth/
data/yrbs/pdf/trends/2015_us_violence_trend_yrbs.pdf. Accessed April
11, 2018.

Cicchetti D, Rogosch FA, Thibodeau EL: The effects of child maltreatment
on early signs of antisocial behavior: genetic moderation by tryptophan
hydroxylase, serotonin transporter, and monoamine oxidase A genes.
Dev Psychopathol 24(3):907–928, 2012 22781862

Connor DF, Glatt SJ, Lopez ID, et al: Psychopharmacology and aggression, I: a meta-analysis of stimulant effects on overt/covert aggression-related behaviors in ADHD. J Am Acad Child Adolesc Psychiatry 41(3):253–261, 2002 11886019

Connor DF, Findling RL, Kollins SH, et al: Effects of guanfacine extended release on oppositional symptoms in children aged 6–12 years with attention-deficit hyperactivity disorder and oppositional symptoms: a randomized, double-blind, placebo-controlled trial. CNS Drugs 24(9):755–768, 2010 20806988

Demmer DH, Hooley M, Sheen J, et al: Sex differences in the prevalence of oppositional defiant disorder during middle childhood: a meta-analysis. J Abnorm Child Psychol 45(2):313–325, 2017 27282758

Federal Bureau of Investigation: Crime in the U.S., 2015. Uniform Crime Reports, U.S. Department of Justice, 2015. Available at: https://ucr.fbi.gov/crime-in-the-u.s/2015/crime-in-the-u.s.-2015. Accessed April 11, 2018.

Ferguson CJ, Dyck D: Paradigm change in aggression research: the time has come to retire the General Aggression Model. Agg Viol Behav 17:220–228, 2012

Ferguson CJ, Rueda SM, Cruz AM: Violent video games and aggression: Causal relationship or byproduct of family violence and intrinsic violence motivation? Crim Justice Behav 35(3):311–332, 2008

Gadow K, Nolan E, Sverd J, et al: Methylphenidate in children with oppositional defiant disorder and both comorbid chronic multiple tic disorder and ADHD. J Child Neurol 23(9):981–990, 2008

Gadow KD, Brown NV, Arnold LE, et al: Severely aggressive children receiving stimulant medication versus stimulant and risperidone: 12-month follow-up of the TOSCA trial. J Am Acad Child Adolesc Psychiatry 55(6):469–478, 2016 27238065

González-Peña P, Egido BD, Carrasco MÁ, et al: Aggressive behavior in children: the role of temperament and family socialization. Span J Psychol 16:E37, 2013 23866232

Hazell P, Sturat J: A randomized controlled trial of clonidine added to psychostimulant medication for hyperactive and aggressive children. J Am Acad Child Adolesc Psychiatry 42(8):886–894, 2003

Holzer B, Lopes V, Lehman R: Combination use of atomoxetine hydrochloride and olanzapine in the treatment of attention-deficit/hyperactivity disorder with comorbid disruptive behavior disorder in children and adolescents 10–18 years of age. J Child Adolesc Psychopharmacol 23(6):415–418, 2013 23952189

Hong JS, Espelage DI: A review of research on bullying and peer victimization in school: an ecological system analysis. Agg Viol Behav 17(4):311–322, 2012

Jensen PS, Youngstrom EA, Steiner H, et al: Consensus report on impulsive aggression as a symptom across diagnostic categories in child psychiatry: implications for medication studies. J Am Acad Child Adolesc Psychiatry 46(3):309–322, 2007 17314717

Kaminski JW, Valle LA, Filene JH, et al: A meta-analytic review of components associated with parent training program effectiveness. J Abnorm Child Psychol 36(4):567–589, 2008 18205039

Kann L, McManus T, Harris WA, et al: Youth risk behavior surveillance—United States, 2015. MMWR Surveill Summ 65(6):1–174, 2016 27280474

Kessler RC, Berglund P, Demler O, et al: Lifetime prevalence and age-of-onset distributions of DSM-IV disorders in the National Comorbidity Survey Replication. Arch Gen Psychiatry 62(6):593–602, 2005 15939837

Klein RG, Abikoff H, Klass E, et al: Clinical efficacy of methylphenidate in conduct disorder with and without attention deficit hyperactivity disorder. Arch Gen Psychiatry 54(12):1073–1080, 1997 9400342

Kronenberger WG, Giauque AL, Lafata DE, et al: Quetiapine addition in methylphenidate treatment-resistant adolescents with comorbid ADHD, conduct/oppositional-defiant disorder, and aggression: a prospective, open-label study. J Child Adolesc Psychopharmacol 17(3):334–347, 2007 17630867

Lei MK, Simons RL, Simons LG, et al: Gender equality and violent behavior: how neighborhood gender equality influences the gender gap in violence. Violence Vict 29(1):89–108, 2014 24672996

Linton D, Barr AM, Honer WG, et al: Antipsychotic and psychostimulant drug combination therapy in attention deficit/hyperactivity and disruptive behavior disorders: a systematic review of efficacy and tolerability. Curr Psychiatry Rep 15(5):355, 2013 23539465

López-Villalobos JA, Andrés-De Llano JM, Rodríguez-Molinero L, et al: Prevalence of oppositional defiant disorder in Spain. Rev Psiquiatr Salud Ment 7(2):80–87, 2014 24161231

Loy JH, Merry SN, Hetrick SE, et al: Atypical antipsychotics for disruptive behaviour disorders in children and youths. Cochrane Database Syst Rev 12(9):CD008559, 2012 22972123

Mann A, Li A, Radwan K, et al: Factors associated with management of teen aggression: child psychiatric clinical decision making. J Child Adolesc Psychopharmacol 27(5):445–450, 2017 26784955

Marsh AA, Finger EC, Fowler KA, et al: Empathic responsiveness in amygdala and anterior cingulate cortex in youths with psychopathic traits. J Child Psychol Psychiatry 54(8):900–910, 2013 23488588

Merikangas KR, He JP, Burstein M, et al: Lifetime prevalence of mental disorders in U.S. adolescents: results from the National Comorbidity Survey Replication—Adolescent Supplement (NCS-A). J Am Acad Child Adol Psychiatry 49(10):980–989, 2010 20855043

Meyer BJ, Byrne M, Parletta N, et al: Fish oil and impulsive aggressive behavior. J Child Adolesc Psychopharmacol 26(8):766, 2016 26217883

Mishra A, Garg SP, Desai SN: Prevalence of oppositional defiant disorder and conduct disorder in primary school children. J Indian Acad Forensic Med 36:246–250, 2014

Multisite Violence Prevention Project: The ecological effects of universal and selective violence prevention programs for middle school students: a randomized trial. J Consult Clin Psychol 77(3):526–542, 2009 19485593

Munshi KR, Oken T, Guild DJ, et al: The use of antiepileptic drugs (AEDs) for the treatment of pediatric aggression and mood disorders. Pharmaceuticals (Basel) 3(9):2986–3004, 2010 27713387

Murakami S, Rappaport N, Penn JV: An overview of juveniles and school violence. Psychiatr Clin North Am 29(3):725–741, 2006 16904508

Newcorn JH, Spencer TJ, Biederman J, et al: Atomoxetine treatment in children and adolescents with attention-deficit/hyperactivity disorder and comorbid oppositional defiant disorder. J Am Acad Child Adolesc Psychiatry 44(3):240–248, 2005 15725968

Park S, Kim BN, Cho SC, et al: Prevalence, correlates, and comorbidities of DSM-IV psychiatric disorders in children in Seoul, Korea. Asia Pac J Public Health 27(2):NP1942–NP1951, 2015 25113525

Portnoy J, Farrington DP: Resting heart rate and antisocial behavior: an updated systematic review and meta-analysis. Agg Viol Behav 22:33–45, 2015

Powis L, Oliver C: The prevalence of aggression in genetic syndromes: a review. Res Dev Disabil 35(5):1051–1071, 2014 24594523

Pringsheim T, Gorman D: Second-generation antipsychotics for the treatment of disruptive behaviour disorders in children: a systematic review. Can J Psychiatry 57(12):722–727, 2012 23228230

Raine A, Cheney RA, Ho R, et al: Nutritional supplementation to reduce child aggression: a randomized, stratified, single-blind, factorial trial. J Child Psychol Psychiatry 57(9):1038–1046, 2016 27166583

Rogers JC, De Brito SA: Cortical and subcortical gray matter volume in youths with conduct problems: a meta-analysis. JAMA Psychiatry 73(1):64–72, 2016 26650724

Takahashi A, Quadros IM, de Almeida RMM, et al: Behavioral and pharmacogenetics of aggressive behavior. Curr Top Behav Neurosci 12:73–138, 2012 22297576

Ttofi MM, Farrington DP: Risk and protective factors, longitudinal research, and bullying prevention. New Dir Youth Dev 2012(133):85–98, 2012 22504793

Verhoeven FEA, Booij L, Kruijt A-W, et al: The effects of MAOA genotype, childhood trauma, and sex on trait and state-dependent aggression. Brain Behav 2(6):806–813, 2012 23170243

Waller R, Gardner F, Hyde LW: What are the associations between parenting, callous-unemotional traits, and antisocial behavior in youth? A systematic review of evidence. Clin Psychol Rev 33(4):593–608, 2013 23583974

Weisz JR, Chorpita BF, Palinkas LA, et al; Research Network on Youth Mental Health: Testing standard and modular designs for psychotherapy treating depression, anxiety, and conduct problems in youth: a randomized effectiveness trial. Arch Gen Psychiatry 69(3):274–282, 2012 22065252

Wilens TE, Bukstein O, Brams M, et al: A controlled trial of extended-release guanfacine and psychostimulants for attention-deficit/hyperactivity disorder. J Am Acad Child Adolesc Psychiatry 51(1):74.e2–85.e2, 2012 22176941

5

Aggression in Primary Psychotic Disorders

Leslie Citrome, M.D., M.P.H.
Jan Volavka, M.D., Ph.D.

Primary psychotic disorders comprise a variety of severe mental disorders that include schizophrenia and schizoaffective disorder. Other severe disorders, such as severe mania, can include psychotic features. In addition to psychosis, these disorders are often accompanied by agitation, aggression, and hostility to others.

Although agitation, aggression, and hostility are related, they are conceptually different. *Agitation* consists of a state of increased arousal manifested by excessive motor or verbal activity and is often distressing to the patient. Agitation can often wax and wane (Lindenmayer 2000). *Aggression* is defined as overt behavior involving intent to inflict noxious stimulation or to behave destructively, and can be verbal, against objects, against self, or against other persons. Persons who are agitated are not necessarily aggressive (Volicer et al. 2017), but agitation can escalate to aggressive behavior (Powell et al. 1994). Physical aggression against other persons is frequently called *violence*. The terms *violence* and *aggression* are sometimes used interchangeably, but the term *aggression* is favored in biomedical or psychological research, and *violence* (or violent crime) is more commonly used in criminology, sociology, law, and public policy. Of note, agitation and aggression are among the most frequent reasons for psychiatric hospitalization. *Hostility* is a term with multiple meanings. In addition to overt aggression, it may include temper tantrums, irritability, refusal to cooperate, jealousy, suspicion, and many other attitudes and behaviors (Buss and Durkee 1957).

Phenomenology

Rating scales that have been used to measure agitation include the single-item Behavioural Activity Rating Scale (BARS; Swift et al. 2002) and the 5-item subset of the Positive and Negative Syndrome Scale (PANSS), called the PANSS Excited Component (PANSS-EC; Montoya et al. 2011), which consists of excitement, hostility, tension, uncooperativeness, and poor impulse control. The single PANSS item of "hostility" is defined as "verbal and nonverbal expressions of anger and resentment, including sarcasm, passive-aggressive behavior, verbal abuse, and assaultiveness" and is rated on a scale of 1 (absent) to 7 (extreme), with mild hostility (a rating of 3) defined as follows: "The patient shows indirect or restrained communication of anger, such as sarcasm, disrespect, hostile expressions and occasional irritability" (Kay et al. 2000, p. 40). More serious behaviors are not captured until the higher end of the scale. However, the principal clinical importance of hostility is its highly statistically significant association with violence (Swanson et al. 2006), and thus the association has led to a widespread use of hostility as a proxy measure of violence (Volavka et al. 2016). Hostility is also associated with nonadherence to medication and treatment discontinuation (Volavka et al. 2016).

Aggression can be measured using the Overt Aggression Scale, which separately assesses verbal aggression and physical aggression against objects, against self, and against others (Yudofsky et al. 1986). For acutely ill psychiatric patients, the Brøset Violence Checklist can be used to predict in-patient violence in the short term (Björkdahl et al. 2006). Violence perpetrated by psychiatric patients in the community can be assessed with the MacArthur Community Violence Interview (Swanson et al. 2006).

Epidemiology

The media is replete with news stories of psychotic individuals committing violent acts. However, most individuals with schizophrenia are not violent, and persons with schizophrenia are more likely to be the victims than the perpetrators of violent crimes. In an epidemiological study conducted using Swedish national registers for all hospital admissions and criminal convictions, the population impact of patients with severe mental illness on violent crime was assessed, and it was found that patients with severe mental illness commited 1 in 20 violent crimes; thus, 19 out of 20 of these crimes were perpetrated by persons without severe mental illness (Fazel and Grann 2006).

However, compared with the general population, there is an elevated risk of violence in persons with schizophrenia. A meta-analysis that included 20 individual studies reporting data from 18,423 individuals with schizophrenia and other psychoses showed a twofold increase of violence risk in schizophrenia without substance abuse comorbidity, and a ninefold increase with that comorbidity (Fazel et al. 2009). This latter increase must be seen in the context of the risk of substance abuse that is approximately four times higher in persons with schizophrenia than in the general population. Thus, what exists is a small subset of persons with schizophrenia who are also aggressive, and they pose a formidable but not insurmountable clinical management challenge.

Psychobiology

The pathways to aggression in schizophrenia will be a starting point to determine the treatment approach for a specific individual (Volavka and Citrome 2011). The underlying neurobiology is complex, and explanations are generally incomplete (see also Chapter 1, "Phenomenology and Psychobiology of Aggression and Intermittent Explosive Disorder,"this volume). Nonmodifiable factors include predisposing risk factors for aggression, such as history of childhood conduct problems, parental violent crime, genotype (e.g., certain polymorphisms of the catechol O-methyltransferase [COMT] gene). Modifiable factors are positive psychotic symptoms (including hostility, "threat/control override" paranoid symptoms, and, to a lesser extent, "command" hallucinations), current substance use, and nonadherence. Other factors include poor impulse control and psychopathy. Interventions targeting impulsivity are not well established, and treatments for psychopathy are very limited. However, long-term treatment programs based on cognitive-behavioral therapy and psychoeducation may reduce aggressive behavior in patients with mental disorders (Haddock et al. 2009; Yates et al. 2010). Aggressive behavior in psychoses may also have characteristics of impulsiveness or premeditation and may be related to psychotic symptoms.

Clinical Approach and Treatment

The heterogeneity among clinical presentations of schizophrenia, and of schizophrenia presenting with aggression, must be acknowledged (Volavka and Citrome 2008). For example, in acute agitation, the concern is that elevated arousal will escalate to aggressive behavior, which in turn can result in violence against another person; however, the psychopharmacological treatment approach will be different if the person with schizophrenia is acutely psychotic or withdrawing from alcohol or sedative misuse. In persistent aggressive behavior, aggression and violence can be related directly to positive psychotic symptoms, or they may be better explained by poor impulse control or may stem from comorbidity with personality disorders, particularly psychopathy. More than one factor may be present for any individual patient, and these may change over time. In this section, the acute treatment of agitation and aggressive behavior will be discussed, as well as strategies to reduce the frequency and/or intensity of future episodes of these behaviors.

Acute Treatment

Acute treatment usually involves the emergency management of agitation before it can escalate to aggressive behaviors. In addition to the early offering of medications, interventions that target agitation include environmental and behavioral approaches, especially verbal de-escalation techniques (Richmond et al. 2012). Goals include calming the agitated patient as rapidly as possible, decreasing the likelihood of harm to self or others, allowing the performance of diagnostic tests and procedures, attenuating psychosis, and decreasing the need for seclusion or restraint (a time where staff and patient injury can occur). The induction of sleep is not desirable during evaluation of a patient; sedation that necessitates constant observation and assistance in toileting places an excessive burden on staff and other resources.

The differential diagnosis of agitation and aggression can be complex, and several factors may be simultaneously present. Ruling out somatic causes for an altered mental status is imperative to avoid missing life-threatening illness (Nordstrom et al. 2012). Moreover, somatic causes of agitation may preclude the use of antipsychotic medication—for example, acute withdrawal from alcohol or benzodiazepines, for which the preferred medication intervention would be a benzodiazepine such as lorazepam; in this instance administration of an antipsychotic may induce a seizure. Substance use is a common clinical consideration; it is estimated that approximately half of all patients with schizophrenia have a comorbid drug or alcohol abuse problem (Hartz et al. 2014; Regier et al. 1990); withdrawal from sedative agents can be seen in the emergency department or soon after admission to an inpatient unit. More unusual, but problematic, would be the presence of an underlying metabolic, toxic, or infectious process resulting in agitated behavior in a person otherwise well known to the provider as a person with a chronic psychotic disorder; clues that the agitation may be due to a somatic cause include the presence of an altered sensorium, a phenomenon not expected in an uncomplicated acute exacerbation of schizophrenia. In general, if there is a somatic cause for the change in mental status, management is usually directed to the treatment of the underlying cause. Another source of diagnostic confusion has been antipsychotic-associated akathisia (Advokat 2010); when unrecognized, akathisia can be interpreted as worsening anxiety, and if additional antipsychotics are used as acute treatment, the akathisia will typically worsen.

The ideal medication intervention is one that is readily accepted by all parties, works rapidly and is well tolerated, and has no troublesome lingering aftereffects. For a medication to be rapid-acting, parenteral administration (usually by intramuscular [IM] injection) is often required, although alternative delivery options may be more agreeable to patients (Zeller and Citrome 2016). In the United States, the Food and Drug Administration (FDA) has approved three different second-generation antipsychotics specifically for agitation associated with schizophrenia: short-acting IM formulations of ziprasidone, olanzapine, and aripiprazole (the latter two are also approved for agitation associated with bipolar mania). The FDA has also approved a rapid-acting inhaled formulation of loxapine for agitation associated with schizophrenia or bipolar mania. Table 5–1 summarizes the evidence supporting these treatments. These options are efficacious and relatively tolerable and minimize the risk of extrapyramidal adverse effects seen with older options such as IM haloperidol. Table 5–2 summarizes interventions that have not been FDA-approved for the management of agitation but for which some evidence exists supporting their use (Wilson et al. 2012; Zeller and Citrome 2016).

Instead of using the rapidly acting interventions summarized in Tables 5–1 and 5–2, orally administered (swallowed) interventions can be also considered under specific circumstances. Orally ingested medication results in entry to the systemic circulation via the gastrointestinal tract and through the hepatic portal vein. Thus, absorption can be erratic, and onset of action is slower than for agents administered via injection, sublingually, intranasally, or by inhalation (Nordstrom and Allen 2013). Although research is available regarding oral therapy for the management of agitation, including liquid formulations (Zeller and Rhoades 2010), such use is probably best reserved for mild degrees of agitation when the patient expresses a preference for a specific medication in which he or she has confidence. In some cases, patients may calm down readily after receiving oral medication for agitation. Of interest when oral medications are being considered instead of an injection, liquid risperidone 2 mg combined with oral lorazepam 2 mg had a comparable therapeutic effect when compared with combined IM lorazepam 2 mg and IM haloperidol 5 mg in a convenience sample of willing participants (Currier and Simpson 2001) and in a larger prospective randomized study (Currier et al. 2004). Oral olanzapine administered initially at a high dose (40 mg on days 1 and 2, 30 mg on days 3 and 4, and 5–20 mg thereafter) was superior in reducing the PANSS-EC at 24 hours to oral olanzapine administered at a lower dose (10 mg) with lorazepam supplementation (Baker et al. 2003). In a post hoc analysis of pooled data from the registration trials of lurasidone, in patients with higher levels of agitation at baseline, lurasidone was associated with significantly greater improvement in PANSS-EC scores vs. placebo, with higher doses having a more robust effect (Allen et al. 2017).

TABLE 5–1. U.S. Food and Drug Administration–approved treatments for agitation

	Generic name			
	Ziprasidone mesylate	Olanzapine	Aripiprazole	Loxapine (inhaled)
U.S. brand name	Geodon	Zyprexa	Abilify	Adasuve
Indication	Agitation associated with schizophrenia	Agitation associated with schizophrenia or bipolar mania	Agitation associated with schizophrenia or bipolar mania	Agitation associated with schizophrenia or bipolar mania
Basis for approval	Two double-blind trials testing 20 mg or 10 mg vs. 2 mg (Daniel et al. 2001; Lesem et al. 2001); about 80% of the subjects had schizophrenia or schizoaffective disorder	Three placebo-controlled trials (Breier et al. 2002; Meehan et al. 2001; Wright et al. 2001); active controls: IM haloperidol 7.5 mg (schizophrenia studies) and IM lorazepam 2 mg (bipolar mania study)	Three placebo-controlled trials (Andrezina et al. 2006; Tran-Johnson et al. 2007; Zimbroff et al. 2007); active controls: IM haloperidol 6.5 or 7.5 mg (schizophrenia studies) and IM lorazepam 2 mg (bipolar mania study)	Three placebo-controlled trials in patients with schizophrenia (Allen et al. 2011; Lesem et al. 2011) or bipolar mania (Kwentus et al. 2012); no active controls
Definition of response	Two-point decrease in BARS score	40% decrease on the PANSS-EC	40% decrease on the PANSS-EC	40% decrease on the PANSS-EC
NNT response at 2 hours[a]	2 (for 20 mg); 4 (for 10 mg)	3 (for 10 mg)	5 (for 9.75 mg)	4 (for 10 mg) (schizophrenia)

TABLE 5–1.   U.S. Food and Drug Administration–approved treatments for agitation *(continued)*

	Generic name			
	Ziprasidone mesylate	Olanzapine	Aripiprazole	Loxapine (inhaled)
Speed of response[b]	15–30 minutes	As fast as 15 minutes (Wright et al. 2001)	45 minutes (vs. 105 minutes for haloperidol 7.5 mg in Tran-Johnson et al. 2007); 1 hour (vs. 45 minutes for haloperidol 6.5 mg in Andrezina et al. 2006); 1 hour (vs. 45 minutes for lorazepam 2 mg in Zimbroff et al. 2007)	10 minutes (first time point measured; see Citrome 2013)
Adverse events[c]	Somnolence, nausea, dizziness, headache, postural hypotension	Somnolence (no adverse event was significantly more frequent for IM olanzapine compared with IM haloperidol or IM lorazepam)	Nausea	Dysgeusia (an unpleasant taste in the mouth)
NNH adverse event and the rates of that event[d]	Somnolence: 9 (for 20 mg) (20% vs. 8%)	Somnolence: 34 (for 10 mg) (6% vs. 3%)	Nausea: 17 (for 9.75 mg) (9% vs. 3%)	Dysgeusia: 11 (for 10 mg) (14% vs. 5%)

TABLE 5–1. U.S. Food and Drug Administration–approved treatments for agitation (*continued*)

	Generic name			
	Ziprasidone mesylate	**Olanzapine**	**Aripiprazole**	**Loxapine (inhaled)**
Additional safety considerations/ comments	Caution in patients with impaired renal function because the cyclodextrin excipient is cleared by renal filtration; prolongation of ECG QTc interval (see also Zimbroff et al. 2005) similar to that observed with IM haloperidol (Miceli et al. 2010)	Simultaneous injection of olanzapine and benzodiazepines is not recommended; in a report of safety data among more than 500,000 patient exposures, there were 29 fatalities; concomitant benzodiazepines or other antipsychotics were reported in 66% and 76% of these cases, respectively (Marder et al. 2010)	As of this writing, short-acting IM aripiprazole is no longer being marketed in the United States[e]	Potential risk of bronchospasm; see Risk Evaluation and Mitigation Strategy program (Galen 2017)

Note.   BARS=Behavioural Activity Rating Scale; ECG=electrocardiogram; IM=intramuscular; NNH=number needed to harm; NNT=number needed to treat; PANSS-EC=Positive and Negative Syndrome Scale–Excited Component.

[a]NNT response *vs.* placebo-control (or in the case of ziprasidone, 2 mg). Lower values of NNT are preferable. Data from Citrome 2007 and Citrome 2012.

[b]Determined by when the medication statistically separated from the placebo control (or in the case of ziprasidone, 2 mg) after medication administration.

[c]Incidence ≥5% and ≥2× for therapeutic dose vs. placebo control (or in the case of ziprasidone, 2 mg). From Table 13 in Pfizer 2017; Table 15 in Eli Lilly and Company 2009; Table 24 in Otsuka Pharmaceutical Company 2018; Table 1 in Galen 2017.

[d]NNH *vs.* placebo control (or in the case of ziprasidone, 2 mg) for the adverse event, with the biggest difference in rates comparing medication with placebo. Higher values of NNH are preferable. Data from Citrome 2007 and Citrome 2013.

[e]See U.S Food and Drug Administration Approved Drug Products, https://www.accessdata.fda.gov/scripts/cder/daf/index.cfm?event= overview.processandAppINo=021866.

TABLE 5–2. Rapidly acting treatments for agitation used off-label

Medication	Comments
Haloperidol IM	Efficacy appears similar to that for short-acting IM olanzapine and aripiprazole, with a NNT vs. placebo of 4 for PANSS-EC response at 2 hours postinjection (Citrome 2007). However, haloperidol has a distinctly unfavorable adverse event profile regarding extrapyramidal symptoms (Citrome 2007). Of concern are acute dystonic reactions, including laryngospasm, oculogyric crisis, and torticollis, which typically can occur 12–24 hours after administration (Jhee et al. 2003) and can lead to a general reluctance on the part of the patient to take similar medications in the future.
IM benzodiazepines (lorazepam, midazolam)	IM lorazepam given as a monotherapy has been used to manage agitation (Foster et al. 1997; Salzman et al. 1991). In studies of agitation associated with bipolar mania in which IM lorazepam 2 mg served as an active control, the NNT for PANSS-EC response for IM lorazepam 2 mg vs. placebo at 2 hours postinjection was 4 (Citrome 2007). Respiratory depression is a potential concern in persons with lung disease or sleep apnea. Of note, lorazepam is not useful for control of psychotic symptoms, and long-term control of aggressive behavior with benzodiazepines is problematic because of tolerance, dependence, and missed doses leading to rebound anxiety, withdrawal, and potential grand mal seizures. However, lorazepam is particularly useful to consider in the presence of alcohol or sedative withdrawal, which may be accompanied by agitation and which may be overlooked in persons known to have psychotic disorders. Another short-acting benzodiazepine, midazolam, has been studied as an antiagitation agent alone and in combination, and is notable for fast onset of action but short duration requiring repeat dosing; it has also been noted to be associated with unexpected oversedation (Parker 2015).

TABLE 5–2. Rapidly acting treatments for agitation used off-label *(continued)*

Medication	Comments
Haloperidol IM combined with lorazepam IM	The combination of haloperidol with lorazepam (usually in the same syringe) is commonly used and supported by a randomized study in which effective symptom reduction was achieved in each treatment group (lorazepam 2 mg, haloperidol 5 mg, or both in combination), with a difference favoring combination treatment at the 1-hour mark (Battaglia et al. 1997). Similar advantages at this time point when using this combination approach have been found by others (Bieniek et al. 1998), but there remains the risk of oversedation (Gillies et al. 2013).
IM antihistamines	Antihistamines such as diphenhydramine and hydroxyzine have also been used in the management of agitation, particularly in children and adolescents (Sonnier and Barzman 2011). Promethazine, a phenothiazine medication with prominent antihistamine activity, has been used adjunctively with haloperidol with success (Huf et al. 2009), but is not available in the United States.
Sublingual asenapine	An additional noninjectable alternative with rapid onset is sublingual asenapine 10 mg, for which efficacy for agitation was evidenced in a single-site placebo-controlled study demonstrating an effect size comparable to that of injectable antipsychotics (Pratts et al. 2014). In contrast to the orally disintegrating tablets of olanzapine, risperidone, and aripiprazole, asenapine is administered sublingually and is absorbed in the oral mucosa, bypassing first-pass metabolism. NNT for response vs. placebo as measured by the PANSS-EC at 2 hours after administration was 3. In routine use, asenapine has been associated with oral hypoesthesia and dysgeusia.

Note. IM=intramuscular; NNT=number needed to treat; PANSS-EC=Positive and Negative Syndrome Scale–Excited Component.

Long-Term Treatment for Persistent Aggressive Behavior

In contrast to the number of approved treatments for agitation, there are no FDA-approved treatments for persistent aggressive behavior. Treatment is thus directed to the underlying cause(s). Persistent aggressive behavior may be related to psychosis, psychopathy, impulsivity, co-occurring substance or alcohol use, cognitive impairments, underlying somatic conditions, or, typically, combinations of several of these factors occurring simultaneously (Volavka and Citrome 2008).

Within this context, oral antipsychotics that were used for acute treatment in an individual with schizophrenia are logical choices for maintenance treatment. It is useful to have multiple formulations to select from, including long-acting injectables (Mohr et al. 2017). Foundational medications will reduce violence risk in populations, as demonstrated by a study of Swedish national registers, which found that violent crime fell by 45% during periods in which patients were taking antipsychotics compared with periods during which patients were not taking medication (Fazel et al. 2014). If aggressivity persists, despite adequate adherence to antipsychotic medication, there is a limited array of evidence-based pharmacological interventions, of which clozapine has the most support.

Clozapine

Clozapine was found to have superior effects when compared with other antipsychotics (in particular, haloperidol) in reducing hostility or overt aggression in double-blind, randomized studies (Citrome et al. 2001; Krakowski et al. 2006; Volavka et al. 2004), and these effects are consistent with those that had been previously observed in uncontrolled studies and in case series (Frogley et al. 2012). The anti-aggressive effect of clozapine appears to be specific in the sense that it is independent of clozapine's effect on positive symptoms of psychosis and it is not mediated by sedation (Topiwala and Fazel 2011). In practice, the full antiaggressive effect of clozapine is not achieved until the dose escalation is completed, and it may take about 3 weeks for the dosage to reach 400 mg/day; a faster rate of dose increase may not be possible because of cardiovascular side effects. The main risk of clozapine is agranulocytosis, developing in approximately 1% of patients, and thus blood monitoring is a requirement (Citrome et al.

2016c). Other adverse effects of clozapine include weight gain, metabolic abnormalities, seizures, and myocarditis. Nonetheless, despite clozapine's tolerability and safety profile, a large epidemiological study has demonstrated that clozapine treatment is associated with a lower mortality rate than any other antipsychotic (Tiihonen et al. 2009).

Overall, clozapine is considered the treatment of choice for persistent aggression and hostility in schizophrenia and schizoaffective patients. In addition, clozapine has received FDA approval for reducing suicidal behavior in patients with schizophrenia or schizoaffective disorder (Novartis Pharmaceuticals Corporation 2015). With regard to comorbid substance use, clozapine is particularly well suited in that clozapine reduces craving (particularly for cocaine) and reduces comorbid substance use in patients with schizophrenia (Murthy and Chand 2012).

Olanzapine

Olanzapine was superior to haloperidol (but inferior to clozapine) in a double-blind, randomized study in aggressive patients with schizophrenia (Krakowski et al. 2006). Olanzapine has demonstrated superior efficacy in comparison with typical antipsychotics against aggression or hostility in other randomized studies that enrolled treatment-refractory patients (Volavka et al. 2004) and chronically ill outpatients (Volavka et al. 2014), and in patients being treated for their first episode of schizophrenia (Volavka et al. 2011). These observed antihostility effects were independent of effects on the positive symptoms of schizophrenia. Olanzapine use is associated with weight gain and metabolic changes (Citrome et al. 2011); the risk of these adverse effects requires monitoring. Overall, olanzapine can be considered a second-choice treatment of persistent aggressive behavior in schizophrenia or schizoaffective disorder, particularly for patients who will not or cannot be treated with clozapine.

Other Atypical Antipsychotics

Risperidone was superior to placebo in reducing hostility in a randomized study (Czobor et al. 1995), but inconsistent results were observed using other study designs enrolling more refractory patients (Beck et al. 1997; Buckley et al. 1997). Ziprasidone's effect against hostility was superior to that of haloperidol only in the first week of a 6-week open-label study (Citrome et al. 2006), and its efficacy against aggression was indistinguishable from that of perphenazine, risperidone, olanzapine, and quetiapine in a randomized trial (Swanson et al. 2008). In the same trial, the efficacy of quetiapine against aggression was indistinguishable from that of risperidone, olanzapine, or ziprasidone, but inferior to that of perphenazine (Swanson et al. 2008). Specific antihostility effect has also been assessed in post hoc analyses of other second-generation antipsychotics, including oral aripiprazole (Volavka et al. 2005), lurasidone (Citrome et al. 2014), and cariprazine (Citrome et al. 2016b), and long-acting injectable aripiprazole lauroxil (Citrome et al. 2016a). In summary, atypical antipsychotics are effective against hostility and aggression in schizophrenia. The most effective among them is clozapine, followed by olanzapine, with more limited information available supporting the use of risperidone, quetiapine, ziprasidone, aripiprazole, lurasidone, and cariprazine, as mainly reported in post hoc analyses examining antihostility effects.

Augmentation Strategies

Beta-adrenergic blockers such as nadolol and pindolol have demonstrated efficacy in the control of aggressive behaviors in patients with organic brain disease and may also be useful in persons with schizophrenia (Alpert et al. 1990; Caspi et al. 2001; Ratey et al. 1992). However, dose escalation of beta-blockers is time-consuming because these compounds significantly reduce blood pressure and pulse rate. Although adjunctive lithium and anticonvulsants are often used in the management of persistent aggressive behavior in persons with schizophrenia, supporting data for this are mixed (Citrome 2009).

Clinical Vignette

AV is a 30-year-old white male who was emergently brought to the local community hospital after getting into a fight in the park with "someone who was looking at me funny." He is convinced that "the antichrist is following me" and has auditory hallucinations commenting on his day-to-day activities. AV is well known to the police and has been admitted to the hospital approximately 20 times over the past 8 years under similar circumstances. AV has been diagnosed with schizophrenia and has used marijuana and cocaine intermittently. He lives in a board-and-care home. He is intermittently adherent with his antipsychotic medications. He states that "the medicines don't work and make me dumb."

In the emergency department AV is agitated and uncomfortable. The staff is fearful that he will hit someone. AV is offered an IM injection but does not want to take it because 5 years ago he had an acute dystonic reaction after an injection of haloperidol 5 mg.

Discussion of Vignette

What is the optimal choice for AV? AV is clearly psychotic and agitated, but he is not in withdrawal from alcohol or sedatives. Although an oral antipsychotic can be offered, speed of response is a concern because of the acuteness of AV's agitation. IM olanzapine 10 mg, ziprasidone 10 or 20 mg, or aripiprazole 9.75 mg, or inhaled loxapine 10 mg, are all FDA-approved interventions that can be used; the use of these over haloperidol will minimize the risk of an acute dystonic reaction. Lorazepam may also reduce AV's level of agitation, but it will not address his psychotic symptoms. Sublingual asenapine 10 mg can also be considered but is not FDA-approved for this purpose.

Once the acute episode is managed, what is the best choice for continued treatment? AV is persistently aggressive, likely because of his psychosis and lack of adherence to his foundational medication. Efforts should be made to discern what AV finds objectionable to the medications he has taken in the past. Ideally the choice of antipsychotic will be based on minimizing those adverse effects he cares most about. A long-acting injectable atypical antipsychotic should be considered. Clozapine or olanzapine would be considered if after a period of good treatment adherence AV continues to have problematic aggressive behavior. Access to other treatment services, such as assertive community treatment, may be helpful.

Summary

Managing aggressive behavior in persons with schizophrenia or psychotic disorders requires both acute and long-term interventions. Acute treatments to address agitation are plentiful and include agents that are FDA-approved for this purpose, including olanzapine, ziprasidone, and aripiprazole given intramuscularly, and inhaled loxapine administered under supervision through a single-use device. Managing persistent aggressive behavior requires an understanding of the pathways involved in the production of these behaviors in the individual person being treated. The three principal factors involved are psychosis, impulsivity, and psychopathy, of which only the first and possibly second factors can reliably be addressed through psychopharmacological interventions. Treatment adherence will need to be considered, given the established links among nonadherence, hostility, aggressive behavior, and relapse in schizophrenia; long-acting injectable formulations of second-generation antipsychotics may be helpful in this regard. Lastly, comorbid substance use and/or personality disorder will require attention and may call for nonpharmacological interventions such as cognitive-behavioral treatment and psychosocial approaches.

Key Clinical Points

▌ With regard to agitation, atypical antipsychotics are efficacious and are substantially less likely to be associated with acute dystonic reactions or akathisia than typical agents such as haloperidol.

▌ Another option is inhaled loxapine; although loxapine is a typical antipsychotic, the dose used in this formulation is low, and this intervention has not been associated with worrisome extrapyramidal side effects.

▌ Another rapidly acting noninjectable alternative is the off-label use of sublingual asenapine; benzodiazepines also have a role in the acute management of agitation, particularly in cases of withdrawal from alcohol.

▌ For the long-term management of individuals with schizophrenia and persistent aggressive behavior, clozapine is the most effective treatment; olanzapine is the second most effective, followed by other second-generation antipsychotics.

▌ Both clozapine and olanzapine require careful monitoring for weight and metabolic abnormalities, with clozapine also requiring monitoring for potential untoward effects on the production of neutrophils and on cardiac muscle.

▌ Because of weak supporting evidence, the routine use of agents such as adjunctive valproate in patients with schizophrenia is not justified; however, time-limited treatment trials in specific patients remain a reasonable option in the face of failure of other strategies.

References

Advokat C: A brief overview of iatrogenic akathisia. Clin Schizophr Relat Psychoses 3(4):226–236, 2010

Allen MH, Feifel D, Lesem MD, et al: Efficacy and safety of loxapine for inhalation in the treatment of agitation in patients with schizophrenia: a randomized, double-blind, placebo-controlled trial. J Clin Psychiatry 72(10):1313–1321, 2011 21294997

Allen MH, Citrome L, Pikalov A, et al: Efficacy of lurasidone in the treatment of agitation: a post hoc analysis of five short-term studies in acutely ill patients with schizophrenia. Gen Hosp Psychiatry 47:75–82, 2017 28807142

Alpert M, Allan ER, Citrome L, et al: A double-blind, placebo-controlled study of adjunctive nadolol in the management of violent psychiatric patients. Psychopharmacol Bull 26(3):367–371, 1990 2274638

Andrezina R, Josiassen RC, Marcus RN, et al: Intramuscular aripiprazole for the treatment of acute agitation in patients with schizophrenia or schizoaffective disorder: a double-blind, placebo-controlled comparison with intramuscular haloperidol. Psychopharmacology (Berl) 188(3):281–292, 2006 16953381

Baker RW, Kinon BJ, Maguire GA, et al: Effectiveness of rapid initial dose escalation of up to forty milligrams per day of oral olanzapine in acute agitation. J Clin Psychopharmacol 23(4):342–348, 2003 12920409

Battaglia J, Moss S, Rush J, et al: Haloperidol, lorazepam, or both for psychotic agitation? A multicenter, prospective, double-blind, emergency department study. Am J Emerg Med 15(4):335–340, 1997 9217519

Beck NC, Greenfield SR, Gotham H, et al: Risperidone in the management of violent, treatment-resistant schizophrenics hospitalized in a maximum security forensic facility. J Am Acad Psychiatry Law 25(4):461–468, 1997 9460034

Bieniek SA, Ownby RL, Penalver A, et al: A double-blind study of lorazepam versus the combination of haloperidol and lorazepam in managing agitation. Pharmacotherapy 18(1):57–62, 1998 9469682

Björkdahl A, Olsson D, Palmstierna T: Nurses' short-term prediction of violence in acute psychiatric intensive care. Acta Psychiatr Scand 113(3):224–229, 2006 16466406

Breier A, Meehan K, Birkett M, et al: A double-blind, placebo-controlled dose-response comparison of intramuscular olanzapine and haloperidol in the treatment of acute agitation in schizophrenia. Arch Gen Psychiatry 59(5):441–448, 2002 11982448

Buckley PF, Ibrahim ZY, Singer B, et al: Aggression and schizophrenia: efficacy of risperidone. J Am Acad Psychiatry Law 25(2):173–181, 1997 9213289

Buss AH, Durkee A: An inventory for assessing different kinds of hostility. J Consult Psychol 21:343–349, 1957

Caspi N, Modai I, Barak P, et al: Pindolol augmentation in aggressive schizophrenic patients: a double-blind crossover randomized study. Int Clin Psychopharmacol 16(2):111–115, 2001 11236069

Citrome L: Comparison of intramuscular ziprasidone, olanzapine, or aripiprazole for agitation: a quantitative review of efficacy and safety. J Clin Psychiatry 68(12):1876–1885, 2007 18162018

Citrome L: Adjunctive lithium and anticonvulsants for the treatment of schizophrenia: what is the evidence? Expert Rev Neurother 9(1):55–71, 2009 19102669

Citrome L: Inhaled loxapine for agitation revisited: focus on effect sizes from 2 Phase III randomised controlled trials in persons with schizophrenia or bipolar disorder. Int J Clin Pract 66(3):318–325, 2012 22226343

Citrome L: Addressing the need for rapid treatment of agitation in schizophrenia and bipolar disorder: focus on inhaled loxapine as an alternative to injectable agents. Ther Clin Risk Manag 9:235–245, 2013 23723707

Citrome L, Volavka J, Czobor P, et al: Effects of clozapine, olanzapine, risperidone, and haloperidol on hostility among patients with schizophrenia. Psychiatr Serv 52(11):1510–1514, 2001 11684748

Citrome L, Volavka J, Czobor P, et al: Efficacy of ziprasidone against hostility in schizophrenia: post hoc analysis of randomized, open-label study data. J Clin Psychiatry 67(4):638–642, 2006 16669729

Citrome L, Holt RI, Walker DJ, et al: Weight gain and changes in metabolic variables following olanzapine treatment in schizophrenia and bipolar disorder. Clin Drug Investig 31(7):455–482, 2011 21495734

Citrome L, Pikalov A, Tocco M, et al: Effects of lurasidone on hostility in patients with an acute exacerbation of schizophrenia: a pooled post hoc analysis of five short-term studies. Neuropsychopharmacology 39 (suppl 1):S379–S380, 2014

Citrome L, Du Y, Risinger R, et al: Effect of aripiprazole lauroxil on agitation and hostility in patients with schizophrenia. Int Clin Psychopharmacol 31(2):69–75, 2016a 26517202

Citrome L, Durgam S, Lu K, et al: The effect of cariprazine on hostility associated with schizophrenia: post hoc analyses from 3 randomized controlled trials. J Clin Psychiatry 77(1):109–115, 2016b 26845266

Citrome L, McEvoy JP, Saklad SR: Guide to the management of clozapine-related tolerability and safety concerns. Clin Schizophr Relat Psychoses 10(3):163–177, 2016c 27732102

Currier GW, Simpson GM: Risperidone liquid concentrate and oral lorazepam versus intramuscular haloperidol and intramuscular lorazepam for treatment of psychotic agitation. J Clin Psychiatry 62(3):153–157, 2001 11305699

Currier GW, Chou JC, Feifel D, et al: Acute treatment of psychotic agitation: a randomized comparison of oral treatment with risperidone and lorazepam versus intramuscular treatment with haloperidol and lorazepam. J Clin Psychiatry 65(3):386–394, 2004 15096079

Czobor P, Volavka J, Meibach RC: Effect of risperidone on hostility in schizophrenia. J Clin Psychopharmacol 15(4):243–249, 1995 7593706

Daniel DG, Potkin SG, Reeves KR, et al: Intramuscular (IM) ziprasidone 20 mg is effective in reducing acute agitation associated with psychosis: a double-blind, randomized trial. Psychopharmacology (Berl) 155(2):128–134, 2001 11401000

Eli Lilly and Company: Zyprexa: U.S. package insert for ZYPREXA (olanzapine) tablet for oral use, ZYPREXA ZYDIS (olanzapine) tablet, orally disintegrating for oral use, ZYPREXA intramuscular (olanzapine) injection, powder, for solution for intramuscular use. 2009. Available at: http://pi.lilly.com/us/zyprexa_relprevv.pdf. Accessed April 12, 2018.

Fazel S, Grann M: The population impact of severe mental illness on violent crime. Am J Psychiatry 163(8):1397–1403, 2006 16877653

Fazel S, Gulati G, Linsell L, et al: Schizophrenia and violence: systematic review and meta-analysis. PLoS Med 6(8):e1000120, 2009 19668362

Fazel S, Zetterqvist J, Larsson H, et al: Antipsychotics, mood stabilisers, and risk of violent crime. Lancet 384(9949):1206–1214, 2014 24816046

Foster S, Kessel J, Berman ME, et al: Efficacy of lorazepam and haloperidol for rapid tranquilization in a psychiatric emergency room setting. Int Clin Psychopharmacol 12(3):175–179, 1997 9248875

Frogley C, Taylor D, Dickens G, et al: A systematic review of the evidence of clozapine's anti-aggressive effects. Int J Neuropsychopharmacol 15(9):1351–1371, 2012 22339930

Galen: Adasuve: U.S. package insert for ADASUVE (loxapine) inhalation powder, for oral inhalation use. Agugust 2017. Available at: http://www.adasuve.com/PDF/AdasuvePI.pdf. Accessed April 12, 2018.

Gillies D, Sampson S, Beck A, et al: Benzodiazepines for psychosis-induced aggression or agitation. Cochrane Database Syst Rev 4:CD003079, 2013 23633309

Haddock G, Barrowclough C, Shaw JJ, et al: Cognitive-behavioural therapy v. social activity therapy for people with psychosis and a history of violence: randomised controlled trial. Br J Psychiatry 194(2):152–157, 2009 19182178

Hartz SM, Pato CN, Medeiros H, et al; Genomic Psychiatry Cohort Consortium: Comorbidity of severe psychotic disorders with measures of substance use. JAMA Psychiatry 71(3):248–254, 2014 24382686

Huf G, Alexander J, Allen MH, et al: Haloperidol plus promethazine for psychosis-induced aggression. Cochrane Database Syst Rev 3(3):CD005146, 2009 19588366

Jhee SS, Zarotsky V, Mohaupt SM, et al: Delayed onset of oculogyric crisis and torticollis with intramuscular haloperidol. Ann Pharmacother 37(10):1434–1437, 2003 14519055

Kay SR, Opler LA, Fiszbein A: Positive and Negative Syndrome Scale Manual. North Tonawanda, NY, Multi-Health Systems, 2000

Krakowski MI, Czobor P, Citrome L, et al: Atypical antipsychotic agents in the treatment of violent patients with schizophrenia and schizoaffective disorder. Arch Gen Psychiatry 63(6):622–629, 2006 16754835

Kwentus J, Riesenberg RA, Marandi M, et al: Rapid acute treatment of agitation in patients with bipolar I disorder: a multicenter, randomized, placebo-controlled clinical trial with inhaled loxapine. Bipolar Disord 14(1):31–40, 2012 22329470

Lesem MD, Zajecka JM, Swift RH, et al: Intramuscular ziprasidone, 2 mg versus 10 mg, in the short-term management of agitated psychotic patients. J Clin Psychiatry 62(1):12–18, 2001 11235922

Lesem MD, Tran-Johnson TK, Riesenberg RA, et al: Rapid acute treatment of agitation in individuals with schizophrenia: multicentre, randomised, placebo-controlled study of inhaled loxapine. Br J Psychiatry 198(1):51–58, 2011 21200077

Lindenmayer JP: The pathophysiology of agitation. J Clin Psychiatry 61(Suppl 14):5–10, 2000 11154018

Marder SR, Sorsaburu S, Dunayevich E, et al: Case reports of postmarketing adverse event experiences with olanzapine intramuscular treatment in patients with agitation. J Clin Psychiatry 71(4):433–441, 2010 20156413

Meehan K, Zhang F, David S, et al: A double-blind, randomized comparison of the efficacy and safety of intramuscular injections of olanzapine, lorazepam, or placebo in treating acutely agitated patients diagnosed with bipolar mania. J Clin Psychopharmacol 21(4):389–397, 2001 11476123

Miceli JJ, Tensfeldt TG, Shiovitz T, et al: Effects of high-dose ziprasidone and haloperidol on the QTc interval after intramuscular administration: a randomized, single-blind, parallel-group study in patients with schizophrenia or schizoaffective disorder. Clin Ther 32(3):472–491, 2010 20399985

Mohr P, Knytl P, Vorácková V, et al: Long-acting injectable antipsychotics for prevention and management of violent behaviour in psychotic patients. Int J Clin Pract 71(9):e12997, 2017 28869705

Montoya A, Valladares A, Lizán L, et al: Validation of the Excited Component of the Positive and Negative Syndrome Scale (PANSS-EC) in a naturalistic sample of 278 patients with acute psychosis and agitation in a psychiatric emergency room. Health Qual Life Outcomes 9(9):18, 2011 21447155

Murthy P, Chand P: Treatment of dual diagnosis disorders. Curr Opin Psychiatry 25(3):194–200, 2012 22395768

Nordstrom K, Allen MH: Alternative delivery systems for agents to treat acute agitation: progress to date. Drugs 73(16):1783–1792, 2013 24151084

Nordstrom K, Zun LS, Wilson MP, et al: Medical evaluation and triage of the agitated patient: consensus statement of the American Association for Emergency Psychiatry Project Beta Medical Evaluation workgroup. West J Emerg Med 13(1):3–10, 2012 22461915

Novartis Pharmaceuticals Corporation: Clozaril: U.S. package insert for CLOZARIL (clozapine) tablets, for oral use. September 2015. Available at: http://clozaril.com/wp-content/themes/eyesite/pi/Clozaril-2015A507-10022015-Approved.pdf. Accessed April 12, 2018.

Otsuka Pharmaceutical Company: Abilify: U.S. package insert for ABILIFY (aripiprazole) tablets, ABILIFY DISCMELT (aripiprazole) orally disintegrating tablets, ABILIFY (aripiprazole) oral solution, ABILIFY (aripiprazole) injection for intramuscular use only. March 2018. Available at: https://www.otsuka-us.com/media/static/Abilify-M-PI.pdf. Accessed April 12, 2018.

Parker C: Midazolam for rapid tranquillisation: its place in practice. J Psychiatr Intensive Care 11(1):66–72, 2015

Pfizer: Geodon: U.S. package insert for Geodon (ziprasidone HCl) capsules and Geodon (ziprasidone mesylate) injection for intramuscular use. February 2017. Available at: http://labeling.pfizer.com/ShowLabeling.aspx?id=584. Accessed April 12, 2018.

Powell G, Caan W, Crowe M: What events precede violent incidents in psychiatric hospitals? Br J Psychiatry 165(1):107–112, 1994 7953012

Pratts M, Citrome L, Grant W, et al: A single-dose, randomized, double-blind, placebo-controlled trial of sublingual asenapine for acute agitation. Acta Psychiatr Scand 130(1):61–68, 2014 24606117

Ratey JJ, Sorgi P, O'Driscoll GA, et al: Nadolol to treat aggression and psychiatric symptomatology in chronic psychiatric inpatients: a double-blind, placebo-controlled study. J Clin Psychiatry 53(2):41–46, 1992 1347291

Regier DA, Farmer ME, Rae DS, et al: Comorbidity of mental disorders with alcohol and other drug abuse. Results from the Epidemiologic Catchment Area (ECA) Study. JAMA 264(19):2511–2518, 1990 2232018

Richmond JS, Berlin JS, Fishkind AB, et al: Verbal de-escalation of the agitated patient: consensus statement of the American Association for Emergency Psychiatry Project BETA De-escalation Workgroup. West J Emerg Med 13(1):17–25, 2012 22461917

Salzman C, Solomon D, Miyawaki E, et al: Parenteral lorazepam versus parenteral haloperidol for the control of psychotic disruptive behavior. J Clin Psychiatry 52(4):177–180, 1991 1673123

Sonnier L, Barzman D: Pharmacologic management of acutely agitated pediatric patients. Paediatr Drugs 13(1):1–10, 2011 21162596

Swanson JW, Swartz MS, Van Dorn RA, et al: A national study of violent behavior in persons with schizophrenia. Arch Gen Psychiatry 63(5):490–499, 2006 16651506

Swanson JW, Swartz MS, Van Dorn RA, et al; CATIE investigators: Comparison of antipsychotic medication effects on reducing violence in people with schizophrenia. Br J Psychiatry 193(1):37–43, 2008 18700216

Swift RH, Harrigan EP, Cappelleri JC, et al: Validation of the Behavioural Activity Rating Scale (BARS): a novel measure of activity in agitated patients. J Psychiatr Res 36(2):87–95, 2002 11777497

Tiihonen J, Lönnqvist J, Wahlbeck K, et al: 11-year follow-up of mortality in patients with schizophrenia: a population-based cohort study (FIN11 study). Lancet 374(9690):620–627, 2009 19595447

Topiwala A, Fazel S: The pharmacological management of violence in schizophrenia: a structured review. Expert Rev Neurother 11(1):53–63, 2011 21158555

Tran-Johnson TK, Sack DA, Marcus RN, et al: Efficacy and safety of intramuscular aripiprazole in patients with acute agitation: a randomized, double-blind, placebo-controlled trial. J Clin Psychiatry 68(1):111–119, 2007 17284138

Volavka J, Citrome L: Heterogeneity of violence in schizophrenia and implications for long-term treatment. Int J Clin Pract 62(8):1237–1245, 2008 18564202

Volavka J, Citrome L: Pathways to aggression in schizophrenia affect results of treatment. Schizophr Bull 37(5):921–929, 2011 21562140

Volavka J, Czobor P, Nolan K, et al: Overt aggression and psychotic symptoms in patients with schizophrenia treated with clozapine, olanzapine, risperidone, or haloperidol. J Clin Psychopharmacol 24(2):225–228, 2004 15206671

Volavka J, Czobor P, Citrome L, et al: Efficacy of aripiprazole against hostility in schizophrenia and schizoaffective disorder: data from 5 double-blind studies. J Clin Psychiatry 66(11):1362–1366, 2005 16420071

Volavka J, Czobor P, Derks EM, et al; EUFEST Study Group: Efficacy of antipsychotic drugs against hostility in the European First-Episode Schizophrenia Trial (EUFEST). J Clin Psychiatry 72(7):955–961, 2011 21824456

Volavka J, Czobor P, Citrome L, et al: Effectiveness of antipsychotic drugs against hostility in patients with schizophrenia in the Clinical Antipsychotic Trials of Intervention Effectiveness (CATIE) study. CNS Spectr 19(5):374–381, 2014 24284234

Volavka J, Van Dorn RA, Citrome L, et al: Hostility in schizophrenia: an integrated analysis of the combined Clinical Antipsychotic Trials of Intervention Effectiveness (CATIE) and the European First Episode Schizophrenia Trial (EUFEST) studies. Eur Psychiatry 31:13–19, 2016 26657597

Volicer L, Citrome L, Volavka J: Measurement of agitation and aggression in adult and aged neuropsychiatric patients: review of definitions and frequently used measurement scales. CNS Spectr 22(5):407–414, 2017 28179043

Wilson MP, Pepper D, Currier GW, et al: The psychopharmacology of agitation: consensus statement of the American Association for Emergency Psychiatry Project Beta Psychopharmacology Workgroup. West J Emerg Med 13(1):26–34, 2012 22461918

Wright P, Birkett M, David SR, et al: Double-blind, placebo-controlled comparison of intramuscular olanzapine and intramuscular haloperidol in the treatment of acute agitation in schizophrenia. Am J Psychiatry 158(7):1149–1151, 2001 11431240

Yates KF, Kunz M, Khan A, et al: Psychiatric patients with histories of aggression and crime five years after discharge from a cognitive-behavioral program. J Forensic Psychiatry Psychol 21(2):167–188, 2010

Yudofsky SC, Silver JM, Jackson W, et al: The Overt Aggression Scale for the objective rating of verbal and physical aggression. Am J Psychiatry 143(1):35–39, 1986 3942284

Zeller SL, Citrome L: Managing agitation associated with schizophrenia and bipolar disorder in the emergency setting. West J Emerg Med 17(2):165–172, 2016 26973742

Zeller SL, Rhoades RW: Systematic reviews of assessment measures and pharmacologic treatments for agitation. Clin Ther 32(3):403–425, 2010 20399981

Zimbroff DL, Allen MH, Battaglia J, et al: Best clinical practice with ziprasidone IM: update after 2 years of experience. CNS Spectr 10(9):1–15, 2005 16247923

Zimbroff DL, Marcus RN, Manos G, et al: Management of acute agitation in patients with bipolar disorder: efficacy and safety of intramuscular aripiprazole. J Clin Psychopharmacol 27(2):171–176, 2007 17414241

6

Aggression in Bipolar Disorders

Susan L. McElroy, M.D.
Brian E. Martens, L.S.W., M.S., C.C.R.C.
Paul E. Keck, Jr., M.D.

A wide range of aggressive behavior occurs in persons with bipolar disorder, including anger attacks, verbal and physical aggression, intimate partner violence, homicide, and sexual aggression (Belete et al. 2016; Crane et al. 2014; Fazel et al. 2007; Perlis et al. 2004; Yoon et al. 2012). For example, among 121 inpatients with bipolar disorder evaluated with the Overt Aggression Scale—Modified (OAS-M) over the past 7 days, the most common type of aggression was verbal (20.4%), followed by, in descending order, physical aggression (19.0%), aggression against property (17.5%), and aggression against self (14.6%) (Belete et al. 2016). Thirty of the patients displayed all four domains of aggression. In a study of 79 outpatients with bipolar or unipolar depression, 62% of the bipolar patients reported having anger attacks as compared with 26% of the unipolar patients; anger attacks were defined as sudden episodes of intense anger and autonomic arousal (Perlis et al. 2004). The authors concluded that anger attacks were a common feature of bipolar depression. In a 22-year study of 219 offenders with bipolar I disorder sentenced to receive treatment at the National Institute of Forensic Psychiatry in South Korea, 62 (28.3%) had killed 79 victims (Yoon et al. 2012). Although the general rate of total offenses was higher in manic than depressive phases (87% vs. 13%), rates of homicide were higher in depressive than in manic phases (90% vs. 19%). Homicide victims were usually family members. Parricide, however, was only committed during the manic phase. In a case-control study examining the comorbidity of severe mental illness and sexual offending behavior, sexual offenders were significantly more likely to have bipolar disorder than the general population (Fazel et al. 2007).

Phenomenology

Few empirical studies, however, have evaluated the nature or phenomenology of aggressive behavior in bipolar disorder—that is, whether aggression is impulsive, reactive, or affective versus planned or premeditated, or whether it is impulsive, psychotic, or instrumental (Látalová 2009). Factor analytic studies indicate that aggression is a core symptom of pure and mixed mania that often co-occurs with irritability, suggesting that manic aggression has an affective component (Cassidy et al. 1998; Sato et al. 2002). Importantly, irritable aggression may be a stable factor across manic episodes (Cassidy et al. 2002; Safer et al. 2012). Another factor analytic study found that aggression was associated with a "negative emotion" factor in patients with remitted bipolar I disorder (Johnson et al. 2016).

Of note, it is often assumed that aggression in bipolar disorder is largely impulsive, but this has received little empirical study (Látalová 2009). In the only study we found that explored this issue, verbal and physical aggression scores from the short-form Buss-Perry Aggression Questionnaire (BPAQ) were correlated with emotion-relevant impulsivity (as assessed with the Positive Urgency Measure) among 58 individuals with remitted bipolar I disorder (Johnson and Carver 2016). Moreover, little is known about psychotic or instrumental aggression in bipolar disorder. For example, though one of the factor analytic studies of manic symptoms noted above found that aggression was associated with paranoia as well as irritability, a separate factor was found for psychosis (Cassidy et al. 1998).

A number of studies have explored correlates of aggression in bipolar disorder. Identified correlates, which are numerous, include presentation in youth, especially preadolescents (Connor et al. 2017; Safer et al. 2012); male sex (Fazel et al. 2010a); co-occurring substance use disorders (Alnıak et al. 2016; Fazel et al. 2010b; Garno et al. 2008; Grunebaum et al. 2006) or current substance use (Belete et al. 2016); co-occurring personality disorders, especially antisocial and borderline disorders (Garno et al. 2008; Látalová et al. 2013); history of suicide attempts (Michaelis et al. 2004; Oquendo et al. 2000); history of childhood trauma (Garno et al. 2008), severe childhood discipline (Yesavage 1983), or verbal or physical abuse (Belete 2017a); previous history of aggression or violent behavior (Alnıak et al. 2016; Belete et al. 2016; Yesavage 1983); poor adherence with psychotropic medication (Belete et al. 2016); involuntary hospital admissions (Schuepbach et al. 2006); and poor social support (Belete et al. 2016).

In particular, the combination of bipolar disorder and substance abuse is associated with aggressive behavior. In one epidemiological study, the risk of violent crime among persons with bipolar disorder and comorbid substance abuse was over 21%, whereas the risk among those without substance abuse was 4.9% (Fazel et al. 2010b). In another study, a logistic regression analysis of demographic and clinical data from 146 patients with bipolar disorder, aggression (evaluated with the Brown-Goodwin Aggression Inventory) was found to be the only variable associated with lifetime substance use disorder (the dependent variable) (Grunebaum et al. 2006). Another study, of 100 male inpatients with bipolar I disorder, found that current substance abuse, but not lifetime substance abuse, was associated with violent behavior (Alnıak et al. 2016).

Epidemiology

Although aggression is not a defining feature of bipolar disorder in nosological systems, epidemiological data have consistently shown that aggressive behavior is more common in individuals with bipolar disorder than in those without bipolar disorder (Fazel et al. 2010a, 2010b; Látalová 2009; Volavka 2013). Persons with bipolar disorder are two to nine times more likely than those in the general population to commit violent crimes (Fazel et al. 2010a) and five times more likely to be jailed, arrested, or convicted of an offense other than drunk driving

(Calabrese et al. 2003). In a recent systematic review of nine epidemiological studies, 9.8% of individuals with bipolar disorder had a history of violent crime compared with 3.0% of those from the general population (Fazel et al. 2010a, 2010b). Even subthreshold bipolar disorder (defined as major depressive disorder with subsyndromal hypomania) may be associated with aggression. In a prospective, 10-year longitudinal study of more than 3,000 randomly selected German residents ages 14–24 years evaluated with structured clinical interviews, respondents with subthreshold bipolar disorder, as well as those with bipolar I and II disorders, had higher odds of reporting criminal acts than those with pure major depressive disorder (Zimmermann et al. 2009).

In addition, epidemiological studies exploring correlates of aggression in bipolar disorder generally find that aggression is equally common in manic versus depressive episodes and in psychotic versus nonpsychotic patients. In a follow-up study of 3,743 individuals with bipolar disorder, 8.4% of whom had committed a violent crime, there were no differences in rates of violent crime by type of mood episode (manic or depressed) or presence or absence of psychotic features (Fazel et al. 2010b). Nonetheless, a large proportion of individuals experience legal involvement during a manic episode. In the 2001–2002 National Epidemiologic Survey on Alcohol and Related Conditions, 13% of respondents meeting criteria for having experienced a manic episode reported criminal justice system involvement during the episode (Christopher et al. 2012). Males, those with a first episode at age 23 years or younger, and persons with mania-associated social indiscretions, excessive spending, or reckless driving and social and occupational impairment were at greatest risk. Indeed, "disruptive-aggressive behavior" is one of 11 items, and one of 4 core items, on the Young Mania Rating Scale (YMRS), a reliable and validated clinician-administered scale commonly used to assess severity of manic symptoms (Young et al. 1978). The scale scores range from 0 to 76; if a patient is assaultive or destructive, he or she receives 8 points.

Clinical studies have similarly found high rates of aggressive behavior in patients with bipolar disorder, especially when they are experiencing mood episodes. In a study of 253 hospitalized psychiatric patients on a locked unit, patients with mania and those with schizophrenia were equally more likely than patients with other diagnoses to have engaged in assaultive behavior in the community before admission (Binder and McNiel 1988). However, in the hospital, patients with mania were more likely to be assaultive (26.1%) than patients with schizophrenia (10.3%) or other diagnoses (10.0%).

During an 18-month period, data on aggressive behavior were collected from 1,268 psychiatric patients hospitalized on four different units in Illawarra, Australia (Barlow et al. 2000). Patients with bipolar disorder had the highest risk of being aggressive (a 2.81 increased risk, compared with a 1.98 increased risk for patients with schizophrenia) and decreased risks (0.44 and 0.54, respectively) for patients with depression or adjustment disorder. In a study evaluating 225 patients with bipolar I or II disorder, 85 patients with nonbipolar psychopathology, and 84 healthy control subjects with the BPAQ, bipolar patients had significantly higher total and subscale BPAQ scores than both nonbipolar and healthy control subjects (Ballester et al. 2012). Bipolar patients in an acute mood episode had higher BPAQ scores than those not in a current episode, although among the former, there were no effects of episode polarity or severity on BPAQ scores. Additionally, those with current psychotic symptoms had higher total BPAQ scores than those without psychosis. In a 4-year follow up of these study participants, patients with bipolar disorder continued to display persistently higher total and subscale BPAQ scores than both nonbipolar patients and healthy controls (Ballester et al. 2014).

In a study of 685 patients experiencing a major depressive episode, those with bipolar I or II disorder had significantly higher Life History of Aggression (LHA) scores as compared with those with unipolar major depressive disorder (Dervic et al. 2015). Patients with bipolar I depression had higher LHA scores as compared with those with bipolar II depression.

In a study of 411 hospitalized patients with bipolar disorder in Ethiopia evaluated over the past 7 days with the OAS-M, the prevalence of aggressive behavior was 29.4% (Belete et al. 2016). Manic, depressive, and psychotic symptoms, among other factors, were all associated with aggression.

Persons with bipolar disorder may also have increased aggression when euthymic. In a study comparing aggression in 24 stable patients with bipolar II disorder and 38 age-matched control subjects, Overt Aggression Scale total and subscale scores were significantly higher in bipolar patients than in controls (Chou et al. 2013). In a study of 67 individuals with remitted bipolar I disorder and 58 control subjects without mood disorders, bipolar individuals had higher measures of verbal and physical aggression (as assessed with the Bryant Aggression Questionnaire) than controls (Johnson et al. 2016). These findings have led to the suggestions that trait aggression may be increased in some persons with bipolar disorder or that aggression might be a trait marker for bipolar disorder. Of note, aggressiveness has also been identified as a prodromal symptom of bipolar disorder, though specificity is low (Skjelstad et al. 2010).

Comorbidity

Persons with bipolar disorder also have elevated comorbidity with other psychiatric disorders specifically characterized by aggression. These disorders include intermittent explosive disorder (IED), borderline and antisocial personality disorders, oppositional defiant and conduct disorders, attention deficit/hyperactivity disorder, and paraphilias (Blanco et al. 2017; Dunsieth et al. 2004; Nierenberg et al. 2005; Saylor and Amann 2016; Scott et al. 2016). Thus, in a cross-national study of the epidemiology of IED, 14.1% of individuals with IED also had a lifetime diagnosis of bipolar disorder (Scott et al. 2016). In an epidemiological study of 36,309 adults from the United States, individuals with bipolar I disorder had significantly higher rates of borderline and antisocial personality disorders than people without bipolar I disorder (Blanco et al. 2017). In another study, involving 84 persons convicted of a sexual offense who had at least one paraphilia and were in a residential treatment program, 41.7% also had a diagnosis of bipolar disorder confirmed by structured clinical interview (Dunsieth et al. 2004). Conversely, of 26 sex offenders without paraphilias in the same program, 15.4% had a diagnosis of bipolar disorder. Thus, for the patient with bipolar disorder and aggression, the aggression needs to be carefully evaluated and its cause attributed to bipolar disorder, trait aggression, and/or a co-occurring aggressive disorder

Psychobiology

Behavioral Genetics

Familial factors, including genetic influence, have been hypothesized to contribute to aggression in bipolar disorder (Manchia and Fanos 2017). In a longitudinal study of 4,059 unaffected siblings of 3,743 individuals with bipolar disorder and 37,429 individuals from the general population, there was an increase in violent crime among the unaffected siblings, though it was less than that seen in the bipolar individuals (Fazel et al. 2010a). In a large population-based cohort study of all persons born in Denmark in 1967 through 1997 followed up from their fifteenth birthday until occurrence of an adverse event or December 31, 2012 (whichever came first), representing 1,743,525 cohort members and a total follow-up of 27.2 million person-years, parental bipolar disorder was found to modestly increase the risk of violent offending (and suicidal behavior) in offspring (Mok et al. 2016). However, it is unknown if the familiality displayed in either of these studies represents heritable versus shared environmental factors.

Neurobiology

The pathophysiology of aggression in bipolar disorder is unknown. In one study, single-photon emission computed tomography showed no difference in serotonin transporter availability between subjects with stable bipolar II disorder and healthy control subjects (Chou et al. 2013). This finding is inconsistent with a relatively large body of literature finding that serotonergic abnormalities are associated with impulsive aggression (see Chapter 1, "Phenomenology and Psychobiology of Aggression and Intermittent Explosive Disorder," in this volume). In another study, activity of the left subgenual anterior cingulate gyrus, right amygdala, left Brodmann area 10, and right thalamus (assessed with functional magnetic resonance imaging) was inversely related with aggression (as measured with the Brief Rating of Aggression by Children and Adolescents [BRACHA]) in 10 adolescents with bipolar disorder (Barzman et al. 2006). Additionally, three tumor necrosis factor gene expressions were inversely correlated with BRACHA score, while another was positively correlated. Because of the small sample size and lack of control group, the relevance of these findings is unclear.

Clinical Approach and Treatment

Differential Diagnosis

There are a variety of disorders to consider when evaluating aggressive individuals who might have bipolar disorder. First is whether the aggression meets criteria for another disorder characterized by aggression rather than a bipolar symptom. The critical issue in this regard is to determine if the aggressive behavior is better accounted for by IED, a substance use disorder, or a personality disorder in the absence of bipolar disorder. The presence of psychosis is also important since the diagnostic boundary between bipolar disorder and psychotic disorders is typically difficult to draw in cross-section. In this case it is important to determine if the aggressive behavior is due primarily to core bipolar symptomatology or to psychosis (e.g., delusional thinking) in the absence of other bipolar symptoms.

After the aggressive behavior is determined to be primarily due to bipolar disorder, pharmacological and psychological treatment strategies are crucial for the treatment of the bipolar patient with aggression. However, to our knowledge, no randomized controlled trials (RCTs) have evaluated any type of treatment in a group of patients with both bipolar disorder and aggressive behavior.

Psychopharmacology

Randomized clinical trials of acute mania find that antipsychotics decrease aggressive behavior when it is measured. For example, participant-level data were pooled from four similarly designed randomized, double-blind, placebo-controlled trials of quetiapine—given as monotherapy or adjunctively with lithium or valproate—in acute bipolar mania (Buckley et al. 2007; McIntyre et al. 2007). Compared with patients receiving placebo, patients receiving quetiapine showed significant decreases in manic symptoms (assessed with the YMRS) as well as significant decreases in aggression (assessed with the Positive and Negative Syndrome Scale [PANSS] supplemental aggression risk subscale). Pooled participant-level data from two positive RCTs in acute mania showed that aripiprazole decreased disruptive-aggressive symptoms as assessed with the YMRS (Frye et al. 2008). Similarly, analysis of pooled participant-level data from three positive RCTs of cariprazine showed that active drug was superior to placebo for reducing all 11 items assessed with the YMRS, including "disruptive-aggressive behavior" (Frye et al. 2008; Vieta et al. 2015). Of note, we were unable to find any RCTs of lithium, valproate, or carbamazepine in acute mania that specifically reported on aggression as an outcome. However, as these drugs are efficacious in acute mania, and the YMRS was often used to assess manic symptoms (which specifically assesses aggression) in the clinical trials testing these agents, it is likely that these compounds also reduce aggression due to mania. For example, in a post hoc analysis of a RCT of valproate versus quetiapine in adolescents with bipolar disorder, disruptive behavioral disorders, and elevated PANSS Excited Component (EC) scores, valproate and quetiapine similarly reduced "impulsivity and reactive aggression" as evaluated with the PANSS-EC, which measures excitement, tension, hostility, uncooperativeness, and poor impulse control (Barzman et al. 2006). Thus, there is no clear evidence suggesting that one drug or drug class is superior to another for the treatment of manic aggression.

Indeed, lithium and a number of antiepileptic drugs have been reported to have therapeutic effects in people with impulsive aggression but without clear-cut bipolar disorder (Citrome and Volavka 2014; Goldstein and Mascitelli 2016; Huband et al. 2010; Jones et al. 2011; Munshi et al. 2010; Worrall et al. 1975). In a meta-analysis of 10 RCTs that compared lithium or an antiepileptic with placebo in patients with repetitive or impulsive aggression (but without intellectual disability, organic brain disorder, or psychotic illness), there was an overall significant reduction in the frequency/severity of aggressive behavior, though heterogeneity was high (Jones et al. 2011). Analysis by drug type found significant reductions in aggression in one lithium trial, two oxcarbazepine/carbamazepine trials, and three phenytoin trials. There was no evidence for reduction of aggression with valproate. In another meta-analysis of antiepileptics in people with impulsive aggression, the authors concluded that carbamazepine, oxcarbazepine, and phenytoin, as well as valproate, had evidence of antiaggressive effects (Huband et al. 2010). Both meta-analyses, however, commented that their conclusions were highly preliminary and in need of further study.

Of note, though phenytoin is not generally regarded as a mood stabilizer, small RCTs suggest it might have antimanic and prophylactic effects in patients with bipolar disorder (Mishory et al. 2000, 2003). Moreover, meta-analyses indicate that lithium is an effective treatment for preventing suicide (Cipriani et al. 2013). Since its antisuicide effect is larger than its effect on mood episodes, it has been hypothesized that lithium has a specific antisuicide effect that may be related to its ability to reduce aggression (Cipriani et al. 2013; Kovacsics et al. 2009).

A wide range of antipsychotics have been shown to be efficacious for rapidly reducing acute agitation, which may be associated with or lead to aggression, in patients with acute mania (Correll et al. 2017; Garriga et al. 2016; Látalová 2009; Volavka 2013; Yu et al. 2016). Accordingly, short-acting intramuscular aripiprazole and olanzapine and inhaled loxapine all have regulatory approval for treatment of agitation in patients with bipolar disorder, and sublingual asenapine has been shown to reduce agitation in acutely ill patients, including those with bipolar disorder (Pratts et al. 2014). Thus, rapid treatment of agitation with antipsychotic medication might prevent escalation into aggression. In contrast, evidence for the efficacy of benzodiazepines in psychosis-associated agitation or aggression is poor (Gillies et al. 2013).

Long-acting injectable (LAI) antipsychotic drugs may reduce aggressive behavior in patients with bipolar disorder over the long term, including those who are noncompliant with their prescribed medication (Vieta et al. 2008). Indeed, one expert-consensus guideline concluded that LAI antipsychotic agents should be considered for patients with severe mental illness who pose a risk to others (Llorca et al. 2013); and LAI formulations of risperidone and aripiprazole have regulatory approval for maintenance treatment of patients with bipolar I disorder (Calabrese et al. 2017; Vieta et al. 2012). Thus, if the aggression is a primary symptom of bipolar disorder, it often responds to appropriate pharmacotherapy and successful mood stabilization—both acutely and over the long term.

Indeed, registry data suggest that treatment with antipsychotics and mood stabilizers reduces violent crime. In a Swedish national registry study that evaluated 82,647 patients prescribed antipsychotics or mood stabilizers over a 4-year period of time (11,918 with bipolar disorder), violent crimes decreased by 45% when patients were receiving antipsychotics and by 24% when patients were receiving mood stabilizers (Fazel et al. 2014). Mood stabilizers, however, were associated with a decreased rate of crime only in patients with bipolar disorder.

Clozapine has been shown to be superior to other antipsychotics in reducing aggression in patients with schizophrenia and schizoaffective disorder (see Chapter 5 in this volume) but has received little empirical attention for treating aggression in bipolar disorder (Frogley et al. 2012; Krakowski et al. 2006). Indeed, in the registry study noted above (Fazel et al. 2014), the use of clozapine was not associated with reduced aggression, but the lack of effect was attributed to the very small sample size of bipolar patients receiving the drug. Because clozapine has been shown to be effective in treatment-resistant patients with a history of mania (Suppes et al. 1999), it should be considered for those aggressive bipolar patients who have failed to respond to standard treatments. Given that clozapine has also been reported to reduce violent behavior in men with antisocial personality disorder and aggression in women with borderline personality disorder, it could be considered for aggressive bipolar patients with either of these comorbid personality disorders (Brown et al. 2014; Frogley et al. 2013).

One important clinical issue is that antidepressants have been reported to trigger aggressive behavior in some patients with bipolar disorder (Ramasubbu 2004), as well as in youth at high risk for bipolar disorder (Strawn et al. 2014). In a study evaluating illness course over 43–227 weeks of antidepressant exposure among 25 youth with depressive or anxiety disorders and at least one parent with bipolar I disorder, 57% had an adverse reaction, with the most common reactions being increased irritability ($n=7$) and aggression ($n=5$) (Strawn et al. 2014). Conversely, anger attacks in adults with bipolar depression may respond to addition of a serotonin reuptake inhibitor to ongoing mood stabilizer therapy (Mammen et al. 2004).

Another important clinical issue is the treatment of bipolar disorder when it co-occurs with another disorder characterized by aggression. In the only randomized clinical trial conducted in such a sample that we are aware of where aggression was measured as an outcome, patients with bipolar II disorder and borderline personality disorder receiving valproate showed significantly less aggression (evaluated with the OAS-M) compared with those receiving placebo (Frankenburg and Zanarini 2002). However, clinical data suggest that in some instances, appropriate treatment of bipolar disorder may not result in resolution of the aggression associated with the co-occurring disorder. For example, in a chart review of all sex offenders participating in a residential rehabilitative program who received valproate for treatment of bipolar disorder, manic symptoms improved with valproate but paraphilic symptoms did not (Nelson et al. 2001). Thus, for some bipolar patients with a co-occurring aggressive disorder, both disorders will need to be a focus of targeted treatment.

Psychotherapeutic Strategies

When bipolar patients are acutely ill and aggressive, de-escalation techniques should be employed, including conducting a risk assessment for aggression, taking patients' threats seriously, calling for support if needed, and maintaining a calm and non-confrontational demeanor (Garriga et al. 2016; Látalová 2009; Volavka 2013). Though widely accepted and practiced, however, there are few empirical data to support such de-escalation techniques. In a comprehensive review of the effectiveness of strategies to de-escalate aggressive behavior in psychiatric patients, only risk assessment was found to decrease subsequent aggression or reduce use of seclusion and restraint (Gaynes et al. 2016). Treatment staff must therefore be ready to employ proper seclusion and restraint and have received adequate training in such techniques. In one study of 400 inpatients with bipolar disorder, 65% had been physically restrained (Belete 2017b).

Once the patient is stabilized, psychoeducation regarding the relationship between bipolar disorder and aggression is crucial, including the importance of adherence with prescribed medications and avoidance of substance misuse to reduce the risk for further aggression. Indeed, psychoeducation has been shown to enhance medication compliance and reduce the risk of relapse (Colom et al. 2003, 2009), including in bipolar patients with co-occurring personality disorders (Colom et al. 2004).

For bipolar patients with apparently elevated trait aggression or a co-occurring disorder characterized by aggression, various evidence-based psychotherapies in addition to psychoeducation could be considered, including cognitive-behavioral therapy, interpersonal and social rhythm therapy, dialectical behavior therapy, mindfulness-based cognitive therapy, and family therapy (Salcedo et al. 2016; Volavka 2013). However, no empirical studies of these treatments have been conducted in such patients.

Clinical Vignette

AC, a 35-year-old successful physician, presented with his wife for assessment of "spikes of anger" out of proportion to precipitating events. The angry outbursts had been occurring every 2–3 months over the past year but had recently increased in frequency and severity. They culminated in an event the day before when AC held a loaded gun to his wife's head in their kitchen.

AC's wife described these outbursts as "rages" and said that during them AC's face is contorted with anger and he cannot be reasoned with. AC reported that the episodes are preceded by 3–4 days of progressively increasing irritable mood, abnormally elevated energy level, racing thoughts, and distractibility. He sometimes also had thoughts that he needs to kill someone. He and his wife denied associated euphoria, grandiosity, increased speech, reduced need for sleep, excessive spending of money, or increase in sex drive. After an outburst, AC feels ashamed, depressed, and drained of energy for at least several days.

Past history was notable for AC having a 2-month long major depressive episode at age 29 years that responded fully to a 2-month course of fluoxetine 20 mg daily prescribed by his family physician. However, AC stopped taking the fluoxetine after 2 months because he thought it was making him very irritable. There was no current or past alcohol or drug use. Both AC and his wife agreed that his normal personality was genial and pleasant. Family history was notable for a paternal uncle with bipolar disorder successfully treated with lithium.

AC's "spikes of anger" were attributed to brief, highly irritable and unpleasant hypomanic episodes. Because of his past major depressive episode, a diagnosis of bipolar II disorder, most recent episode hypomanic, was made. Because he and his wife reported that he had had at least four 4-day hypomanic episodes in the last year, his diagnosis was further specified as with rapid cycling. A safety plan was developed (which included giving the gun and ammunition to another family member), and because of the family history of positive lithium response, lithium was begun. At follow-up 2 weeks later, his wife, who accompanied him, was noted to be crying in the waiting room. During the visit, she said she was crying with happiness because AC was "a different man." He continued taking lithium monotherapy (serum levels=0.7–0.8 mEq/mL) with no further hypomanic or rage episodes or homicidal ideation.

Discussion of Vignette

This case demonstrates how an individual with bipolar disorder can present with aggressive behavior and how the aggression resolves once the bipolar disorder is properly treated. More specifically, this patient's aggression appeared to be impulsive and similar to the angry outbursts of IED. It was only after careful questioning that it was discovered his aggressive outbursts were accompanied by hypomanic symptoms and thus better accounted for by a bipolar disorder diagnosis. This case also illustrates that there may be some phenomenological overlap between IED anger outbursts and irritable hypomanic episodes.

Summary

Aggressive behavior is common in persons with bipolar disorder and may manifest as anger attacks, verbal and physical aggression, intimate partner violence, homicide, and sexual aggression. The aggressive behavior can be a primary bipolar symptom, a trait that may be present when the patient is euthymic, or a symptom related to a co-occurring condition that is also characterized by aggression. While aggression representing a primary bipolar symptom should respond to appropriate treatment of bipolar disorder, additional targeted treatment needs to be provided to those bipolar patients with aggression due to a personality trait or a comorbid disorder.

Key Clinical Points

▌ All patients presenting with any type of aggressive behavior should be carefully assessed for bipolar disorder.

▌ Any patient presenting with bipolar disorder should be evaluated for current and past aggressive behavior.

▌ For bipolar patients with aggressive behavior, the behavior should be characterized as impulsive, psychotic, or planned or as having a combination of these components.

▌ For bipolar patients with aggressive behavior, it should also be determined if the aggression is predominantly a manic, hypomanic, depressive, mixed-state, rapid-cycling, and/or psychotic symptom (i.e., a primary bipolar symptom); a trait that may be present when the patient is euthymic; or a symptom related to a co-occurring condition also characterized by aggression (i.e., intermittent explosive disorder, substance abuse, or borderline or antisocial personality disorder).

■ For patients in whom aggression represents a primary bipolar symptom, the goal of treatment is complete mood stabilization and maintenance of euthymia.

■ Since substance abuse is such a strong correlate of aggressive behavior in bipolar disorder, the presence or absence of a co-occurring substance use disorder must be determined; if a substance use disorder is present, appropriate targeted treatment must be provided.

■ For those with aggression representing a trait or related to a comorbid disorder, that trait or disorder needs to be optimally treated in conjunction with mood stabilization.

References

Alnıak I, Erkıran M, Mutlu E: Substance use is a risk factor for violent behavior in male patients with bipolar disorder. J Affect Disord 193:89–93, 2016 26771949

Ballester J, Goldstein T, Goldstein B, et al: Is bipolar disorder specifically associated with aggression? Bipolar Disord 14(3):283–290, 2012 22548901

Ballester J, Goldstein B, Goldstein TR, et al: Prospective longitudinal course of aggression among adults with bipolar disorder. Bipolar Disord 16(3):262–269, 2014 24372913

Barlow K, Grenyer B, Ilkiw-Lavalle O: Prevalence and precipitants of aggression in psychiatric inpatient units. Aust N Z J Psychiatry 34(6):967–974, 2000 11127627

Barzman DH, DelBello MP, Adler CM, et al: The efficacy and tolerability of quetiapine versus divalproex for the treatment of impulsivity and reactive aggression in adolescents with co-occurring bipolar disorder and disruptive behavior disorder(s). J Child Adolesc Psychopharmacol 16(6):665–670, 2006 17201610

Belete H: Leveling and abuse among patients with bipolar disorder at psychiatric outpatient departments in Ethiopia. Ann Gen Psychiatry 16:29, 2017a 28702070

Belete H: Use of physical restraints among patients with bipolar disorder in Ethiopian Mental Specialized Hospital, outpatient department: cross-sectional study. Int J Bipolar Disord 5(1):17, 2017b 28332124

Belete H, Mulat H, Fanta T, et al: Magnitude and associated factors of aggressive behaviour among patients with bipolar disorder at Amanual

Mental Specialized Hospital, outpatient department, Addis Ababa, Ethiopia: cross-sectional study. BMC Psychiatry 16(1):443, 2016 27955659

Binder RL, McNiel DE: Effects of diagnosis and context on dangerousness. Am J Psychiatry 145(6):728–732, 1988 3369561

Blanco C, Compton WM, Saha TD, et al: Epidemiology of DSM-5 bipolar I disorder: results from the National Epidemiologic Survey on Alcohol and Related Conditions—III. J Psychiatr Res 84:310–317, 2017 27814503

Brown D, Larkin F, Sengupta S, et al: Clozapine: an effective treatment for seriously violent and psychopathic men with antisocial personality disorder in a UK high-security hospital. CNS Spectr 19(5):391–402, 2014 24698103

Buckley PF, Paulsson B, Brecher M: Treatment of agitation and aggression in bipolar mania: efficacy of quetiapine. J Affect Disord 100 (suppl 1):S33–S43, 2007 17376537

Calabrese JR, Hirschfeld RM, Reed M, et al: Impact of bipolar disorder on a U.S. community sample. J Clin Psychiatry 64(4):425–432, 2003 12716245

Calabrese JR, Sanchez R, Jin N, et al: Efficacy and safety of aripiprazole once-monthly in the maintenance treatment of bipolar I disorder: a double-blind, placebo-controlled, 52-week randomized withdrawal study. J Clin Psychiatry 78(3):324–331, 2017 28146613

Cassidy F, Forest K, Murry E, et al: A factor analysis of the signs and symptoms of mania. Arch Gen Psychiatry 55(1):27–32, 1998 9435757

Cassidy F, Ahearn EP, Carroll BJ: Symptom profile consistency in recurrent manic episodes. Compr Psychiatry 43(3):179–181, 2002 11994834

Chou YH, Lin CL, Wang SJ, et al: Aggression in bipolar II disorder and its relation to the serotonin transporter. J Affect Disord 147(1–3):59–63, 2013 23123132

Christopher PP, McCabe PJ, Fisher WH: Prevalence of involvement in the criminal justice system during severe mania and associated symptomatology. Psychiatr Serv 63(1):33–39, 2012 22227757

Cipriani A, Hawton K, Stockton S, et al: Lithium in the prevention of suicide in mood disorders: updated systematic review and meta-analysis. BMJ 346:f3646, 2013 23814104

Citrome L, Volavka J: The psychopharmacology of violence: making sensible decisions. CNS Spectr 19(5):411–418, 2014 24571828

Colom F, Vieta E, Martinez-Aran A, et al: A randomized trial on the efficacy of group psychoeducation in the prophylaxis of recurrences in bipolar patients whose disease is in remission. Arch Gen Psychiatry 60(4):402–407, 2003 12695318

Colom F, Vieta E, Sánchez-Moreno J, et al: Psychoeducation in bipolar patients with comorbid personality disorders. Bipolar Disord 6(4):294–298, 2004 15225146

Colom F, Vieta E, Sánchez-Moreno J, et al: Group psychoeducation for stabilised bipolar disorders: 5-year outcome of a randomised clinical trial. Br J Psychiatry 194(3):260–265, 2009 19252157

Connor DF, Ford JD, Pearson GS, et al: Early onset bipolar disorder: characteristics and outcomes in the clinic. J Child Adolesc Psychopharmacol 27(10):875–883, 2017 28829159

Correll CU, Yu X, Xiang Y, et al: Biological treatment of acute agitation or aggression with schizophrenia or bipolar disorder in the inpatient setting. Ann Clin Psychiatry 29(2):92–107, 2017 28463343

Crane CA, Hawes SW, Devine S, et al: Axis I psychopathology and the perpetration of intimate partner violence. J Clin Psychol 70(3):238–247, 2014 23824500

Dervic K, Garcia-Amador M, Sudol K, et al: Bipolar I and II versus unipolar depression: clinical differences and impulsivity/aggression traits. Eur Psychiatry 30(1):106–113, 2015 25280430

Dunsieth NWJr, Nelson EB, Brusman-Lovins LA, et al: Psychiatric and legal features of 113 men convicted of sexual offenses. J Clin Psychiatry 65(3):293–300, 2004 15096066

Fazel S, Sjöstedt G, Långström N, et al: Severe mental illness and risk of sexual offending in men: a case-control study based on Swedish national registers. J Clin Psychiatry 68(4):588–596, 2007 17474815

Fazel S, Lichtenstein P, Frisell T, et al: Bipolar disorder and violent crime: time at risk reanalysis. Arch Gen Psychiatry 67(12):1325–1326, 2010a 21135334

Fazel S, Lichtenstein P, Grann M, et al: Bipolar disorder and violent crime: new evidence from population-based longitudinal studies and systematic review. Arch Gen Psychiatry 67(9):931–938, 2010b 20819987

Fazel S, Zetterqvist J, Larsson H, et al: Antipsychotics, mood stabilisers, and risk of violent crime. Lancet 384(9949):1206–1214, 2014 24816046

Frankenburg FR, Zanarini MC: Divalproex sodium treatment of women with borderline personality disorder and bipolar II disorder: a double-blind placebo-controlled pilot study. J Clin Psychiatry 63(5):442–446, 2002 12019669

Frogley C, Taylor D, Dickens G, et al: A systematic review of the evidence of clozapine's anti-aggressive effects. Int J Neuropsychopharmacol 15(9):1351–1371, 2012 22339930

Frogley C, Anagnostakis K, Mitchell S, et al: A case series of clozapine for borderline personality disorder. Ann Clin Psychiatry 25(2):125–134, 2013 23638443

Frye MA, Eudicone J, Pikalov A, et al: Aripiprazole efficacy in irritability and disruptive-aggressive symptoms: Young Mania Rating Scale line analysis from two, randomized, double-blind, placebo-controlled trials. J Clin Psychopharmacol 28(2):243–245, 2008 18344741

Garno JL, Gunawardane N, Goldberg JF: Predictors of trait aggression in bipolar disorder. Bipolar Disord 10(2):285–292, 2008 18271908

Garriga M, Pacchiarotti I, Kasper S, et al: Assessment and management of agitation in psychiatry: expert consensus. World J Biol Psychiatry 17(2):86–128, 2016 26912127

Gaynes BN, Brown C, Lux LJ, et al: Strategies to de-escalate aggressive behavior in psychiatric patients (Comparative Effectiveness Review, No 180; AHRQ Publ No 16-EHC032EF). Agency for Healthcare Research and Quality, July 2016. Available at: https://www.ncbi.nlm.nih.gov/books/NBK379399/pdf/Bookshelf_NBK379399.pdf. Accessed April 12, 2018.

Gillies D, Sampson S, Beck A, et al: Benzodiazepines for psychosis-induced aggression or agitation. Cochrane Database Syst Rev 9:CD003079, 2013 24049046

Goldstein MR, Mascitelli L: Is violence in part a lithium deficiency state? Med Hypotheses 89:40–42, 2016 26968907

Grunebaum MF, Galfalvy HC, Nichols CM, et al: Aggression and substance abuse in bipolar disorder. Bipolar Disord 8(5 Pt 1):496–502, 2006 17042888

Huband N, Ferriter M, Nathan R, et al: Antiepileptics for aggression and associated impulsivity. Cochrane Database Syst Rev (2):CD003499, 2010 20166067

Johnson SL, Carver CS: Emotion-relevant impulsivity predicts sustained anger and aggression after remission in bipolar I disorder. J Affect Disord 189:169–175, 2016 26437231

Johnson SL, Tharp JA, Peckham AD, et al: Emotion in bipolar I disorder: implications for functional and symptom outcomes. J Abnorm Psychol 125(1):40–52, 2016 26480234

Jones RM, Arlidge J, Gillham R, et al: Efficacy of mood stabilisers in the treatment of impulsive or repetitive aggression: systematic review and meta-analysis. Br J Psychiatry 198(2):93–98, 2011 21282779

Kovacsics CE, Gottesman II, Gould TD: Lithium's antisuicidal efficacy: elucidation of neurobiological targets using endophenotype strategies. Annu Rev Pharmacol Toxicol 49:175–198, 2009 18834309

Krakowski MI, Czobor P, Citrome L, et al: Atypical antipsychotic agents in the treatment of violent patients with schizophrenia and schizoaffective disorder. Arch Gen Psychiatry 63(6):622–629, 2006 16754835

Látalová K: Bipolar disorder and aggression. Int J Clin Pract 63(6):889–899, 2009 19490199

Látalová K, Prasko J, Kamaradova D, et al: Comorbidity bipolar disorder and personality disorders. Neuroendocrinol Lett 34(1):1–8, 2013 23524617

Llorca PM, Abbar M, Courtet P, et al: Guidelines for the use and management of long-acting injectable antipsychotics in serious mental illness. BMC Psychiatry 13:340, 2013 24359031

Mammen OK, Pilkonis PA, Chengappa KN, et al: Anger attacks in bipolar depression: predictors and response to citalopram added to mood stabilizers. J Clin Psychiatry 65(5):627–633, 2004 15163248

Manchia M, Fanos V: Targeting aggression in severe mental illness: the predictive role of genetic, epigenetic, and metabolomic markers. Prog Neuropsychopharmacol Biol Psychiatry 77:32–41, 2017 28372995

McIntyre RS, Konarski JZ, Jones M, et al: Quetiapine in the treatment of acute bipolar mania: efficacy across a broad range of symptoms. J Affect Disord 100(Suppl 1):S5–S14, 2007 17391773

Michaelis BH, Goldberg JF, Davis GP, et al: Dimensions of impulsivity and aggression associated with suicide attempts among bipolar patients: a preliminary study. Suicide Life Threat Behav 34(2):172–176, 2004 15191273

Mishory A, Yaroslavsky Y, Bersudsky Y, et al: Phenytoin as an antimanic anticonvulsant: a controlled study. Am J Psychiatry 157(3):463–465, 2000 10698828

Mishory A, Winokur M, Bersudsky Y: Prophylactic effect of phenytoin in bipolar disorder: a controlled study. Bipolar Disord 5(6):464–467, 2003 14636372

Mok PL, Pedersen CB, Springate D, et al: Parental psychiatric disease and risks of attempted suicide and violent criminal offending in offspring: a population-based cohort study. JAMA Psychiatry 73(10):1015–1022, 2016 27580483

Munshi KR, Oken T, Guild DJ, et al: The use of antiepileptic drugs (AEDs) for the treatment of pediatric aggression and mood disorders. Pharmaceuticals (Basel) 3(9):2986–3004, 2010 27713387

Nelson E, Brusman L, Holcomb J, et al: Divalproex sodium in sex offenders with bipolar disorders and comorbid paraphilias: an open retrospective study. J Affect Disord 64(2–3):249–255, 2001 11313091

Nierenberg AA, Miyahara S, Spencer T, et al; STEP-BD Investigators: Clinical and diagnostic implications of lifetime attention-deficit/hyperactivity disorder comorbidity in adults with bipolar disorder: data from the first 1000 STEP-BD participants. Biol Psychiatry 57(11):1467–1473, 2005 15950022

Oquendo MA, Waternaux C, Brodsky B, et al: Suicidal behavior in bipolar mood disorder: clinical characteristics of attempters and nonattempters. J Affect Disord 59(2):107–117, 2000 10837879

Perlis RH, Smoller JW, Fava M, et al: The prevalence and clinical correlates of anger attacks during depressive episodes in bipolar disorder. J Affect Disord 79(1–3):291–295, 2004 15023510

Pratts M, Citrome L, Grant W, et al: A single-dose, randomized, double-blind, placebo-controlled trial of sublingual asenapine for acute agitation. Acta Psychiatr Scand 130(1):61–68, 2014 24606117

Ramasubbu R: Antidepressant treatment-associated behavioural expression of hypomania: a case series. Prog Neuropsychopharmacol Biol Psychiatry 28(7):1201–1207, 2004 15610935

Safer DJ, Magno Zito J, Safer AM: Age-grouped differences in bipolar mania. Compr Psychiatry 53(8):1110–1117, 2012 22682679

Salcedo S, Gold AK, Sheikh S, et al: Empirically supported psychosocial interventions for bipolar disorder: current state of the research. J Affect Disord 201:203–214, 2016 27243619

Sato T, Bottlender R, Kleindienst N, et al: Syndromes and phenomenological subtypes underlying acute mania: a factor analytic study of 576 manic patients. Am J Psychiatry 159(6):968–974, 2002 12042185

Saylor KE, Amann BH: Impulsive aggression as a comorbidity of attention-deficit/hyperactivity disorder in children and adolescents. J Child Adolesc Psychopharmacol 26(1):19–25, 2016 26744906

Schuepbach D, Goetz I, Boeker H, et al: Voluntary vs. involuntary hospital admission in acute mania of bipolar disorder: results from the Swiss sample of the EMBLEM study. J Affect Disord 90(1):57–61, 2006 16324749

Scott KM, Lim CC, Hwang I, et al: The cross-national epidemiology of DSM-IV intermittent explosive disorder. Psychol Med 46(15):3161–3172, 2016 27572872

Skjelstad DV, Malt UF, Holte A: Symptoms and signs of the initial prodrome of bipolar disorder: a systematic review. J Affect Disord 126(1–2):1–13, 2010 19883943

Strawn JR, Adler CM, McNamara RK, et al: Antidepressant tolerability in anxious and depressed youth at high risk for bipolar disorder: a prospective naturalistic treatment study. Bipolar Disord 16(5):523–530, 2014 23937313

Suppes T, Webb A, Paul B, et al: Clinical outcome in a randomized 1-year trial of clozapine versus treatment as usual for patients with treatment-resistant illness and a history of mania. Am J Psychiatry 156(8):1164–1169, 1999 10450255

Vieta E, Nieto E, Autet A, et al: A long-term prospective study on the outcome of bipolar patients treated with long-acting injectable risperidone. World J Biol Psychiatry 9(3):219–224, 2008 18609430

Vieta E, Montgomery S, Sulaiman AH, et al: A randomized, double-blind, placebo-controlled trial to assess prevention of mood episodes with risperidone long-acting injectable in patients with bipolar I disorder. Eur Neuropsychopharmacol 22(11):825–835, 2012 22503488

Vieta E, Durgam S, Lu K, et al: Effect of cariprazine across the symptoms of mania in bipolar I disorder: analyses of pooled data from phase II/III trials. Eur Neuropsychopharmacol 25(11):1882–1891, 2015 26419293

Volavka J: Violence in schizophrenia and bipolar disorder. Psychiatr Danub 25(1):24–33, 2013 23470603

Worrall EP, Moody JP, Naylor GJ: Lithium in non-manic-depressives: anti-aggressive effect and red blood cell lithium values. Br J Psychiatry 126:464–468, 1975 1092398

Yesavage JA: Bipolar illness: correlates of dangerous inpatient behaviour. Br J Psychiatry 143:554–557, 1983 6661598

Yoon JH, Kim JH, Choi SS, et al: Homicide and bipolar I disorder: a 22-year study. Forensic Sci Int 217(1–3):113–118, 2012 22093701

Young RC, Biggs JT, Ziegler VE, et al: A rating scale for mania: reliability, validity and sensitivity. Br J Psychiatry 133:429–435, 1978 728692

Yu X, Correll CU, Xiang YT, et al: Efficacy of atypical antipsychotics in the management of acute agitation and aggression in hospitalized patients with schizophrenia or bipolar disorder: results from a systematic review. Shanghai Jingshen Yixue 28(5):241–252, 2016 28638198

Zimmermann P, Brückl T, Nocon A, et al: Heterogeneity of DSM-IV major depressive disorder as a consequence of subthreshold bipolarity. Arch Gen Psychiatry 66(12):1341–1352, 2009 19996039

7

Anger and Aggression in Depressive Disorders

Maurizio Fava, M.D.
Ellen Leibenluft, M.D.

Unipolar Depressive Disorders

The idea that a depressive syndrome may be associated with anger and aggression has been with us for some time (Snaith and Taylor 1985). In fact, the presence of irritability was part of the "A" criterion for a major depressive episode (MDE) when the Research Diagnostic Criteria (Spitzer et al. 1978) were first established. Irritability, in this context, was characterized as readiness to express anger and/or annoyance to minor provocations. Irritability continued to be an important criterion for major depressive disorder (MDD) in children and adolescents in DSM-III (American Psychiatric Association 1980), DSM-III-R (American Psychiatric Association 1987), and DSM-IV (American Psychiatric Association 1994). Similarly, with DSM-5, irritability was included as a diagnostic criterion for MDD in youth only, even though irritability remains an observable feature of adults with MDD (American Psychiatric Association 2013).

Phenomenology

One of the first reports, by Giovanni Fava and colleagues in Italy, highlighting a potential difference among depressed patients as a function of anger/hostility was published in the early 1980s (Fava et al. 1982). In this report 40 inpatients with MDE were assessed for depression, hostility, and psychosocial loss. MDE study participants without a reported history of loss displayed higher scores of hostility than those of comparable participants with a reported history of loss. At about the same time a group in Boston noted that several depressed patients displayed "anger attacks" that were similar to panic attacks but without panic-like anxiety. This group reported on its first case series of anger attacks in adult patients with MDE in 1990, describing this phenomenon in detail in four cases (Fava et al. 1990). In each case, anger attacks resolved with the depression after treatment with desipramine (two cases) or clomipramine (two cases). This series led these investigators to develop a self-report questionnaire—the Anger Attacks Questionnaire (AAQ; Fava et al. 1991)—that allowed the field to focus research on an "anger attack" subgroup of MDE patients.

In brief, anger attacks are characterized by sudden spells of anger accompanied by symptoms of autonomic activation such as tachycardia, sweating, hot flashes, and tightness of the chest that resemble panic attacks but lack the predominant affects of fear and anxiety. Notably, anger attacks are often experienced as uncharacteristic of the patient and inappropriate to the situations in which they had occurred (Fava et al. 1990). Given these features, and the finding that antidepressant treatment produced marked improvement in behavior in many cases, Fava and colleagues (1990) hypothesized that anger attacks are variants of MDD, as opposed to a primary disorder of aggression such as intermittent explosive disorder (IED) (see Coccaro 2012 and Chapter 1, "Phenomenology and Psychobiology of Aggression and Intermittent Explosive Disorder," in this volume). In later studies using the AAQ, patients were classified as having anger attacks, in addition to depression, if they exhibited four criteria: (A) irritability during the previous 6 months, (B) overreaction to minor annoyances, (C) occurrence of at least one anger attack during the previous month, and (D) experience during at least one of the attacks of four or more of the following: tachycardia, hot flashes, chest tightness, paresthesia, dizziness, shortness of breath, sweating, trembling, panic, feeling out of control, feeling like attacking others, attacking physically or verbally, and throwing or destroying objects (Fava et al. 1991).

Epidemiology

In clinical studies using the AAQ, the prevalence of anger attacks during depressive episodes has been reported to range from 30% to 50% (Fava et al. 1991, 1993; Gould et al. 1996; Sayar et al. 2000). Although the National Comorbidity Survey–Replication (NCS-R; Kessler et al. 2005) included irritability/"anger attacks" in its interview assessment, in that study the anger attacks were targeted at others and did not require individuals to have autonomic arousal. That said, we re-examined that publicly available data set and found that the prevalence of current irritability/anger attacks, among all individuals with current MDE, was 18.8% (it should be noted that none of these individuals had a diagnosis of IED). Although less than the 30%–50% figure cited above, the NCS-R data are from a community survey, and the prevalence derived from that data set is more likely to represent the true prevalence of MDE with anger attacks in the general population.

Comorbidity

In a clinical study of 306 outpatients, MDE patients with anger attacks reported similar rates of comorbidity as a function of syndromal (formerly Axis I) disorders but significantly higher rates of dependent, avoidant, narcissistic, borderline, and antisocial personality (formerly Axis II) disorders, compared with MDE patients without anger attacks (Tedlow et al. 1999). Reanalysis of the NCS-R community survey data, however, found statistically significant comorbidity between current MDE patients with irritability/anger attacks and current IED (20.3% vs. 0.0%, $P < 0.001$), current bulimia (3.3% vs. 0.2%, $P = 0.005$), and current attention-deficit/hyperactivity disorder (ADHD; 13.8% vs. 4.1%, $P < 0.001$) compared with current MDE patients without anger attacks. Removing current IED subjects from the analysis did not change the results observed with current bulimia (4.1% vs. 0.2%, $P < 0.002$) or with current ADHD (16.3% vs. 4.1%, $P < 0.001$). These results are consistent with the idea that the presence of anger attacks in MDE patients is associated with reduced impulse control as seen in IED, bulimia, and ADHD.

Psychobiology

Neurobiology

A small study examining the potential role of thyrotropin-releasing hormone (TRH) stimulation found that depressed patients with anger attacks had lower prolactin responses to TRH compared with similar patients without anger attacks (Rosenbaum et al. 1993). Since chronic treatment with fluoxetine for 8 weeks was followed by a significant increase in the prolactin response to TRH in those with (but not in those without) anger attacks, the authors suggested that depressed patients with anger attacks may have a relatively greater serotonergic dysregulation than depressed patients without such attacks. However, since acute enhancement of central serotonin (5-HT) function does not affect TSH levels in healthy humans (Coccaro et al. 1988), it is unclear how this finding can explain these results in terms of 5-HT.

A clearer test of this hypothesis was reported in 2000, at which time Fava and colleagues conducted *d,l*-fenfluramine challenge studies in 37 patients with MDE with ($n=17$) and without ($n=20$) history of anger attacks. Fenfluramine is an amphetamine analogue that selectively releases 5-HT and blocks its uptake, leading to an acute pulse of 5-HT to directly stimulate postsynaptic 5-HT receptors, in turn leading to a downstream, dose-dependent release of prolactin. While there were no significant differences in age, gender, or fenfluramine/norfenfluramine blood levels as a function of anger attacks, depressed patients with anger attacks displayed a significantly blunted prolactin response to *d,l*-fenfluramine challenge compared with patients without anger attacks associated with anger/aggression proneness even in the presence of a current depression. This finding is directly comparable to findings from other studies with fenfluramine and other 5-HT probes that demonstrate an inverse correlation between central 5-HT function and impulsivity and aggression (Duke et al. 2013).

Neuroimaging

Neuroimaging studies in patients with MDD and anger attacks also report anomalies of structure and dysfunction of corticolimbic brain regions compared with control patients and/or MDD patients without anger attacks. Specifically, MDD patients with anger attacks have been reported to have greater severity of white matter hyperintensities on structural magnetic resonance imaging (MRI) scans in subcortical areas, suggesting that subcortical brain vascular lesions may be more prevalent, or severe, in MDD patients with anger attacks compared with those without anger attacks (Iosifescu et al. 2007). MDD patients with anger attacks have also been reported to have reduced striatal dopamine$_1$ (D$_1$) receptor binding in patients, suggesting striatal D$_1$ receptor dysfunction in these patients (Dougherty et al. 2006). Finally, MDD patients with anger attacks have been reported to have reduced regional cerebral blood flow increases in the left ventromedial prefrontal cortex during anger induction compared with control subjects (Dougherty et al. 2004). Notably, the study authors observed an inverse relationship in anger-induced cerebral blood flow changes in left ventromedial prefrontal cortex and in left amygdala in controls, but a positive relationship in MDE patients with anger attacks; no such relationship was observed in MDE patients without anger attacks. This suggests important differences in the brain's response to anger, in which the more that anger is induced in control subjects, the less active corticolimbic regions become, while the reverse may be true for MDE patients with anger attacks. In this situation, reduction in corticolimbic activation in control subjects is adaptive, whereas increased corticolimbic activation in MDE patients with anger attacks works to facilitate brain mechanisms underlying anger.

Clinical Approach and Treatment

Differential Diagnosis

The differential diagnosis for anger attacks in MDD includes IED as well as medical conditions, or conditions with pharmacological etiologies (e.g., drugs of abuse), that increase the risk for aggressive behavior. The critical point is that the anger attacks occur only during an episode of depression and are not due to a medical or pharmacologically induced condition. Of course, anger attacks as defined above occur in those with a current diagnosis of IED. We administered the AAQ to 239 study participants (90 healthy control subjects, 63 non–currently depressed psychiatric control subjects, and 86 individuals with current IED without current depression) and found that anger attacks as defined above were present in most (72%) nondepressed IED study participants but in only a few healthy (2.2%) or nondepressed psychiatric (6.3%) controls. The critical issue is that in the context of IED, anger attacks also occur when the individuals are not in an episode of depression.

Treatment

Antidepressant treatment has been associated with a reduction in both irritability and frequency of anger attacks among MDD patients. In particular, two studies (Fava et al. 1993, 1996) administered the AAQ to two large cohorts of consecutive patients who were diagnosed as having MDD and treated openly with fluoxetine, 20 mg/day for 8 weeks. At baseline, 42% of these patients reported having anger attacks according to our criteria; 101 (68%) of the 149 depressed patients with anger attacks at baseline did not report anger attacks following fluoxetine treatment. The degree of improvement in depressive symptoms after antidepressant treatment is comparable in depressed patients with and without anger attacks. In a subsequent study (Fava et al. 1997), depressed outpatients were randomly assigned to receive sertraline ($n=56$), imipramine ($n=52$), or placebo ($n=60$) and were administered the AAQ before and after treatment. Anger attacks ceased in 53% of the patients receiving sertraline, 57% of those receiving imipramine, and 37% of those in the placebo group. These findings suggest that sertraline and imipramine may be more effective than placebo in reducing the number of anger attacks following treatment, although the differences were not statistically significant (the number needed to treat was 5). These studies suggest that antidepressant monotherapy is helpful in the majority of MDD patients with anger attacks.

What to do next when MDD patients with anger attacks do not respond adequately to antidepressants has not been adequately studied. The use the atypical antipsychotic brexpiprazole is promising (Fava et al. 2016), as shown in a study in which patients diagnosed with MDD who had an inadequate response to antidepressant treatment and with irritability received 6 weeks of open-label treatment with their current antidepressant at the same dose and adjunctive brexpiprazole (target dosage: 3 mg/day). At week 6, clinically relevant improvements were observed in Sheehan Irritability Scale Total and Kellner Symptom Questionnaire Anger-Hostility subscale scores. More (15 patients) stopped than developed (5 patients) anger attacks during treatment, as measured by the AAQ. This study suggests that adjunctive treatment with brexpiprazole may represent a strategy for patients with MDD and inadequate response to antidepressant treatment who have symptoms of irritability. In practice, many adjunctive treatments commonly used for treatment-resistant depression (Otte et al. 2016), such as buspirone, lithium, and mirtazapine, are utilized to treat MDD with anger attacks when there is an inadequate response to antidepressants.

Clinical Vignette

> HF, a 45-year-old man, presented with a history of depressed mood, irritability, oversleeping, increased appetite, fatigue, and lack of concentration for several months. He reported prior episodes of MDD since his teens but no history of mania or hypomania. During his depressive episodes, HF complained of having frequent anger attacks, when he would lose his temper and experience signs of autonomic hyperarousal. Occasionally, during the anger attacks, he would throw things around and/or yell at others. He felt remorseful about these attacks and reported that these attacks were uncharacteristic of him. HF also reported that his father was known to have "a temper" and to lose it during periods of depression. No significant history of medical disorders was reported. After being evaluated by a psychiatrist, HF was prescribed a selective serotonin reuptake inhibitor (SSRI), with significant improvement in depressive symptoms and reduction in the frequency of anger attacks. However, irritability and some of his other depressive symptoms persisted, and buspirone was added to the SSRI, with complete resolution of the symptoms.

Discussion of Vignette

This case is typical for patients with depression-related aggression in that we generally see a person with a stable inter-episode temperament that shifts into anger proneness in the context of active depressive symptomatology. The report that HF's father also displayed this type of behavior when depressed is consistent with this clinical presentation. SSRIs tend to work well in treating both depression and irritability, though additional serotonergic activation is needed to achieve optimal results. Buspirone is a 5-HT$_{1A}$ receptor agonist and as such is likely boosting 5-HT signaling by stimulating postsynaptic 5-HT$_{1A}$ receptors that appear to be downregulated in human subjects as a function of aggression (Almeida et al. 2010).

Disruptive Mood Dysregulation Disorder

In addition to anger and aggression occurring in the course of a unipolar depressive episode, recent work has noted that the display of irritability (anger proneness) and aggression may indicate the presence of a unipolar, not bipolar, mood disorder on its own, especially in children. This is critically important because irritability is one of the most common reasons children are first brought to the attention of psychiatrists and/or psychologists (Peterson et al. 1996).

Starting in the 1990s, intramural investigators at the National Institute of Mental Health began to look at the presence of irritability and aggression in children as a form of severe mood instability. This work began around the same time as the diagnosis of pediatric bipolar disorder (Biederman et al. 1998; Leibenluft et al. 2003) was becoming an important focus in child psychiatry. A controversy arose as to whether bipolar disorder in youth presents with distinct episodes of mania, as in adults, or, alternatively, whether there is a unique pediatric presentation of bipolar disorder characterized by severe, chronic irritability and symptoms similar to those of ADHD. Subsequently, a series of longitudinal (Stringaris et al. 2010), family (Brotman et al. 23007), behavioral (Dickstein et al. 2007; Guyer et al. 2007; Rich et al. 2008), and neurobiological (Adleman et al. 2011, 2012; Rich et al. 2007; Thomas et al. 2012) studies have shown that classically defined episodic pediatric bipolar disorder does differ from chronic irritability without distinct manic or hypomanic episodes (Leibenluft et al. 2003), now referred to as *disruptive mood dysregulation disorder* (DMDD; American Psychiatric Association 2013). Importantly, longitudinal studies demonstrate that youth with chronic irritability (and without defined episodes of mania) are at increased risk to develop unipolar depression or anxiety, but not bipolar disorder, as they age (for a meta-analysis, see Vidal-Ribas et al. 2016). Further, twin data suggest that the longitudinal association among irritability, unipolar depression, and anxiety is mediated in part by genetic factors (Savage et al. 2015).

Phenomenology

In the context of DMDD, *irritability* is defined as proneness to anger relative to developmental peers (Leibenluft and Stoddard 2013; Vidal-Ribas et al. 2016). Proneness to anger is a dimensional, relatively stable trait. Some individuals have a low proneness to anger, whereas others, at the extreme end, have a proneness to anger that is quite high and is associated with distress and impairment. DMDD represents the point at which high proneness to anger is associated with frequent temper outbursts and distress and impairment requiring evaluation and treatment (Leibenluft 2011).

DSM-5 describes youth with DMDD as having severe, frequent temper outbursts that occur in contexts that their developmental peers would tolerate without significant distress (Berkowitz 1989; Roy et al. 2014; Wakschlag et al. 2010, 2012, 2015). Most commonly, such outbursts occur in contexts that induce *frustration*, defined as the emotional state that occurs when goal attainment is blocked (Amsel 1958). Although the temper outburst may include aggression toward people, this is relatively rare, with the vast majority of outbursts entailing verbal aggression and potentially aggression against property. Children with DMDD also have a persistent angry mood and display sullen nonverbal behaviors most of the day, on most days. Because temper outbursts are frequently seen in preschool children or in early childhood (Dougherty et al. 2014, 2016; Wiggins et al. 2014), the diagnosis of DMDD requires that the temper outbursts be developmentally nonnormative (Copeland et al. 2015; Wakschlag et al. 2018). Given the normative nature of temper outbursts in young children, settling on a lower age cut-point for DMDD is challenging, and currently the DSM sets a limit of 6 years (American Psychiatric Association 2013). However, recent data elucidate how normative, versus nonnormative, temper outbursts can be distinguished in the preschool years.

Epidemiology

There have been no large community surveys that have formally assessed the presence of DMDD. Estimates of "severe irritability" in community samples of children and adolescents range from 0.12% to 5% (Althoff et al. 2016) when post hoc operationalized criteria for irritability are used on the NCS-R sample. The rate of DMDD in clinically referred samples is higher (Axelson et al. 2012; Martin et al. 2017).

Comorbidity

The primary potential comorbidities that appear with DMDD are the disruptive behavior and anxiety disorders (Copeland et al. 2013; see

Chapter 4, "Aggression in Disruptive Behavioral Disorders Beginning in Childhood," in this volume). These include ADHD, oppositional defiant disorder (ODD), and multiple anxiety disorders (e.g., generalized anxiety disorder, separation anxiety disorder, social anxiety disorder [social phobia]). Despite the possible presence of these comorbidities, DMDD is distinguished by the presence of severe, chronic irritability, and persistent angry mood in between temper outbursts, above and beyond what is observed in the other disorders. For example, about 15% of youth diagnosed with ODD have severe enough irritability to also be diagnosed with DMDD (Brotman et al. 2017).

Psychobiology

Behavioral Genetics

Given that irritability is a behavioral trait, it is not surprising that its heritability is estimated as being 30%–40% (Coccaro et al. 1997; Stringaris et al. 2012). The expression of irritability is not static in early development (Roberson-Nay et al. 2015), however, as both additive genetic and unique environmental effects (Hudziak et al. 2005) also play a role in its expression. For example, genetic effects on irritability may increase with development in males but decrease in females (Roberson-Nay et al. 2015). From an environmental perspective, twin studies report that 70% of the variance in irritability is explained by environmental factors that work to make twins less like each other (nonshared environment; Stringaris et al. 2012). For irritability, one important environmental factor is the content of children's instrumental learning from parents. Irritable children often live in environments that deliver inconsistent rewards and punishments, which may unintentionally encourage disruptive behavior (Becht et al. 2016). Not surprisingly, inconsistent parenting behaviors have also been associated with anger, aggression, and externalizing problems in children (Shortt et al. 2010). Parenting interventions train parents to stop rewarding maladaptive behavior and start rewarding adaptive behavior (e.g., Comer et al. 2013; Waxmonsky et al. 2016), as discussed later in this section.

Neurobiology

Irritability occurs in response to a social threat (i.e., hostility by an outside entity) or to frustration in obtaining a reward or attaining a goal (Amsel 1958). Thus, the neurobiology of irritability can be thought of as being due to aberrant emotional and behavioral responding to threat and/or frustration (Brotman et al. 2017; Rolls 2014), two concepts discussed in detail below.

Clinical Neuroscience

Aberrant threat processing. Threat processing involves several components, including attention to threat, attribution bias, and labeling emotional cues. Data suggest that irritable youth have deficits in each of these domains. First, youth with severe irritability tend to have a bias to attend more toward threatening, angry faces than to neutral faces (Hommer et al. 2014). In addition, trait anger is linked to altered attention to threatening faces (Van Honk et al. 2001), words (Smith and Waterman 2004), and images (Wilkowski et al. 2007). Second, hostile attribution bias has been associated with high levels of self-reported anger, relational aggression, and physical aggression (Coccaro et al. 2016; Dodge et al. 2003; Nelson et al. 2008). Third, irritable youth rate neutral faces as more fear producing and exhibit amygdala dysfunction when making these behavioral ratings (Brotman et al. 2010). In addition, irritable youth make more errors than healthy youth and need more intense emotional information to make correct identifications (Rich et al. 2008). In support of this, irritable youth show poor modulation of amygdala activity in response to increasingly intense face emotions, specifically anger and possibly happiness (Brotman et al. 2010; Thomas et al. 2012). In addition, irritable children demonstrate amygdala hyperactivity relative to healthy subjects even when processing emotion in an implicit (i.e., label gender rather than emotion) design (Thomas et al. 2013).

Aberrant reward processing. Irritable youth are particularly vulnerable to experience frustration because of aberrant reward processing. Reward processing involves reward learning (i.e., when to expect rewards and how to adjust one's behavior when it is not forthcoming), prediction error (i.e., difference between expected outcome and received outcome), and sensitivity to reward or its omission. Reward learning is mediated by prefrontal cortex, cingulate gyrus, inferior frontal gyrus, and caudate nucleus (Blair 2010). Irritable youth exhibit deficits in the initial learning of reward contingencies, and in reversal learning when reward contingencies change and behavior must be adjusted (Adleman et al. 2011; Dickstein et al. 2007). Moreover, irritable children have inferior frontal gyrus and caudate dysfunction during reward learning (Adleman et al. 2011). In addition, youth with disorders involving irritability (ADHD/ODD/conduct disorder) show less orbitofrontal cortical responsiveness during reward learning relative to healthy peers (Finger et al. 2011), as well as reduced striatal and inferior frontal gyrus modulation as a function of the expected reward value of a stimulus (White et al. 2016). Positive prediction errors occur when a reward is better than expected, whereas negative prediction errors occur when a reward is worse than expected. These errors are thought to be mediated by the cingulate, inferior frontal gyrus, and caudate (Blair 2010). Event-related electroencephalographic studies suggest that irritable youth exhibit striatal hypoactivation to the omission of an expected reward (i.e., enhanced negative prediction error; Deveney et al. 2013) and irritable (Rich et al. 2008) and aggressive (Lamm et al. 2011) youth show anomalies in the neural correlates of inhibition, which is highly related to anger proneness.

Sensitivity to reward and omission of reward are also critical to understanding irritability. For example, irritable children report a more positive mood to a tangible reward than nonirritable children and display increased activation in the middle frontal and anterior cingulate gyri (Perlman et al. 2015). Others have reported greater middle but lower ventrolateral prefrontal cortical activity to reward in children with emotional/behavioral dysregulation (Bebko et al. 2014), as well as enhanced neural processing of reward in irritable toddlers (Kessel et al. 2016), suggesting aberrant reward sensitivity.

There may also be a higher sensitivity to frustration (i.e., blocked rewards or objectives) in irritable youth. In paradigms of frustration, higher trait irritability and aggression are associated with higher levels of self-reported frustration (Deveney et al. 2013; Pawliczek et al. 2013; Rich et al. 2007, 2008, 2011). In healthy individuals, the absence of an expected reward is associated with prefrontal and striatal activity (O'Doherty et al. 2004). In contrast, irritable children display diminished recruitment of regions mediating attention (frontal, parietal), salience (amygdala), and reward functioning (striatal, amygdala) (Perlman et al. 2014, 2015) when frustrated. In addition, irritable children exhibit a decreased ability to shift their attention following reward omission, along with amygdala, striatal, parietal, and posterior cingulate dysfunction. Anterior cingulate cortical and striatal dysfunction has also been shown for irritable children following reward omission (Perlman et al. 2014, 2015).

Clinical Approach and Treatment

Differential Diagnosis

One important differential diagnosis for severe chronic irritability in children is between DMDD and pediatric bipolar disorder. The distinction is critical because long-term outcome and treatment options for the two disorders may be quite different. It is critical to rule out the presence of frank manic or hypomanic episodes that are present in pediatric bipolar disorder but not present in DMDD. In fact, the DSM-5 criteria for mania/hypomania specify that there must be a distinct period of abnormal mood (i.e., euphoria or irritability), different from baseline, and that the "B" criterion items must either have their onset at the same time as the onset of abnormal mood or worsen significantly concurrently with the abnormal mood. Indeed, recent work shows that DMDD differs from pediatric bipolar disorders in several ways. First, although chronically irritable children are at elevated risk for later depression and anxiety, they are not at elevated risk for manic episodes (as are children with pediatric bipolar disorder; see, e.g., Leibenluft et al. 2006; Stringaris and Goodman 2009; Stringaris et al. 2010; Vidal-Ribas et al. 2016). Second, behavioral and functional MRI studies have found that while both youth with bipolar disorder and those with DMDD have impairments in labeling face emotions (Guyer et al. 2007; Rich et al. 2008), the neural correlates of this deficit differ between the two groups (Brotman et al. 2010; Thomas et al. 2012; Wiggins et al. 2016). In fact, recent evidence indicates that the neurobiological correlates of irritability differ, as a trait, between bipolar disorder and DMDD (Wiggins et al. 2016).

Another differential is IED, which also appears phenotypically similar to DMDD. Although the DSM-5 criteria for IED and DMDD are very similar, they were developed for different patient populations (i.e., IED for adolescents and adults, DMDD for children). DMDD and IED both involve highly aggressive behavior, but the two disorders differ in several ways, the most important of which is that DMDD is characterized by persistent mood dysregulation (i.e., anger) and IED is not. Recent data from the laboratory of Coccaro (2018) indicate that very few (8%) of adults with IED report periods of postoutburst anger lasting more than 50% of the interoutburst time, whereas this is required for the DSM-5 diagnosis of DMDD.

Pharmacological Treatment

Pharmacological interventions for irritability include stimulants (Blader et al. 2016), SSRIs (see, e.g., Kim and Boylan 2016), and atypical antipsychotics (Krieger et al. 2011) and are of variable effectiveness. Given that our treatment focus is on children (and their families), nonpharmacological intervention may be as effective and more practical in younger individuals.

Nonpharmacological Treatment

Nonpharmacological interventions include parenting interventions, cognitive-behavioral therapy (CBT), and experimental interventions focused on aberrant threat and reward processing.

Inconsistent parenting behaviors have been associated with anger, aggression, and externalizing problems in children (Becht et al. 2016; Knapp et al. 2012; Shortt et al. 2010). Thus, parenting interventions to train parents to stop rewarding maladaptive behavior and start rewarding adaptive behavior may represent an effective intervention in some, if not many, cases (see, e.g., Comer et al. 2013; Waxmonsky et al. 2016). A recent meta-analysis found that a critical aspect of such treatments was increased parental consistency in the delivery of consequences for child behavior (Kaminski et al. 2008).

CBT for aggression and irritability can also be used in treating irritability in childhood and adolescence. As such, CBT is designed to reduce hostile attribution and provide socially appropriate coping skills to reduce aggression and irritability, and it appears to do so in adults with IED (McCloskey et al. 2008). Recently, a manualized CBT for anger and aggression for children has been developed (Sukhodolsky and Scahill 2012), as has a parent and child group psychotherapy to improve irritable children's ability to assess the potential consequences of their behavior before responding to social situations and thus select more adaptive behaviors (Waxmonsky et al. 2016).

Most interestingly, there are preliminary data supporting the efficacy of computer-based cognitive interventions for irritability through a paradigm (Penton-Voak et al. 2013) whereby irritable youth are trained to attribute less anger to emotional faces that are morphed between angry and happy emotional faces (Wilkowski et al. 2007). These investigators trained irritable youth to report a more positive, less hostile interpretation of ambiguous faces and reported less overt aggressive behavior over the 4 weeks of the trial.

Clinical Vignette

A 10-year-old boy, ZG, presented with a history of frequent and intense temper tantrums since the time he was about 5 years of age. These tantrums were typically triggered by frustration in not being recognized in class by his teacher and by threats of social rejection by his peers. Although ZG was medically healthy, his parents reported periods of his being sad and sullen alternating with temper outbursts that were present both at school and at home. The temper outbursts varied from multiple times daily to three or more a week and resulted in ZG being asked to leave two different schools. At the time of evaluation, he was on leave from his current school pending psychiatric evaluation. Despite his difficulties at school and home, ZG was reported to have empathy for others and was not known to engage any type of bullying behaviors. ZG's symptoms also met criteria for ADHD. ZG was started on stimulant treatment for ADHD, which resulted in remission of his ADHD symptoms and some diminution of his irritability. He and his family were then referred for a parent-child intervention. Within a few weeks of the start of combined treatment, ZG's outbursts slowly diminished with time so that after 6 months, his outbursts were occurring only one to two times per week.

Discussion of Vignette

This case illustrates what is often observed in prepubertal children with frequent temper tantrums persisting after the age of 6. ZG is highly irritable and disruptive to others around him both at home and in school. His dysphoric mood is intense but, while possibly suggestive of bipolar disorder, is not associated with symptoms of bipolar disorder. The comorbidity of ADHD is common in many of these patients, and ZG's positive response to stimulants confirms that ADHD contributes, though does not fully explain, his impulsive aggressive outbursts. Accordingly, simply reducing ZG's ADHD symptomatology was not sufficient for optimal therapeutic response; parent-child intervention was a necessary, and critical, addition to his treatment plan. The presence of empathy and the absence of bullying behaviors indicate that ZG does not have conduct disorder, which is associated with premediated aggression and later development of antisocial personality disorder and/or psychopathy.

Key Clinical Points

Unipolar Depressive Disorders

▋ Anger attacks are sudden spells of anger accompanied by symptoms of autonomic activation, such as tachycardia, sweating, flushing, and tightness of the chest, and are experienced as uncharacteristic for the individual in question.

▋ Anger attacks are typically reported by about one-third of patients with major depressive disorder (MDD) in clinical settings.

▋ MDD patients with anger attacks often have clinical features that meet criteria for several of the personality disorders.

▋ Anger attacks subside in the majority of depressed outpatients treated with antidepressants, and the degree of improvement in depressive symptoms after antidepressant treatment is comparable in depressed patients with and without anger attacks.

Disruptive Mood Dysregulation Disorder

▋ Although temper tantrums are common in children, frequent and intense temper outbursts are not normative after the age of 6 years.

▋ Children with disruptive mood dysregulation disorder (DMDD) appear to have aberrations in neural threat and reward processing so that ambiguous cues can be viewed as threatening and the absence of reward (when otherwise expected) is tolerated poorly.

▋ Children should receive the diagnosis of bipolar disorder only when they have a clear history of a manic or hypomanic episode. During the episode, which must last at least 4 days, their irritability must be significantly worse than at baseline and must be accompanied by the onset, or worsening, of the "B" criterion items in DSM-5.

▋ Treatment should be centered on ameliorating aberrations of threat and reward processing and on increasing the threshold at which individuals with DMDD have temper outbursts in the context of social threat and/or frustration.

References

Adleman NE, Kayser R, Dickstein D, et al: Neural correlates of reversal learning in severe mood dysregulation and pediatric bipolar disorder. J Am Acad Child Adolesc Psychiatry 50(11):1173–1185.e2, 2011 22024005

Adleman NE, Fromm SJ, Razdan V, et al: Cross-sectional and longitudinal abnormalities in brain structure in children with severe mood dysregulation or bipolar disorder. J Child Psychol Psychiatry 53(11):1149–1156, 2012 22650379

Almeida M, Lee R, Coccaro EF: Cortisol responses to ipsapirone challenge correlate with aggression, while basal cortisol levels correlate with impulsivity, in personality disorder and healthy volunteer subjects. J Psychiatr Res 44(14):874–880, 2010 20378126

Althoff RR, Crehan ET, He JP, et al: Disruptive mood dysregulation disorder at ages 13–18: results from the National Comorbidity Survey–Adolescent Supplement. J Child Adolesc Psychopharmacol 26(2):107–113, 2016 26771536

American Psychiatric Association: Diagnostic and Statistical Manual of Mental Disorders, 3rd Edition. Washington, DC American Psychiatric Association, 1980

American Psychiatric Association: Diagnostic and Statistical Manual of Mental Disorders, 3rd Edition, Revised. Washington, DC American Psychiatric Association, 1987

American Psychiatric Association: Diagnostic and Statistical Manual of Mental Disorders, 4th Edition. Washington, DC American Psychiatric Association, 1994

American Psychiatric Association: Diagnostic and Statistical Manual of Mental Disorders, 5th Edition. Arlington, VA, American Psychiatric Association, 2013

Amsel A: The role of frustrative nonreward in noncontinuous reward situations. Psychol Bull 55(2):102–119, 1958 13527595

Axelson D, Findling RL, Fristad MA, et al: Examining the proposed disruptive mood dysregulation disorder diagnosis in children in the Longitudinal Assessment of Manic Symptoms study. J Clin Psychiatry 73(10):1342–1350, 2012 23140653

Bebko G, Bertocci MA, Fournier JC, et al: Parsing dimensional vs diagnostic category-related patterns of reward circuitry function in behaviorally and emotionally dysregulated youth in the Longitudinal Assessment of Manic Symptoms study. JAMA Psychiatry 71(1):71–80, 2014 24285346

Becht AI, Prinzie P, Dekovic M, et al: Child personality facets and overreactive parenting as predictors of aggression and rule-breaking trajectories from childhood to adolescence. Dev Psychopathol 28(2):399–413, 2016 26198735

Berkowitz L: Frustration-aggression hypothesis: examination and reformulation. Psychol Bull 106(1):59–73, 1989 2667009

Biederman J, Klein RG, Pine DS, et al: Resolved: mania is mistaken for ADHD in prepubertal children. J Am Acad Child Adolesc Psychiatry 37(10):1091–1096, discussion 1096–1099, 1998 9785721

Blader JC, Pliszka SR, Kafantaris V, et al: Prevalence and treatment outcomes of persistent negative mood among children with attention-deficit/hyperactivity disorder and aggressive behavior. J Child Adolesc Psychopharmacol 26(2):164–173, 2016 26745211

Blair RJ: Psychopathy, frustration, and reactive aggression: the role of ventromedial prefrontal cortex. Br J Psychol 101(Pt 3):383–399, 2010 19321035

Brotman MA, Kassem L, Reising MM, et al: Parental diagnoses in youth with narrow phenotype bipolar disorder or severe mood dysregulation. Am J Psychiatry 164(8):1238–1241, 2007 17671287

Brotman MA, Rich BA, Guyer AE, et al: Amygdala activation during emotion processing of neutral faces in children with severe mood dysregulation versus ADHD or bipolar disorder. Am J Psychiatry 167(1):61–69, 2010 19917597

Brotman MA, Kircanski K, Stringaris A, et al: Irritability in youths: a translational model. Am J Psychiatry 174(6):520–532, 2017 28103715

Coccaro EF: Intermittent explosive disorder as a disorder of impulsive aggression for DSM-5. Am J Psychiatry 169(6):577–588, 2012 22535310

Coccaro EF: DSM-5 intermittent explosive disorder: relationship with disruptive mood dysregulation disorder. Compr Psychiatry 84:118–121, 2018 29753187

Coccaro EF, Siever LJ, Kourides IA, et al: Central serotoninergic stimulation by fenfluramine challenge does not affect plasma thyrotropin-stimulating hormone levels in man. Neuroendocrinology 47(4):273–276, 1988 3374753

Coccaro EF, Bergeman CS, Kavoussi RJ, et al: Heritability of aggression and irritability: a twin study of the Buss-Durkee aggression scales in adult male subjects. Biol Psychiatry 41(3):273–284, 1997 9024950

Coccaro EF, Fanning JR, Keedy SK, et al: Social cognition in Intermittent Explosive Disorder and aggression. J Psychiatr Res 83:140–150, 2016 27621104

Comer JS, Chow C, Chan PT, et al: Psychosocial treatment efficacy for disruptive behavior problems in very young children: a meta-analytic examination. J Am Acad Child Adolesc Psychiatry 52(1):26–36, 2013 23265631

Copeland WE, Angold A, Costello EJ, et al: Prevalence, comorbidity, and correlates of DSM-5 proposed disruptive mood dysregulation disorder. Am J Psychiatry 170(2):173–179, 2013 23377638

Copeland WE, Brotman MA, Costello EJ: Normative irritability in youth: developmental findings from the Great Smoky Mountains Study. J Am Acad Child Adolesc Psychiatry 54(8):635–642, 2015 26210332

Deveney CM, Connolly ME, Haring CT, et al: Neural mechanisms of frustration in chronically irritable children. Am J Psychiatry 170(10):1186–1194, 2013 23732841

Dickstein DP, Nelson EE, McClure EB, et al: Cognitive flexibility in phenotypes of pediatric bipolar disorder. J Am Acad Child Adolesc Psychiatry 46(3):341–355, 2007 17314720

Dodge KA, Lansford JE, Burks VS, et al: Peer rejection and social information-processing factors in the development of aggressive behavior problems in children. Child Dev 74(2):374–393, 2003 12705561

Dougherty DD, Rauch SL, Deckersbach T, et al: Ventromedial prefrontal cortex and amygdala dysfunction during an anger induction positron emission tomography study in patients with major depressive disorder with anger attacks. Arch Gen Psychiatry 61(8):795–804, 2004 15289278

Dougherty DD, Bonab AA, Ottowitz WE, et al: Decreased striatal D1 binding as measured using PET and [11C]SCH 23,390 in patients with major depression with anger attacks. Depress Anxiety 23(3):175–177, 2006 16528700

Dougherty LR, Smith VC, Bufferd SJ, et al: DSM-5 disruptive mood dysregulation disorder: correlates and predictors in young children. Psychol Med 44(11):2339–2350, 2014 24443797

Dougherty LR, Smith VC, Bufferd SJ, et al: Disruptive mood dysregulation disorder at the age of 6 years and clinical and functional outcomes 3 years later. Psychol Med 46(5):1103–1114, 2016 26786551

Duke AA, Bègue L, Bell R, et al: Revisiting the serotonin-aggression relation in humans: a meta-analysis. Psychol Bull 139(5):1148–1172, 2013 23379963

Fava GA, Kellner R, Munari F, et al: Losses, hostility, and depression. J Nerv Ment Dis 170(8):474–478, 1982 7097264

Fava M, Anderson K, Rosenbaum JF: "Anger attacks": possible variants of panic and major depressive disorders. Am J Psychiatry 147(7):867–870, 1990 2356872

Fava M, Rosenbaum JF, McCarthy M, et al: Anger attacks in depressed out-patients and their response to fluoxetine. Psychopharmacol Bull 27(3):275–279, 1991 1775598

Fava M, Rosenbaum JF, Pava JA, et al: Anger attacks in unipolar depression, Part 1: clinical correlates and response to fluoxetine treatment. Am J Psychiatry 150(8):1158–1163, 1993 7848377

Fava M, Alpert J, Nierenberg AA, et al: Fluoxetine treatment of anger attacks: a replication study. Ann Clin Psychiatry 8(1):7–10, 1996 8743642

Fava M, Nierenberg AA, Quitkin FM, et al: A preliminary study on the efficacy of sertraline and imipramine on anger attacks in atypical depression and dysthymia. Psychopharmacol Bull 33(1):101–103, 1997 9133758

Fava M, Vuolo RD, Wright EC, et al: Fenfluramine challenge in unipolar depression with and without anger attacks. Psychiatry Res 94(1):9–18, 2000 10788673

Fava M, Ménard F, Davidsen CK, et al: Adjunctive brexpiprazole in patients with major depressive disorder and irritability: an exploratory study. J Clin Psychiatry 77(12):1695–1701, 2016 27379823

Finger EC, Marsh AA, Blair KS, et al: Disrupted reinforcement signaling in the orbitofrontal cortex and caudate in youths with conduct disorder or oppositional defiant disorder and a high level of psychopathic traits. Am J Psychiatry 168(2):152–162, 2011 21078707

Gould RA, Ball S, Kaspi SP, et al: Prevalence and correlates of anger attacks: a two site study. J Affect Disord 39(1):31–38, 1996 8835651

Guyer AE, McClure EB, Adler AD, et al: Specificity of facial expression labeling deficits in childhood psychopathology. J Child Psychol Psychiatry 48(9):863–871, 2007 17714371

Hommer RE, Meyer A, Stoddard J, et al: Attention bias to threat faces in severe mood dysregulation. Depress Anxiety 31(7):559–565, 2014 23798350

Hudziak JJ, Derks EM, Althoff RR, et al: The genetic and environmental contributions to oppositional defiant behavior: a multi-informant twin study. J Am Acad Child Adolesc Psychiatry 44(9):907–914, 2005 16113619

Iosifescu DV, Renshaw PF, Dougherty DD, et al: Major depressive disorder with anger attacks and subcortical MRI white matter hyperintensities. J Nerv Ment Dis 195(2):175–178, 2007 17299307

Kaminski JW, Valle LA, Filene JH, et al: A meta-analytic review of components associated with parent training program effectiveness. J Abnorm Child Psychol 36(4):567–589, 2008 18205039

Kessel EM, Dougherty LR, Kujawa A, et al: Longitudinal associations between preschool disruptive mood dysregulation disorder symptoms and neural reactivity to monetary reward during preadolescence. J Child Adolesc Psychopharmacol 26(2):131–137, 2016 26771832

Kessler RC, Chiu WT, Demler O, et al: Prevalence, severity, and comorbidity of 12-month DSM-IV disorders in the National Comorbidity Survey Replication. Arch Gen Psychiatry 62(6):617–627, 2005 15939839

Kim S, Boylan K: Effectiveness of antidepressant medications for symptoms of irritability and disruptive behaviors in children and adolescents. J Child Adolesc Psychopharmacol 26(8):694–704, 2016 27482998

Knapp P, Chait A, Pappadopulos E, et al; T-MAY Steering Group: Treatment of maladaptive aggression in youth: CERT guidelines I. Engagement, assessment, and management. Pediatrics 129(6):e1562–e1576, 2012 22641762

Krieger FV, Pheula GF, Coelho R, et al: An open-label trial of risperidone in children and adolescents with severe mood dysregulation. J Child Adolesc Psychopharmacol 21(3):237–243, 2011 21663426

Lamm C, Granic I, Zelazo PD, et al: Magnitude and chronometry of neural mechanisms of emotion regulation in subtypes of aggressive children. Brain Cogn 77(2):159–169, 2011 21940093

Leibenluft E: Severe mood dysregulation, irritability, and the diagnostic boundaries of bipolar disorder in youths. Am J Psychiatry 168(2):129–142, 2011 21123313

Leibenluft E, Stoddard J: The developmental psychopathology of irritability. Dev Psychopathol 25(4 Pt 2):1473–1487, 2013 24342851

Leibenluft E, Charney DS, Towbin KE, et al: Defining clinical phenotypes of juvenile mania. Am J Psychiatry 160(3):430–437, 2003 12611821

Leibenluft E, Cohen P, Gorrindo T, et al: Chronic versus episodic irritability in youth: a community-based, longitudinal study of clinical and diagnostic associations. J Child Adolesc Psychopharmacol 16(4):456–466, 2006 16958570

Martin SE, Hunt JI, Mernick LR, et al: Temper loss and persistent irritability in preschoolers: implications for diagnosing disruptive mood dysregulation disorder in early childhood. Child Psychiatry Hum Dev 48(3):498–508, 2017 27510439

McCloskey MS, Noblett KL, Deffenbacher JL, et al: Cognitive-behavioral therapy for intermittent explosive disorder: a pilot randomized clinical trial. J Consult Clin Psychol 76(5):876–886, 2008 18837604

Nelson DA, Mitchell C, Yang C: Intent attributions and aggression: a study of children and their parents. J Abnorm Child Psychol 36(6):793–806, 2008 18256923

O'Doherty J, Dayan P, Schultz J, et al: Dissociable roles of ventral and dorsal striatum in instrumental conditioning. Science 304(5669):452–454, 2004 15087550

Otte C, Gold SM, Penninx BW, et al: Major depressive disorder. Nat Rev Dis Primers 2:16065, 2016 27629598

Pawliczek CM, Derntl B, Kellermann T, et al: Anger under control: neural correlates of frustration as a function of trait aggression. PLoS One 8(10):e78503, 2013 24205247

Penton-Voak IS, Thomas J, Gage SH, et al: Increasing recognition of happiness in ambiguous facial expressions reduces anger and aggressive behavior. Psychol Sci 24(5):688–697, 2013 23531485

Perlman SB, Hein TC, Stepp SD et al: Emotional reactivity and its impact on neural circuitry for attention-emotion interaction in childhood and adolescence. Dev Cogn Neurosci 8:100–109, 2014 24055416

Perlman SB, Jones BM, Wakschlag LS, et al: Neural substrates of child irritability in typically developing and psychiatric populations. Dev Cogn Neurosci 14:71–80, 2015 26218424

Peterson BS, Zhang H, Santa Lucia R, et al: Risk factors for presenting problems in child psychiatric emergencies. J Am Acad Child Adolesc Psychiatry 35(9):1162–1173, 1996 8824060

Rich BA, Schmajuk M, Perez-Edgar KE, et al: Different psychophysiological and behavioral responses elicited by frustration in pediatric bipolar disorder and severe mood dysregulation. Am J Psychiatry 164(2):309–317, 2007 17267795

Rich BA, Grimley ME, Schmajuk M, et al: Face emotion labeling deficits in children with bipolar disorder and severe mood dysregulation. Dev Psychopathol 20(2):529–546, 2008 18423093

Rich BA, Carver FW, Holroyd T, et al: Different neural pathways to negative affect in youth with pediatric bipolar disorder and severe mood dysregulation. J Psychiatr Res 45(10):1283–1294, 2011 21561628

Roberson-Nay R, Leibenluft E, Brotman MA, et al: Longitudinal stability of genetic and environmental influences on irritability: from childhood to young adulthood. Am J Psychiatry 172(7):657–664, 2015 25906668

Rolls ET: Emotion and Decision Making Explained. Oxford, UK, Oxford University Press, 2014

Rosenbaum JF, Fava M, Pava JA, et al: Anger attacks in unipolar depression, Part 2: neuroendocrine correlates and changes following fluoxetine treatment. Am J Psychiatry 150(8):1164–1168, 1993 8328558

Roy AK, Lopes V, Klein RG: Disruptive mood dysregulation disorder: a new diagnostic approach to chronic irritability in youth. Am J Psychiatry 171(9):918–924, 2014 25178749

Savage J, Verhulst B, Copeland W, et al: A genetically informed study of the longitudinal relation between irritability and anxious/depressed symptoms. J Am Acad Child Adolesc Psychiatry 54(5):377–384, 2015 25901774

Sayar K, Guzelhan Y, Solmaz M, et al: Anger attacks in depressed Turkish outpatients. Ann Clin Psychiatry 12(4):213–218, 2000 11140922

Shortt JW, Stoolmiller M, Smith-Shine JN, et al: Maternal emotion coaching, adolescent anger regulation, and siblings' externalizing symptoms. J Child Psychol Psychiatry 51(7):799–808, 2010 20059622

Smith P, Waterman M: Role of experience in processing bias for aggressive words in forensic and non-forensic populations. Aggress Behav 30:105–122, 2004

Snaith RP, Taylor CM: Irritability: definition, assessment and associated factors. Br J Psychiatry 147:127–136, 1985 3840045

Spitzer RL, Endicott J, Robins E: Research diagnostic criteria: rationale and reliability. Arch Gen Psychiatry 35(6):773–782, 1978 655775

Stringaris A, Goodman R: Longitudinal outcome of youth oppositionality: irritable, headstrong, and hurtful behaviors have distinctive predictions. J Am Acad Child Adolesc Psychiatry 48(4):404–412, 2009 19318881

Stringaris A, Baroni A, Haimm C, et al: Pediatric bipolar disorder versus severe mood dysregulation: risk for manic episodes on follow-up. J Am Acad Child Adolesc Psychiatry 49(4):397–405, 2010 20410732

Stringaris A, Zavos H, Leibenluft E, et al: Adolescent irritability: phenotypic associations and genetic links with depressed mood. Am J Psychiatry 169(1):47–54, 2012 22193524

Sukhodolsky DG, Scahill L: Cognitive-Behavioral Therapy for Anger and Aggression in Children. New York, Guilford, 2012

Tedlow J, Leslie V, Keefe BR, et al: Axis I and Axis II disorder comorbidity in unipolar depression with anger attacks. J Affect Disord 52(1–3):217–223, 1999 10357036

Thomas LA, Brotman MA, Muhrer EJ, et al: Parametric modulation of neural activity by emotion in youth with bipolar disorder, youth with severe mood dysregulation, and healthy volunteers. Arch Gen Psychiatry 69(12):1257–1266, 2012 23026912

Thomas LA, Kim P, Bones BL, et al: Elevated amygdala responses to emotional faces in youths with chronic irritability or bipolar disorder: elevated amygdala responses to emotional faces in youths with chronic irritability or bipolar disorder. Neuroimage Clin 2:637–645, 2013 23977455

Van Honk J, Tuiten A, de Haan E, et al: Attentional biases for angry faces: relationships to trait anger and anxiety. Cogn Emotion 15:279–297, 2001

Vidal-Ribas P, Brotman MA, Valdivieso I, et al: The status of irritability in psychiatry: a conceptual and quantitative review. J Am Acad Child Adolesc Psychiatry 55(7):556–570, 2016 27343883

Wakschlag LS, Tolan PH, Leventhal BL: Research review: "Ain't misbehaving": towards a developmentally specified nosology for preschool disruptive behavior. J Child Psychol Psychiatry 51(1):3–22, 2010 19874427

Wakschlag LS, Choi SW, Carter AS, et al: Defining the developmental parameters of temper loss in early childhood: implications for developmental psychopathology. J Child Psychol Psychiatry 53(11):1099–1108, 2012 22928674

Wakschlag LS, Estabrook R, Petitclerc A, et al: Clinical implications of a dimensional approach: the normal:abnormal spectrum of early irritability. J Am Acad Child Adolesc Psychiatry 54(8):626–634, 2015 26210331

Wakschlag LS, Perlman SB, Blair RJ, et al: The neurodevelopmental basis of early childhood disruptive behavior: irritable and callous phenotypes as exemplars. Am J Psychiatry 175(2):114–130, 2018 29145753

Waxmonsky JG, Waschbusch DA, Belin P, et al: A randomized clinical trial of an integrative group therapy for children with severe mood dysregulation. J Am Acad Child Adolesc Psychiatry 55(3):196–207, 2016 26903253

White SF, Tyler PM, Erway AK, et al: Dysfunctional representation of expected value is associated with reinforcement-based decision-making deficits in adolescents with conduct problems. J Child Psychol Psychiatry 57(8):938–946, 2016 27062170

Wiggins JL, Mitchell C, Stringaris A, et al: Developmental trajectories of irritability and bidirectional associations with maternal depression. J Am Acad Child Adolesc Psychiatry 53(11):1191–1205, 1205.e1–1205.e4, 2014 25440309

Wiggins JL, Brotman MA, Adleman NE, et al: Neural correlates of irritability in disruptive mood dysregulation and bipolar disorders. Am J Psychiatry 173(7):722–730, 2016 26892942

Wilkowski BM, Robinson MD, Gordon RD, et al: Tracking the evil eye: trait anger and selective attention within ambiguously hostile scenes. J Res Pers 41(3):650–666, 2007 24920865

8

Aggression in Anxiety Disorders

Emily B. O'Day, B.A.
Richard G. Heimberg, Ph.D.

Aggression, hostility, irritability, and anger are often evident in persons with anxiety disorders. These constructs are similar insofar as they represent reactivity to negative stimuli. However, whereas anger, hostility, and irritability are displeasing or unfriendly emotional states, aggression may also constitute an intent to harm (Fernandez and Johnson 2016; Snaith and Taylor 1985). For individuals with anxiety, aggression appears to be closely related to the expression of anger and may present verbally, physically, or in the form of an anger attack (or the expression of angry feelings may be suppressed). Any attempt to understand the nature of aggressive thoughts, feelings, and behaviors across the anxiety disorders, including social anxiety disorder (SAD), panic disorder (PD), and generalized anxiety disorder (GAD), must address the multifaceted presentation of aggression in these disorders.

Individuals with anxiety disorders engage in a "fight-or flight" response in the presence of threatening stimuli (Barlow 2002). Anxiety may be considered an antecedent to anger, because anxiety may lead individuals to respond in either an avoidant or an angry/aggressive manner to fend off a threatening stimulus (Hawkins and Cougle 2011; Rothenberg 1971). Thus, avoidance and anger/aggression can both be conceptualized as motivated responses to fear or anxiety (Carver and Harmon-Jones 2009). In response to threatening stimuli, some individuals may be prone to engage avoidant motivational systems to distance themselves from threat, whereas others may be more likely to engage approach-oriented motivational systems that lead them toward aggression (Carver and Harmon-Jones 2009).

Individuals with anxiety disorders experience heightened levels of anger, hostility, or irritability, which may lead to aggressive behavior (Moscovitch et al. 2008). Individuals with anxiety and related disorders report higher levels of experienced anger than nonanxious control subjects (Moscovitch et al. 2008). Anger experience in the last 30 days is also uniquely associated with anxiety disorders, even after adjustment for bipolar disorder, substance use disorder, and borderline personality disorder (Hawkins and Cougle 2011).

It should come as little surprise that anxious individuals, who demonstrate elevated levels of anger experience, also exhibit heightened levels of expression of anger (i.e., verbally or physically aggressive behavior directed toward other people or objects) (Moscovitch et al. 2008). *Anger attacks*, defined as sudden loss of control that results in a verbally and/or physically aggressive outburst, are common forms of anger/aggression expression in the anxiety disorders (Keyes et al. 2016). Individuals with a lifetime diagnosis of an anxiety disorder are more likely to have recurrent anger attacks that are considered out-of-control and out of proportion to the situation, compared with individuals without a lifetime anxiety disorder (Keyes et al. 2016). Many anxious individuals also suppress the expression of anger, such that they experience heightened levels of anger but do not allow themselves to express it outwardly (Moscovitch et al. 2008). However, continuously attempting to suppress the expression of negative emotions may contribute to emotional outbursts over time (Gross 1998).

Individuals with anxiety disorders may be at increased risk of exhibiting aggressive behaviors because of a genetic sensitivity to stress (Barlow 2002). Serotonin dysregulation appears to be a shared biological risk factor among individuals with anxiety and those who act aggressively, and this may play a key role in maintaining heightened sensitivity to stress among these individuals (Apter et al. 1990; Kahn et al. 1988). Recent research also suggests that there may be shared genetic vulnerability between anxiety disorders and intermittent explosive disorder (IED), and there is growing evidence that inflammation processes may account for some of the association between anger/ aggression and psychiatric disorders like anxiety disorders (see Boylan and Ryff 2013; Coccaro 2010; Hettema et al. 2001). In a recent neuroimaging study, irritability and anxiety jointly influenced left amygdala-to-left medial prefrontal cortex connectivity during viewing of emotional faces, highlighting that anxious and irritable characteristics may share biological pathways that influence behavior (Stoddard et al. 2017). Thus, because of genetic sensitivity to stress and shared biological pathways between anxiety and aggression, anxious individuals may be at elevated risk of acting aggressively in response to threat.

Phenomenology

Social Anxiety Disorder

The hallmark symptom of SAD is fear of negative evaluation in social situations, such as meeting new people, giving a speech or presentation, or eating or drinking in public (American Psychiatric Association 2013). Individuals with SAD typically overestimate the amount of threat in their social environment, which may lead them to avoid social interactions. They brace for the worst and consider every social interaction to be a threatening encounter (DeWall et al. 2010). As a result of this negative worldview, socially anxious individuals experience anger and increased self-criticism in response to social rejection (Breen and Kashdan 2011). Thus, social rejection can be considered a precursor to anger and hostility (Kashdan and McKnight 2010; Leary et al. 2006). However, the majority of those with social anxiety do not express their anger outwardly or act in a verbally or physically aggressive manner for fear of negative evaluation or rejection by others (DeWall et al. 2010). Furthermore, individuals with social anxiety often believe that emotional expression is a sign of weakness and that they should control their emotional states at all times (Spokas et al. 2009). Thus, although a given situation may lead individuals with social anxiety to feel angry or hostile toward others, they do not necessarily act aggressively.

The majority of individuals with SAD are shy and inhibited and suppress the expression of negative emotions, just as they use behavioral avoidance to remove themselves from threat or negative evaluation. Compared with control subjects, individuals with SAD have higher levels of trait anger but are more likely to suppress their expression of anger, than to display it outwardly through verbal and physical aggression (Erwin et al. 2003). Additionally, socially anxious individuals engage in more generalized suppression of their emotional expression than nonanxious peers in order to avoid unwanted emotional experiences (Breen and Kashdan 2011; Spokas et al. 2009). However, individuals with SAD who feel heightened levels of anger paired with a greater tendency to suppress the expression of their anger have the greatest level of distress and general impairment among treatment-seeking individuals with SAD (Versella et al. 2016).

In addition to suppressing the expression of their anger and aggression, socially anxious individuals are also more likely to engage in maladaptive emotion regulation strategies such as rumination about negative mood states. In one study, greater use of rumination mediated the relationships between social anxiety and trait anger, anger expression, and suppression of anger expression, although the last-mentioned relationship was no longer significant when depression was taken into account (Trew and Alden 2009). Further research must identify how maladaptive coping strategies, such as rumination, may affect anger experience and expression in clinical samples of individuals with SAD with and without comorbid disorders.

Although the majority of socially anxious individuals suppress their outward expression of anger, there appears to be a subset of individuals with SAD who exhibit novelty-seeking, disinhibited, risk-prone, and outwardly aggressive behaviors (Kashdan and Hofmann 2008; Kashdan and McKnight 2010; Kashdan et al. 2009). Approximately one-fifth of individuals with SAD appear to fit this profile and exhibit high levels of anger as well as outward aggression (Kashdan and McKnight 2010). Aggression in this group of persons includes endorsing a desire to hit, push, or hurt someone or to break or intentionally damage things that belong to others. These individuals also engage in activities just for fun or thrills despite others thinking it is a waste of time, participate in risky and more frequent sexual behavior, and demonstrate heightened levels of substance use despite it causing interpersonal problems (Kashdan and Hofmann 2008; Kashdan and McKnight 2010; Kashdan et al. 2009). Additionally, they experience greater functional impairment and psychiatric comorbidities compared with typical individuals with SAD, as well as increased interpersonal problems related to their angry, hostile behavior (Kachin et al. 2001; Kashdan et al. 2009). Because of their fear of rejection, these individuals act aggressively, attacking other people before others have a chance to negatively evaluate or reject them (Kashdan and McKnight 2010). It is also possible that socially anxious persons who exhibit novelty-seeking, disinhibited, risk-prone, and outwardly aggressive behaviors act according to the norms of a deviant peer group in order to gain acceptance and respect from that group, as well as to prevent a loss in social status (Leary et al. 2006). However, this aggressive behavior only provides short-term relief from the threat of social rejection, and eventually individuals with this atypical presentation of SAD report more difficulty managing negative emotions, increased hostile impulses, poorer psychological flexibility to cope with changing situations and demands, and lower levels of social support compared with a more prototypical group of persons with SAD (Kashdan and McKnight 2010).

There also appears to be an association between SAD and antisocial personality disorder (ASPD), similarly characterized by risk-prone, impulsive, disinhibited behavior. Longitudinal research found that adolescent boys with generalized SAD, characterized by fear of most or all social situations, compared with adolescent boys with nongeneralized SAD, who feared only performance or other specific social situations, were more likely to develop ASPD (Tillfors et al. 2009). Furthermore, analysis of data from the National Epidemiologic Survey on Alcohol and Related Conditions found that 6.5% of individuals with SAD had presentations that also met criteria for ASPD (Galbraith et al. 2014). Interestingly, the SAD-ASPD group endorsed more interpersonal problems (e.g., more difficulty with a boss or coworker; more serious problems with neighbors, friends, or relatives; and higher rates of divorce or separation from their spouses) than did those with SAD alone, lending support to the notion that this subgroup of individuals with SAD may exhibit more aggressive behaviors because of increased conflict (Galbraith et al. 2014). Of note, the SAD-ASPD group also endorsed being more likely to hurt or be cruel to an animal or pet on purpose compared with the group with ASPD alone (Galbraith et al. 2014).

Panic Disorder

PD is marked by recurrent, unexpected panic attacks, which are periods of sudden, intense physical sensations (e.g., sweating, numbness, trembling or shaking, or heart palpitations). In addition to panic attacks, individuals with PD experience at least 1 month of persistent worry or concern about the recurrence of these panic attacks and their consequences, or significant, maladaptive behavior change as a result of the attacks (American Psychiatric Association 2013).[1] For individuals with PD, the persistent, intense fear of losing control over their physical sensations and the perceived unpredictability and dangerousness of panic attacks increase their sensitivity to threat, which in turn makes them susceptible to experience both heightened anger and elevated anger expression (Moscovitch et al. 2008). Thus, because of their threat-sensitive nature, individuals with PD appear to have deficits in the ability to effectively express their emotions, leading them either to lash out and act more aggressively or to try to control their emotions by bottling up and suppressing the expression of their anger (Baker et al. 2004).

PD is associated with increased feelings of anger and hostile attitudes and behaviors directed toward others, suggesting that anger experience and aggression may play a role in the maintenance of PD (Baker et al. 2004; Cassiello-Robbins et al. 2015; Fava et al. 1993, 1990; George et al. 1989). Early research on PD and aggression examined the relationship between panic attacks and anger attacks, hypothesizing that they both arose from a common physiological substrate and were similarly unexpected and unwanted (Fava et al. 1990).

---

[1]Some of the individuals included in the studies described in this chapter had symptoms that met criteria for PD with or without agoraphobia according to DSM-IV (American Psychiatric Association 1994) because of the historical context in which most studies were conducted (agoraphobia is a distinct diagnosis in DSM-5). In most instances in the current chapter, we refer to anyone who received a diagnosis of PD with or without agoraphobia as simply having PD.

Further, individuals with PD may endorse feeling hostile and irritable toward others in response to feelings of panic, which may lead individuals to experience anger attacks or engage in other aggressive behaviors (Fava et al. 1993). However, although anger attacks seem be related to panic attacks, individuals who experience anger attacks do not necessarily report anxiety or fear associated with their aggressive outbursts, suggesting panic attacks and anger attacks are related yet distinct constructs that may both develop in the context of PD (Fava et al. 1990).

More recent research highlights that, in addition to anger expression through anger attacks and other aggressive behaviors, the tendency to suppress the expression of anger is also an important emotional processing difficulty among individuals with PD (Baker et al. 2004; Cassiello-Robbins et al. 2015). In one study, compared with control subjects, individuals with PD exhibited an increased tendency to suppress the expression of anger, which was associated with significantly higher baseline levels of anxiety and functional impairment (Baker et al. 2004). Thus, while earlier research highlights that individuals with PD may commonly express their anger through anger attacks or other aggressive behaviors, individuals with PD may also suppress their expression of anger.

Generalized Anxiety Disorder

GAD is defined primarily by excessive worry and thoughts about the future (American Psychiatric Association 2013). Individuals with GAD spend the majority of their time worrying about everyday things, such as their health, family, relationships, career, and finances (American Psychiatric Association 2013). Conceptualized from an emotion dysregulation framework, individuals with GAD do not develop the necessary emotion regulation skills to cope with distress because they allocate so much time and attention to worrying (Mennin et al. 2005). Lacking the necessary coping skills to regulate their emotions, individuals with GAD have greater difficulty managing negative emotions like anger, such that they have a heightened sensitivity to the experience of negative emotions, fear the consequences of experiencing negative emotions, and are unable to self-soothe when they are upset (Asberg 2013; Mennin et al. 2005). We can hypothesize, then, that when individuals with GAD feel angry, they are not able to effectively express how they feel, leading them to either lash out aggressively toward others or suppress the expression of their anger.

Research examining anger expression in GAD suggests that many of the cognitive vulnerabilities that can lead to increased anger experience and suppression of anger expression, such as intolerance of uncertainty, biases toward threatening stimuli, and irritability, are also seen in GAD (Deschênes et al. 2012). When compared with individuals without GAD, those with GAD had significantly higher levels of anger and hostility, as well as greater suppression of anger expression, all of which predicted GAD symptom severity (Deschênes et al. 2012). In another sample, individuals with GAD, compared with those with PD and control subjects, were more likely to consider angry faces as threats and consequently react, showing faster and more accurate detection of angry faces compared with happy faces in response to attentional bias paradigms (Ashwin et al. 2012). Further, irritability, defined in this study as a low threshold for anger that commonly leads to aggression, was found to be predictive of GAD among adolescents, suggesting there may be a shared vulnerability between irritability and GAD that may influence later aggressive tendencies (Stringaris et al. 2009).

With regard to specific aspects of anger, one study found that individuals with GAD had greater levels of trait anger, suppression of anger expression, and externalized anger expression than nonanxious individuals, all of which suggest there may be individual differences in how those with GAD either express or suppress their aggression (Erdem et al. 2008). When other psychiatric comorbidity is controlled for, there also seems to be a unique relationship between GAD symptoms, anger experience, and anger expression, signifying that anger and aggression should be specifically addressed within this clinical population (Hawkins and Cougle 2011). Additionally, some individuals with GAD exhibit heightened levels of cold and vindictive behavior, which may be a presentation of anger experience and aggression among these individuals (Przeworski et al. 2011; Salzer et al. 2008). Research to date has not directly measured the relationship between GAD and outward verbal and physical aggression, yet there appears to be preliminary evidence that irritability, coldness-vindictiveness, heightened anger experience, and suppression of anger expression may occur within a subgroup of individuals with GAD.

Multiple Anxiety and Related Disorders

A few studies have compared hostility, anger experience, anger expression, and aggression across anxiety disorders. An early study examined the relationship between hostility and anxiety disorders among individuals with SAD, GAD, and PD and found no significant differences in expression of hostility directed toward others (Dadds et al. 1993). In a more recent study, Moscovitch et al. (2008) examined anger experience, anger expression, and aggression among individuals with PD, SAD, obsessive-compulsive disorder (OCD), and specific phobia (SP) and control subjects. Individuals with PD, OCD, and SAD reported significantly higher levels of anger experience and hostility than control subjects (Moscovitch et al. 2008). Although Moscovitch et al. (2008) found no significant differences in physical aggression between groups, when compared with controls, individuals with PD had higher "anger aggression" (i.e., a combination of anger experience and verbal aggression), individuals with SAD had lower verbal aggression, and individuals with SP did not differ in anger experience or anger expression. After the study authors controlled for depression within this sample, some of these findings became nonsignificant. However, even after depression was controlled for, individuals with PD remained more likely to experience and express their anger than those with OCD, and individuals with SAD continued to demonstrate lower verbal aggression than controls, highlighting that some relationship exists between PD and aggression and that individuals with SAD are likely to suppress their desire to verbally retaliate when provoked (Moscovitch et al. 2008).

Hawkins and Cougle (2011) examined anger experience and expression in a population study across individuals with PD, SAD, SP, GAD, and posttraumatic stress disorder and found that each disorder was uniquely related to anger experience. Additionally, despite numerous studies supporting the association between SAD and suppression of anger expression, anger expression was associated with all lifetime and 12-month anxiety disorders except for lifetime SAD (Hawkins and Cougle 2011). In a later population study examining the prevalence and burden of anger and aggressive tendencies across the anxiety disorder spectrum, Keyes et al. (2016) found that individuals with SAD, PD, and GAD were likely to have recurrent anger attacks throughout their lifetime as well as increased risk for the development of IED, a disorder characterized by increased anger and aggressive outbursts. Keyes et al. (2016) additionally found that adolescents with a lifetime history of SAD and PD were particularly at risk for the onset of anger attacks and the development of IED, suggesting that lifetime experiences of SAD and PD may be risk factors for the onset of later aggressive behavior. Nonetheless, it is evident that despite some conflicting results across studies, each anxiety disorder has a unique relationship with anger experience and expression and that further research must continue to disentangle the different relationships that exist between these disorders and aggressive behaviors.

Summary

Aggression seems to arise in individuals with anxiety disorders as one of several possible responses to threatening stimuli, representing the "fight" portion of the "fight-or-flight" response. In response to overestimates of threats in their environment, most individuals with SAD experience high levels of anger but often suppress their aggressive response because they fear negative evaluation and rejection (Breen and Kashdan 2011; DeWall et al. 2010; Erwin et al. 2003). However, a significant subgroup of individuals with SAD display more overt aggressive behavior (Kashdan and McKnight 2010). Among those with PD, an intense fear of losing control of physical sensations has been associated with increased angry feelings and aggression toward others, which may manifest in the form of anger attacks (Baker et al. 2004; Cassiello-Robbins et al. 2015; Fava et al. 1990, 1993; George et al. 1989). Because of the incessant worry that characterizes GAD, individuals with GAD do not develop the necessary emotion regulation strategies to cope with negative emotions, leading them to suppress the expression of their anger or act aggressively toward others through cold or vindictive behavior (Erdem et al. 2008; Mennin et al. 2005; Przeworski et al. 2011; Salzer et al. 2008). Further research must look at the overlapping comorbidity across anxiety disorders and explore how this comorbidity influences the multifaceted presentation of aggression in this population.

Clinical Approach and Treatment

To date, cognitive-behavioral therapy (CBT) has proved effective for treating anxiety disorders and may simultaneously, yet indirectly, target some of the maladaptive coping strategies associated with anger expression and aggressive behavior (Cassiello-Robbins et al. 2015; Erwin et al. 2003). Few studies have examined how to directly target anger expression and aggression in the context of anxiety treatment. Although research to date has not examined aggression among treatment-seeking individuals with GAD, research conducted across samples of treatment-seeking individuals with SAD and PD may shed light on clinical approaches and treatment models for aggression seen in this population.

In a study by Erwin et al. (2003), higher trait anger (especially the inclination to express anger when criticized, evaluated negatively, or treated unfairly by others) was associated with premature dropout from CBT for SAD. Both state and trait anger, as well as suppression of angry feelings, were associated with higher posttreatment scores on measures of social anxiety and depression. Interestingly, even though they were not directly targeted in treatment, trait anger and suppression of angry feelings were both reduced after CBT. Erwin et al. (2003) recommend that treatments for socially anxious patients should address individuals' ability to appropriately express and cope with anger in order to improve treatment outcomes.

Although the majority of individuals with SAD will suppress their expression of angry and aggressive thoughts and behaviors as mentioned above, the subset of individuals with SAD who do exhibit aggressive tendencies when faced with social threat may be overlooked in clinical settings. For this disinhibited, impulsive, aggressive subset of individuals with SAD, research suggests that treatment should incorporate emotion regulation strategies and training to increase self-control (Kashdan and McKnight 2010). Furthermore, the aggressive, hostile behavior seen among these socially anxious individuals may lead to interpersonal conflicts, and this is important to consider and target as a component of treatment (Kachin et al. 2001). Because individuals with SAD vary in their presentations of anger expression and aggression, it is important to carefully consider what may be the best course of treatment for their tendencies toward aggression.

Anger attacks as well as other aggressive behaviors directed toward others have been examined among treatment-seeking individuals with PD. In one study, Bond et al. (1995) examined the aggressive feelings and behaviors of individuals with PD in the context of a medication trial. Aggression was measured using a competitive reaction time task developed by Taylor (1967), which has been shown to be a valid measure of aggression in laboratory settings (Bond and Lader 1986; Giancola and Zeichner 1995). Interestingly, while patients with PD treated with benzodiazepines reported reduced feelings of panic and hostility, they behaved more aggressively in response to provocation on the competitive reaction time task, compared with those not treated with a benzodiazepine. It is possible that medications may reduce feelings of anger and hostility among individuals with PD without decreasing (or maybe even increasing) one's willingness to engage in aggressive behavior. By using a behavioral task to measure aggression, this study shed light on the relationship between PD, heightened anger experience, and aggression.

Additionally, individuals with PD who exhibited more aggressive behaviors had lower rates of improvement in anxiety over the course of CBT for PD than those exhibiting less aggressive behaviors (Cassiello-Robbins et al. 2015). Aggressive thoughts and behaviors were also associated with decreased therapist adherence and competence, suggesting that aggression may have an adverse impact on the therapeutic alliance (Boswell et al. 2013; Cassiello-Robbins et al. 2015). As was the case in SAD, aggression was also associated with higher attrition from treatment; however, when highly aggressive individuals remained in treatment, they saw some reduction in their symptoms (Cassiello-Robbins et al. 2015). These findings highlight the importance of creating a strong therapeutic alliance in the beginning stages of treatment to maximize patient retention and outcomes (Boswell et al. 2013; Cassiello-Robbins et al. 2015).

Clinical Vignette

JN is a 27-year-old man with SAD. He fears most social situations in which he thinks he will be negatively evaluated or rejected, such as going to parties, giving presentations at work, starting one-on-one conversations, and eating or drinking in public. He reports that as a child, he tried to make friends with the "popular" crowd, but this resulted in being bullied and ridiculed, so he learned to keep to himself, believing that others would treat him poorly if he were to approach. Presently, he reports the greatest impairment in multiple aspects of his work environment, but he experiences substantial impairment in the social domain as well. He has difficulty giving presentations and recently turned down a promotion because it would require him to give frequent committee reports at staff meetings. He handles work-related conversations with coworkers without great difficulty, but he reacts angrily to any personal questions, which he believes will be "used against" him. Additionally, he reports difficultly interacting with authority figures at work and responds angrily to his boss when he receives critical feedback. Thus, although he gets along well enough with his coworkers, his relationship with his boss is sometimes contentious. His social relationships at work (and elsewhere) tend to be quite superficial, and he spends most evenings and weekends alone. His coworkers often spend time at bars together on nights or weekends, but because of his social anxiety, he avoids going out to these social events. He is ashamed of his avoidance and very angry at his coworkers since they are constantly inviting him to come join them, which he views as a source of unrelenting social pressure. On the rare occasion when he has joined his coworkers at a bar, he has tended to sit silently, initiating little and feeling very awkward and alone. When a coworker makes an overture, he responds with an angry tone, punishing the coworker for the approach behavior. On one such occasion, the coworker persisted, and JN physically pushed him away.

Discussion of Vignette

JN received individual CBT for SAD (Hope et al. 2010), which, in this case, consisted of cognitive restructuring of his negative cognitions about himself and others and exposures to feared situations both in session and as homework tasks to be completed between sessions. Because his fear of rejection resulted in difficulty expressing his feelings to others and letting things build up until he lashed out in anger, assertive behavior (expressing one's thoughts and feelings without violating the rights of others to be treated with respect) was prominently featured in his fear and avoidance hierarchy and was addressed in several situations in his work and social life. Specifically, exposures were designed to address his angry, verbal outbursts in response to personal questions or critical feedback from coworkers and authority figures in order to identify and practice more positive forms of communication.

Over the course of his treatment, JN worked on making small-talk conversations, extending these conversations to include increasingly personal details, responding to personal questions from others, stating his preference to not talk about specific topics in a socially appropriate manner, responding in a nondefensive manner to good-natured teasing, and joining in the good-natured teasing of others as well. Most of these behaviors were addressed first in the workplace and later on in social settings that would expand the potential for JN to develop meaningful personal relationships.

Key Clinical Points

- Cognitive-behavioral therapy (CBT) has proved effective for treatment of anxiety disorders, and many CBT treatments can be modified to additionally target anger expression and aggressive behavior.

- Because there is room for flexibility within treatments such as CBT, assertiveness training for those with a variety of anxiety disorders who either exhibit aggression or appear to suppress the expression of their anger may be a beneficial aspect of treatment (Swee et al. 2018).

- Emotion regulation difficulties additionally appear to maintain and perpetuate hostile attitudes and aggressive behaviors across the anxiety disorders. These should be seen as key targets for clinical intervention, with strategies dependent on a patient's clinical presentation and symptoms.

- Clinicians should find ways to target maladaptive anger expression and develop a strong therapeutic alliance early in treatment.

  - Clinicians treating individuals with social anxiety disorder (SAD) must pay close attention to the different presentations of SAD symptoms. As mentioned previously, most individuals with SAD present as shy, inhibited patients who are likely to suppress the expression of their anger. One way clinicians can help patients with typically presenting SAD to alleviate their distress may be to help them effectively access and express their anger, rather than suppress emotional expression (Erwin et al. 2003; Swee et al. 2018). More impulsive, risk-prone socially anxious individuals, who may be more likely to lash out and direct their aggression toward others, are more likely to be misdiagnosed in clinical settings, since this presentation is less common and contrary to "typical" social anxiety. In the treatment of these disinhibited individuals, it is important to improve self-control capacities and help them to inhibit negative impulses to act aggressively toward others (Kashdan and McKnight 2010).

▋ Individuals with panic disorder (PD) may possibly be at increased risk of lashing out aggressively through anger attacks or other forms of aggression as well as suppressing anger expression, all of which should be addressed in treatment. Because aggression has been found to be associated with poorer treatment outcomes among those with PD, clinicians must identify how individuals with PD may present their aggression in the beginning of treatment to see reductions in both anxiety symptoms and aggressive tendencies throughout treatment (Cassiello-Robbins et al. 2015). Further, clinicians should find ways to engage their patients and establish a therapeutic alliance to address anger attacks and expressive suppression, since these behaviors may have an impact on therapeutic adherence and patient attrition (Boswell et al. 2013; Cassiello-Robbins et al. 2015).

▋ Patients with generalized anxiety disorder (GAD) may exhibit many of the cognitive vulnerabilities that put them at risk for increased anger experience and expression, so it is important to identify how excessive worry and other maladaptive emotion regulation strategies may be inhibiting their ability to effectively express negative emotions like anger (Deschênes et al. 2012; Mennin et al. 2005). Further, clinicians should note if patients with GAD endorse irritability as one of their symptoms, because irritability may be the feature of their GAD that puts them at increased risk for aggressive behavior (Stringaris et al. 2009). Additionally, some individuals with GAD may exhibit cold or vindictive behaviors, which may possibly be presentations of anger expression or aggression that should be addressed in treatment (Przeworski et al. 2011; Salzer et al. 2008).

▌ It is important to note that many of the anxiety disorders covered in this chapter will be comorbid among clinical populations, so clinicians must assess their patients for a variety of manifestations of anger expression and aggressive behaviors early in treatment and create a treatment plan to fully address each patient's maladaptive aggressive behaviors.

References

American Psychiatric Association: Diagnostic and Statistical Manual of Mental Disorders, 4th Edition. Washington, DC, American Psychiatric Association, 1994

American Psychiatric Association: Diagnostic and Statistical Manual of Mental Disorders, 5th Edition. Arlington, VA, American Psychiatric Association, 2013

Apter A, van Praag HM, Plutchik R, et al: Interrelationships among anxiety, aggression, impulsivity, and mood: a serotonergically linked cluster? Psychiatry Res 32(2):191–199, 1990 2367604

Asberg K: Hostility/anger as a mediator between college students' emotion regulation abilities and symptoms of depression, social anxiety, and generalized anxiety. J Psychol 147(5):469–490, 2013 24003591

Ashwin C, Holas P, Broadhurst S, et al: Enhanced anger superiority effect in generalized anxiety disorder and panic disorder. J Anxiety Disord 26(2):329–336, 2012 22196167

Baker R, Holloway J, Thomas PW, et al: Emotional processing and panic. Behav Res Ther 42(11):1271–1287, 2004 15381438

Barlow DH: Anxiety and Its Disorders: The Nature and Treatment of Anxiety and Panic, 2nd Edition. New York, Guilford, 2002

Bond A, Lader M: A method to elicit aggressive feelings and behaviour via provocation. Biol Psychol 22(1):69–79, 1986 3697459

Bond AJ, Curran HV, Bruce MS, et al: Behavioural aggression in panic disorder after 8 weeks' treatment with alprazolam. J Affect Disord 35(3):117–123, 1995 8749839

Boswell JF, Gallagher MW, Sauer-Zavala SE, et al: Patient characteristics and variability in adherence and competence in cognitive-behavioral therapy for panic disorder. J Consult Clin Psychol 81(3):443–454, 2013 23339537

Boylan JM, Ryff CD: Varieties of anger and the inverse link between education and inflammation: toward an integrative framework. Psychosom Med 75(6):566–574, 2013 23766379

Breen WE, Kashdan TB: Anger suppression after imagined rejection among individuals with social anxiety. J Anxiety Disord 25(7):879–887, 2011 21636245

Carver CS, Harmon-Jones E: Anger is an approach-related affect: evidence and implications. Psychol Bull 135(2):183–204, 2009 19254075

Cassiello-Robbins C, Conklin LR, Anakwenze U, et al: The effects of aggression on symptom severity and treatment response in a trial of cognitive behavioral therapy for panic disorder. Compr Psychiatry 60:1–8, 2015 25987198

Coccaro EF: A family history study of intermittent explosive disorder. J Psychiatr Res 44(15):1101–1105, 2010 20488459

Dadds MR, Gaffney LR, Kenardy J, et al: An exploration of the relationship between expression of hostility and the anxiety disorders. J Psychiatr Res 27(1):17–26, 1993 8515385

Deschênes SS, Dugas MJ, Fracalanza K, et al: The role of anger in generalized anxiety disorder. Cogn Behav Ther 41(3):261–271, 2012 22429207

DeWall CN, Buckner JD, Lambert NM, et al: Bracing for the worst, but behaving the best: social anxiety, hostility, and behavioral aggression. J Anxiety Disord 24(2):260–268, 2010 20079603

Erdem M, Celik C, Yetkin S, et al: Anger level and anger expression in generalized anxiety disorder. Anatolian Journal of Psychiatry 9:203–207, 2008

Erwin BA, Heimberg RG, Schneier FR, et al: Anger experience and expression in social anxiety disorder: pretreatment profile and predictors of attrition and response to cognitive-behavioral treatment. Behav Ther 34:331–350, 2003

Fava GA, Grandi S, Rafanelli C, et al: Hostility and irritable mood in panic disorder with agoraphobia. J Affect Disord 29(4):213–217, 1993 8126308

Fava M, Anderson K, Rosenbaum JF: "Anger attacks": possible variants of panic and major depressive disorders. Am J Psychiatry 147(7):867–870, 1990 2356872

Fernandez E, Johnson SL: Anger in psychological disorders: prevalence, presentation, etiology and prognostic implications. Clin Psychol Rev 46:124–135, 2016 27188635

Galbraith T, Heimberg RG, Wang S, et al: Comorbidity of social anxiety disorder and antisocial personality disorder in the National Epidemiological Survey on Alcohol and Related Conditions (NESARC). J Anxiety Disord 28(1):57–66, 2014 24384071

George DT, Anderson P, Nutt DJ, et al: Aggressive thoughts and behavior: another symptom of panic disorder? Acta Psychiatr Scand 79(5):500–502, 1989 2750551

Giancola PR, Zeichner A: Construct validity of a competitive reaction-time aggression paradigm. Aggress Behav 21:199–204, 1995

Gross JJ: Antecedent- and response-focused emotion regulation: divergent consequences for experience, expression, and physiology. J Pers Soc Psychol 74(1):224–237, 1998 9457784

Hawkins KA, Cougle JR: Anger problems across the anxiety disorders: findings from a population-based study. Depress Anxiety 28(2):145–152, 2011 21284067

Hettema JM, Neale MC, Kendler KS: A review and meta-analysis of the genetic epidemiology of anxiety disorders. Am J Psychiatry 158(10):1568–1578, 2001 11578982

Hope DA, Heimberg RG, Turk CL: Managing Social Anxiety: A Cognitive-Behavioral Therapy Approach, Client Workbook, 2nd Edition. New York, Oxford University Press, 2010

Kachin KE, Newman MG, Pincus AL: An interpersonal problem approach to the division of social phobia subtypes. Behavior Therapy 32:479–501, 2001

Kahn RS, van Praag HM, Wetzler S, et al: Serotonin and anxiety revisited. Biol Psychiatry 23(2):189–208, 1988 3275471

Kashdan TB, Hofmann SG: The high-novelty-seeking, impulsive subtype of generalized social anxiety disorder. Depress Anxiety 25(6):535–541, 2008 17935217

Kashdan TB, McKnight PE: The darker side of social anxiety: when aggressive impulsivity prevails over shy inhibition. Curr Dir Psychol Sci 19:47–50, 2010

Kashdan TB, McKnight PE, Richey JA, et al: When social anxiety disorder co-exists with risk-prone, approach behavior: investigating a neglected, meaningful subset of people in the National Comorbidity Survey—Replication. Behav Res Ther 47(7):559–568, 2009 19345933

Keyes KM, McLaughlin KA, Vo T, et al: Anxious and aggressive: the co-occurrence of IED with anxiety disorders. Depress Anxiety 33(2):101–111, 2016 26422701

Leary MR, Twenge JM, Quinlivan E: Interpersonal rejection as a determinant of anger and aggression. Pers Soc Psychol Rev 10(2):111–132, 2006 16768650

Mennin DS, Heimberg RG, Turk CL, et al: Preliminary evidence for an emotion dysregulation model of generalized anxiety disorder. Behav Res Ther 43(10):1281–1310, 2005 16086981

Moscovitch DA, McCabe RE, Antony MM, et al: Anger experience and expression across the anxiety disorders. Depress Anxiety 25(2):107–113, 2008 17311254

Przeworski A, Newman MG, Pincus AL, et al: Interpersonal pathoplasticity in individuals with generalized anxiety disorder. J Abnorm Psychol 120(2):286–298, 2011 21553942

Rothenberg A: On anger. Am J Psychiatry 128(4):454–460, 1971 5098611

Salzer S, Pincus AL, Hoyer J, et al: Interpersonal subtypes within generalized anxiety disorder. J Pers Assess 90(3):292–299, 2008 18444126

Snaith RP, Taylor CM: Irritability: definition, assessment and associated factors. Br J Psychiatry 147:127–136, 1985 3840045

Spokas M, Luterek JA, Heimberg RG: Social anxiety and emotional suppression: the mediating role of beliefs. J Behav Ther Exp Psychiatry 40(2):283–291, 2009 19135648

Stoddard J, Tseng WL, Kim P, et al: Association of irritability and anxiety with the neural mechanisms of implicit face emotion processing in youths with psychopathology. JAMA Psychiatry 74(1):95–103, 2017 27902832

Stringaris A, Cohen P, Pine DS, et al: Adult outcomes of youth irritability: a 20-year prospective community-based study. Am J Psychiatry 166(9):1048–1054, 2009 19570932

Swee MB, Kaplan SC, Heimberg RG: Assertive behavior and assertion training as important foci in a clinical context: the case of social anxiety disorder. Clin Psychol Sci Pract 25:e12222, 2018

Taylor SP: Aggressive behavior and physiological arousal as a function of provocation and the tendency to inhibit aggression. J Pers 35(2):297–310, 1967 6059850

Tillfors M, El-Khouri B, Stein MB, et al: Relationships between social anxiety, depressive symptoms, and antisocial behaviors: evidence from a prospective study of adolescent boys. J Anxiety Disord 23(5):718–724, 2009 19304451

Trew JL, Alden LE: Predicting anger in social anxiety: the mediating role of rumination. Behav Res Ther 47(12):1079–1084, 2009 19679302

Versella MV, Piccirillo ML, Potter CM, et al: Anger profiles in social anxiety disorder. J Anxiety Disord 37:21–29, 2016 26590429

9

Aggression in Obsessive-Compulsive Disorder

Jon E. Grant, J.D., M.D., M.P.H.
Samuel R. Chamberlain, M.B./B.Chir., Ph.D., M.R.C.Psych.

Obsessive-compulsive disorder (OCD) is characterized by unwanted intrusive thoughts, impulses, or images (obsessions) and/or repetitive, often ritualistic behaviors with the purpose of neutralizing the obsessive content or preventing an unlikely event (American Psychiatric Association 2013). The content of obsessions can vary widely. Common themes of obsessions involve aggression and contamination, as well as sexual or blasphemous thoughts. Compulsions are equally diverse and involve overt behaviors (e.g., washing, checking, ordering) and/or covert internal rituals (e.g., saying certain phrases or prayers). A meta-analysis of 21 studies involving 5,124 participants with OCD found that OCD symptoms grouped according to four factors: 1) symmetry (symmetry obsessions and repeating, ordering, and counting compulsions), 2) forbidden thoughts (aggression, sexual, religious, and somatic obsessions and checking compulsions), 3) cleaning (cleaning and contamination), and 4) hoarding (hoarding obsessions and compulsions) (Bloch et al. 2008). Aggressive obsessions are often a symptom of OCD. Examples of aggressive obsessions in OCD include thoughts of strangling, stabbing, punching, or driving into someone. In OCD, these thoughts are ego-dystonic—the individual does not undertake the aggressive act, and in fact finds the thought of it repulsive and distressing. He or she may go to great lengths to neutralize these thoughts. For example, an individual with the obsessional aggressive thought of running someone down in their car may repeatedly check their mirror and repeatedly drive back to previous locations.

Phenomenology

The nature of aggression in OCD is complex. In some respects, OCD may resemble disorders with clinically prominent impulsive aggressive behaviors (e.g., intermittent explosive disorder [IED]). For example, individuals with OCD often report difficulties resisting the ego-dystonic urge to engage in specific behaviors (e.g., cleaning, ordering, or other ritualistic behaviors) that interfere with functioning. Whereas individuals with IED act out aggressive urges, OCD patients undertake nonaggressive compulsions in an effort to "neutralize" ego-dystonic aggressive obsessional thoughts. Conversely, substantial differences between the two types of disorders exist. For example, IED is characterized by recurrent episodes of aggression that are out of proportion to psychosocial stressors and/or provocation (American Psychiatric Association 2013). Impulsive aggressive behavior may be repetitive, persistent, and recurrent as in OCD, but it is often episodic. Unlike compulsions in OCD, aggressive outbursts in IED do not typically occur in response to an obsession. Such aggression is typically unplanned and occurs without substantial forethought (Grant and Potenza 2006). Aggression in IED also differs from compulsions in OCD in that it may be gratifying and accompanied by excitement rather than by anxiety reduction; however, like OCD compulsions, aggressive acts can be perceived as distressing (McElroy et al. 1998).

IED and OCD have been conceptualized to lie along an impulsive/compulsive spectrum, with disorders with high harm avoidance like OCD positioned closer to the more compulsive end and those with low harm avoidance like IED positioned closer to the more impulsive end (Hollander and Wong 1995). Heterogeneities in OCD and in IED and possible changes that occur during the course of these disorders, however, may complicate comparisons, particularly because investigations concurrently examining OCD and IED are scarce. Although data indicate that individuals with OCD score high on measures of harm avoidance, many adults with OCD demonstrate high levels of cognitive impulsiveness, as measured by the Barratt Impulsiveness Scale (Ettelt et al. 2007). In fact, an association between measures of cognitive impulsiveness and aggressive obsessions and checking suggests that impulsiveness may be particularly relevant to specific subgroups of individuals with OCD (Ettelt et al. 2007). Individuals with IED appear to score high on measures of impulsivity and related measures like novelty seeking, but also score high on measures of harm avoidance (Phan et al. 2011).

Our understanding of the inconsistencies in the clinical similarities and differences between OCD and IED is likely complicated by the heterogeneity of OCD. One study found that obsessive-compulsive spectrum disorders in subjects with OCD clustered into three groups: 1) a "reward deficiency" group that included trichotillomania, gambling, Tourette's disorder, and hypersexual disorder; 2) an "impulsivity" group that included kleptomania, IED, compulsive shopping, and self-injurious behaviors; and 3) a "somatic" group that included body dysmorphic disorder and hypochondriasis (Lochner et al. 2005). The different clusters correlated with different clinical features of OCD. The reward deficiency cluster was associated with early age at onset of OCD and the presence of tics, the impulsivity cluster with female gender and childhood trauma, and the somatic cluster with poor insight. These findings highlight an important point—that IED might be a particularly common comorbidity but only in a specific subset of OCD. Additionally, factor analytic studies have suggested that OCD subtypes may represent biologically distinct disorders (Leckman et al. 2001; Rauch et al. 1998). Thus, IED may be particularly relevant to a specific subtype of OCD (e.g., the impulsivity subtype).

Comorbidity

Studies using samples of convenience have found that IED and OCD frequently co-occur. One study using a clinical sample of IED patients reported co-occurring OCD in 22% (McElroy et al. 1998). Conversely, estimates of IED in clinical samples of subjects with OCD have ranged from about 2% to 10% (du Toit et al. 2005; Fontenelle et al. 2005).

Is there an impulsive subtype of OCD that includes co-occurring problems with aggression? One study of 153 subjects with OCD found that 7% had IED. OCD subjects with elevated impulsivity were more likely to have more behavioral dysregulation, conduct disturbance in childhood, and a greater range of psychopathology in adulthood (Matsunaga et al. 2005). Impulsive aggressive features have been found in OCD patients with neurologically based disorders such as tic disorders or pervasive developmental disorders, and in patients with early-onset OCD (Nikolajsen et al. 2011). Swedo and colleagues (1989) found that 33% of their pediatric OCD sample either had a disruptive disorder or abused a substance, and that 24% of them had a specific developmental disability. Similarly, Fontenelle and colleagues (2005) found that individuals with OCD and an impulse-control disorder (10% had IED) were characterized by an earlier age at onset of OCD, a more insidious appearance of obsessive–compulsive symptoms, a greater number and severity of compulsive symptoms, and a higher number of therapeutic trials with different serotonin reuptake inhibitors (SRIs) during long-term follow-up.

There are several (and not mutually exclusive) pathways through which OCD and IED may relate to each other: either OCD or IED may be the primary phenomenon, or, alternatively, OCD and IED may both result from a common underlying psychopathological and/or neurobiological process (e.g., these disorders may reflect behaviors used to cope with increased levels of anxiety and distress).

One possible explanation is that the compulsive symptoms of OCD may be conceptualized as attempts to control impulses during times of heightened anxiety. For instance, Hoehn-Saric and Barksdale (1983) found that acting-out behavior preceded OCD symptoms in impulsive patients with OCD. Similarly, impulsivity scores, as measured by the Barratt Impulsiveness Scale, correlated positively with aggressive and sexual symptoms in OCD subjects (Sahmelikoglu Onur et al. 2016). Thus, it may be possible that some OCD patients with aggressive obsessions suffer primarily from an impulsivity problem and that in these cases the obsessions may reflect an attempt to control the underlying impulsivity. The hyperfrontality found routinely in neuroimaging studies of OCD might reflect a compensatory mechanism rather than a primary pathology.

Conversely, impulsive acts such as aggression may be a response to OCD. Studies have suggested a link between disruptive/impulsive behavior and increased OCD symptomatology and imply that in at least some cases the impulsive behaviors are secondary to OCD (Lebowitz et al. 2011; Shoval et al. 2006). Finally, because both impulsive and compulsive symptoms often develop during times of heightened anxiety and distress, they may be interpreted as different ways to try to manage uncomfortable and distressing feelings or as different consequences of a general inability to suppress repetitive behaviors. The coexistence of compulsivity and impulsivity may be explained, in part, for example, by unstable dopamine and glutamate systems fluctuating between hyperactivity and hypoactivity (Fineberg et al. 2014).

In addition, cognitive models posit that obsessions partly arise due to cognitive biases. One of these cognitive biases is a pathological sense of responsibility, by which individuals evaluate thoughts in terms of potential harm to themselves or others for which they are personally responsible (Salkovskis 1985, 1989). This inflated sense of responsibility has been associated with several subtypes of OCD, particularly checking compulsions (Foa et al. 2001). Rachman (1993) further proposed that this pathological sense of responsibility is often associated with higher anger scores, as people with OCD assign the blame for their obsessional thoughts internally rather than externally.

Students scoring high in obsessive-compulsive traits as well as patients with OCD reported a greater tendency to suppress or internalize their anger compared with healthy control subjects (Moscovitch et al. 2008; Whiteside and Abramowitz 2005). Inflated latent aggression toward others was assessed first in an online study, and then in person, in individuals with OCD compared with healthy and psychiatric control subjects (Moritz et al. 2011). Individuals with OCD showed higher scores on latent aggression compared with healthy controls (Moritz et al. 2011). The suppression of anger was associated with the cognitive distortion that bad thoughts have moral significance or increase the risk of harm (Whiteside and Abramowitz 2005).

Psychobiology

Neurobiology

Many neurotransmitter systems and brain regions contribute to aggression. Animal models have implicated numerous biological systems and neurotransmitters, including those involving testosterone, γ-aminobutyric acid, nitric oxide, monoamine oxidase, glutamate, dopamine, and serotonin (5-HT) (Korff and Harvey 2006). Data implicate the serotonin 5-HT$_{1B}$ receptor in impulsive aggression in mice; knockout mice lacking the receptor show marked physical aggression (Saudou et al. 1994). Although some of the same systems (e.g., 5-HT, dopamine) are relevant to both IED and OCD, they seem involved in different ways. For example, disruption of the genes encoding the 5-HT$_{2C}$ receptor and the dopamine transporter generates stereotypic behaviors resembling OCD (Korff and Harvey 2006), as compared with the 5-HT$_{1B}$ receptor manipulation more relevant to IED. Genetic variations in commonly occurring 5-HT-related gene variants (e.g., of the 5-HT transporter) influence 5-HT measures associated with impulsive aggression (Mannelli et al. 2006).

Although 5-HT systems have been implicated in OCD, the nature of the involvement differs. Administration of the serotonergic drugs *m*-chlorophenylpiperazine (m-CPP, a 5-HT$_1$ and 5-HT$_2$ receptor agonist) and fenfluramine (a drug inducing 5-HT release and having postsynaptic 5-HT action) is associated with an exacerbation of OCD symptoms and enhanced prolactin release in subjects with OCD (Gross-Isseroff et al. 2004; Hollander et al. 1991). However, groups of children and adults characterized by impulsive aggression exhibit a blunted prolactin response to m-CPP and fenfluramine (New et al. 2004).

Neuroimaging

Brain imaging studies have yielded insight into the pathophysiology of impulsive aggression in humans. Individuals with impulsive aggression show relatively diminished activation of ventromedial prefrontal cortex (vmPFC). Aspects of vmPFC function as related to impulsive aggression appear linked to 5-HT function. Individuals with impulsive aggression as compared with those without show blunted hemodynamic responses to the serotonergic drugs fenfluramine (Siever et al. 1999) and m-CPP (New et al. 2002). Individuals with impulsive aggression also show diminished 5-HT availability in the anterior cingulate cortex, including within the ventral portion included in the vmPFC (Frankle et al. 2005). A functional magnetic resonance imaging (fMRI) study demonstrated increased activation of the amygdala and reduced activation of the orbitofrontal cortex in response to angry faces in subjects with IED (Coccaro et al. 2007; McCloskey et al. 2016).

In apparent contrast to the relatively specific neural abnormalities in IED (diminished vmPFC activity associated with impulsive aggression), OCD has been associated with distributed structural and functional abnormalities of frontostriatal circuitry, which is, in part, responsible for habit learning and top-down control. Notable implicated brain regions include the ventral and dorsal striatum (accumbens and caudate/putamen) and frontal cortex sectors (orbitofrontal and dorsolateral) (Chamberlain and Menzies 2009; Korff and Harvey 2006; Mataix-Cols and van den Heuvel 2006). Additionally, specific subgroups of individuals with OCD show differential activation of this circuitry. During an fMRI symptom provocation study, individuals with washing OCD showed increased activation of vmPFC and caudate, and those with checking showed increased activation of putamen/globus pallidus, thalamus, and dorsal cortical areas (Mataix-Cols et al. 2004). Two large studies, by Pujol et al. (2004) and van den Heuvel et al. (2009), found significant associations between aggression/checking symptoms and temporolimbic volume reductions, including the amygdala, while greater severity of contamination/cleaning symptoms and symmetry/ordering symptoms predicted decreased volume of the dorsal caudate nucleus and sensorimotor cortex, respectively. In both studies, these dimensional effects were anatomically distinct from brain structural differences that characterized patients as a whole, including changes in the orbitofrontal cortex and ventral striatum. In addition, OCD patients with more aggression symptoms have shown relatively greater connectivity with the ventromedial frontal cortex and decreased connectivity with the amygdala (Harrison et al. 2013). This latter finding implies that a relationship may exist with aggression symptoms, which, unlike some other dimensions, appear more overtly related to heightened fear and threat estimation processes.

Behavioral Genetics

Several lines of research have identified familial sociopathy and aggression as risk factors for the persistence of childhood aggression into adolescence and adulthood (Cadoret et al. 1995; Frick et al. 1992). The family history of individuals with IED is characterized by high rates of mood, substance use, and other impulse-control disorders (McElroy et al. 1998). By contrast, the family history of individuals with OCD consists of high rates of OCD, anxiety disorders, and depression (Black et al. 2013; Rasmussen and Tsuang 1986).

Molecular Genetics

A genetic linkage study found an association between an allelic variant of the 5-HT$_{1B}$ receptor gene and alcoholism in aggressive/impulsive individuals whose presentations met criteria for either antisocial personality disorder or IED (Lappalainen et al. 1998). In contrast, the 5-HT$_{1B}$ receptor has not been implicated in genetic studies of OCD, although two other 5-HT-related genes (i.e., those encoding the 5-HT2$_A$ receptor [HTR2A] and the 5-HT transporter [SLC6A4]) have been implicated in OCD (Taylor 2013).

Clinical Approach and Treatment

Assessment

The diagnosis of OCD requires a comprehensive clinical evaluation, focusing on the history of illness, co-occurring mental and physical health issues, a review of medical and mental health systems, medication history, family and social histories, and current mental status examination. Careful risk assessment is also needed: people with OCD can become overwhelmed by their symptoms, prompting suicidal thoughts and behaviors. OCD has a moderate to high association with suicidality, especially in cases of comorbid depressive/anxiety symptoms, high severity of obsessions, and pervasive feelings of hopelessness (Angelakis et al. 2015).

The OCD interview should include initial open questions, such as whether the patient has any thoughts that are intrusive, troubling, or distressing; and whether the patient has any repetitive thoughts or behaviors that are hard to stop. The interview should then hone in on the particular nature of these thoughts and/or behaviors. For aggressive thoughts, it is important to clarify whether the individual has ever acted on these thoughts—OCD patients will typically have undertaken nonaggressive "neutralizing" or avoidance behaviors. People with OCD commonly experience multiple types of symptoms, and use of diagnostic instruments such as the Yale-Brown Obsessive Compulsive Scale (Y-BOCS; Goodman et al. 1989) checklist can be helpful. The interviewer should ask about age at onset of symptoms and whether the symptoms have gotten better or worse with time; whether there has ever been a period without obsessive thoughts; factors that make symptoms better or worse (e.g., exercise, drugs, stress, poor sleep); and any family history. OCD shows relatively high heritability (Hettema et al. 2001).

If the person has a history of actually acting out aggressive behaviors (as opposed to troubling obsessions of aggression as in the case of uncomplicated OCD), then the diagnostic assessment should assess for the presence of co-occurring IED. When OCD and IED co-occur, pharmacotherapy in the form of selective serotonin reuptake inhibitors (SSRIs) has the potential to address both problems simultaneously, as discussed later in this section. If psychotherapy is used, however, cognitive-behavioral therapy (CBT) for IED differs from that for OCD, and so the clinician may need to decide whether to treat the disorders sequentially or simultaneously, depending on which is more interfering or distressing to the person.

Close care should be given to differentiation of OCD from other mental disorders. Specifically, depressive and anxiety disorders often involve ruminations, as do eating disorders. Patients with psychosis may have bizarre obsessional thoughts that on superficial inspection may appear to be like OCD (e.g., the belief that they can contract HIV from a door handle). Of course, such disorders can be comorbid with OCD. OCD and other psychiatric disorders can be reliably diagnosed using the Structured Clinical Interview for DSM-5 (SCID-5; First et al. 2016), a clinician-administered instrument that may take up to 90 minutes if the clinician is screening for all psychiatric disorders. However, the module for OCD can be used on its own in clinical practice to make a reliable and valid diagnosis of OCD. The Mini-International Neuropsychiatric Interview (Sheehan et al. 1998) can also be used to diagnose OCD and certain other psychiatric disorders. Again, the OCD questions could be used on their own to help with the diagnosis, when clinicians are comfortable with other mental disorders but less familiar with OCD.

OCD symptom severity should be measured using the gold standard, Y-BOCS; its supplementary checklist can be used to identify the full range of specific symptom types (Goodman et al. 1989). In addition, the Padua Inventory, a self-report questionnaire developed for measuring obsessive-compulsive tendencies in normative and patient populations (Sanavio 1988), and a recently developed transdiagnostic severity tool for compulsivity, the Cambridge-Chicago Trait Scale (Chamberlain and Grant, in press), may also be used.

Medical evaluation is a key part of the thorough assessment process for OCD. Most cases of OCD symptoms are not attributable to a specific focus of brain pathology; however, case reports have documented OCD (and other obsessive-compulsive and impulse symptoms) occurring secondary to seizures, cerebrovascular infarcts, head injury, Parkinson's disease, and certain medications (e.g., dopamine agonists used in certain neurological conditions) (Grant et al. 2014).

Pharmacotherapy

While there are no studies targeting aggression in those with OCD, strong evidence supports the efficacy of pharmacotherapy on OCD symptoms with SRIs, including the tricyclic antidepressant clomipramine as well as the SSRIs) in OCD (Bandelow et al. 2012). Some 40%–60% of OCD patients experience symptom improvement from an SRI, and the mean improvement of symptoms is about 20%–40%. However, the probability of full remission of OCD is only about 12%. Relapse rates after medication discontinuation are approximately 90%. Although clomipramine has yielded a larger effect size than the SSRIs, many patients have trouble tolerating its side effects. Adjunctive low-dose antipsychotic medication can be considered in treatment-resistant OCD. Three placebo-controlled studies support the use of risperidone for OCD and demonstrated efficacy for aripiprazole, but the use of quetiapine and olanzapine has produced only mixed results.

Thus, in cases in which aggression co-occurs with OCD—whether as a form of an obsession, as a maladaptive response to not being able to perform compulsions (see clinical vignette), or as an independent comorbidity such as IED—the use of SSRIs should be the first-line approach. Unlike typical use of SSRIs for depression or even IED, however, the use of these agents in OCD often necessitates higher doses (e.g., up to 100 mg/day of fluoxetine or 300–400 mg/day of sertraline; Grant 2014).

Psychotherapeutic Treatment

CBT also shows efficacy in OCD (Öst et al. 2015). The form of CBT that seems to work well for OCD is exposure and response prevention (ERP). This involves prolonged exposure to obsessional cues and strict prevention of rituals, with the support of a therapist. ERP entails exposing oneself to situations that provoke obsessive anxiety and then abstaining from rituals. Response rates to ERP range from 63% to 90%, with an average reduction of 48% of OCD symptoms. Relapse rates after ERP are relatively low, but refusal rates are 25%–30% and dropout rates are about 28%. Typically, ERP is conducted on a weekly basis, although severity of the disorder may necessitate more frequent sessions. ERP has shown benefit in many different frequency formats, and anywhere from 10 to 16 sessions (each usually lasting 90 minutes) may be helpful. Each session begins with a check on homework progress and ends with a new homework/exposure assignment. ERP has shown effectiveness when the theme of the obsessions is aggression, but in cases in which aggression occurs in response to OCD or as an independent disorder, such as with IED, then the individual may benefit from additional behavioral psychotherapy focusing on his or her aggression.

Clinical Vignette

DF is a 29-year-old man who washes his hands 100 times a day, will not touch anything that has been touched by someone else without scrubbing it first, and has an intense fear of germs. In addition, DF's girlfriend describes verbally violent outbursts that DF has at least once a day, most often directed at her. Upon further inquiry, DF reports that he only gets angry when prevented from washing his hands immediately when he "feels" germs. He recognizes that his anger is out of control but feels it would subside if the obsessions would go away. In fact, after 8 weeks of taking fluoxetine 80 mg/day, DF reported a minimal level of obsessive thinking about germs and as a result, experienced no further anger outbursts.

Discussion of Vignette

This case illustrates the fact that aggression may be secondary to the frustration of OCD. Therefore, focusing treatment on OCD may also result in reduction of aggressive symptoms.

Summary

Although OCD and disorders of impulsive aggression (e.g., IED) usually occur separately, they can occur in tandem in a substantial minority of individuals, and teasing apart symptoms of OCD and IED requires careful thought on the part of the clinician, incorporating a comprehensive psychiatric assessment and use of appropriate clinical instruments. Aggressive intrusive obsessional thoughts are common in OCD; such thoughts are ego-dystonic, and the affected individual is unlikely to act on them in an aggressive way—rather, they are likely to undertake "neutralizing" compulsions (e.g., checking, counting). By contrast, the individual with IED shows aggressive external behavior, not typically driven by intrusive thoughts.

Much more research has been undertaken in relation to the neurobiology and treatment of OCD than in the area of IED or aggression. Based on available findings, OCD appears to involve a broader array of neural changes than observed in others with prominent histories of impulsive aggression IED, extending in OCD to frontal and temporal brain regions, as well as to basal ganglia. Abnormalities of the 5-HT transmitter system may occur in both conditions. SRIs constitute a first-line pharmacological treatment for OCD, and these medications also have some evidence of efficacy in IED. In OCD, SRIs often need to be used in high dose, but it is not yet clear whether high dosing regimens are also needed for treating impulsive aggression in IED. Risk issues are also different; both OCD and IED are associated with increased risk of suicidality, whereas only IED is associated with markedly elevated risk of aggression to others. In comorbid cases of OCD and IED, we recommend treating as for severe OCD, with close risk monitoring.

Although psychiatry traditionally focuses on overt symptomatology, it is increasingly recognized that it is necessary to identify intermediate markers, or latent traits, that predispose toward a range of overt psychiatric pathologies. Future work should consider whether the existence of impulsive aggression in OCD and IED is explained by common latent predisposing traits, such as impulsive or compulsive tendencies. In addition, impulsive aggression may have a compulsive element in some individuals—a sense that the aggressive act needs to be undertaken in a particular way or according to rigid rules. Therefore, when speaking of impulsive aggression and OCD, we can examine this at the level of a trait of aggression in OCD or at the syndromal level of IED and its association with OCD.

Key Clinical Points

▋ Careful screening is necessary to identify obsessive-compulsive disorder (OCD) and the complex relationship between OCD and aggression (i.e., whether aggression is a form of an obsession, a response to the OCD, or an independent disorder such as intermittent explosive disorder [IED]).

▋ Pharmacologically, when OCD and aggression co-occur, serotonin reuptake inhibitors may be an effective option for both the aggression and the OCD, although it may be necessary to titrate to doses higher than used in the treatment of other disorders.

▋ Cognitive-behavioral therapy—especially exposure and response prevention (ERP)—is the first-line psychotherapy intervention for OCD. When aggression co-occurs with OCD, however, additional psychotherapy other than ERP may be necessary.

References

American Psychiatric Association: Diagnostic and Statistical Manual of Mental Disorders, 5th Edition. Arlington, VA, American Psychiatric Association, 2013

Angelakis I, Gooding P, Tarrier N, et al: Suicidality in obsessive compulsive disorder (OCD): a systematic review and meta-analysis. Clin Psychol Rev 39:1–15, 2015 25875222

Bandelow B, Sher L, Bunevicius R, et al; WFSBP Task Force on Mental Disorders in Primary Care; WFSBP Task Force on Anxiety Disorders, OCD and PTSD: Guidelines for the pharmacological treatment of anxiety disorders, obsessive-compulsive disorder and posttraumatic stress disorder in primary care. Int J Psychiatry Clin Pract 16(2):77–84, 2012 22540422

Black DW, Stumpf A, McCormick B, et al: A blind re-analysis of the Iowa family study of obsessive-compulsive disorder. Psychiatry Res 209(2):202–206, 2013 23676614

Bloch MH, Landeros-Weisenberger A, Rosario MC, et al: Meta-analysis of the symptom structure of obsessive-compulsive disorder. Am J Psychiatry 165(12):1532–1542, 2008 18923068

Cadoret RJ, Yates WR, Troughton E, et al: Genetic-environmental interaction in the genesis of aggressivity and conduct disorders. Arch Gen Psychiatry 52(11):916–924, 1995 7487340

Chamberlain SR, Grant JG: Initial validation of a transdiagnostic compulsivity questionnaire: the Cambridge-Chicago Compulsivity Trait Scale. CNS Spectr (in press)

Chamberlain SR, Menzies L: Endophenotypes of obsessive-compulsive disorder: rationale, evidence and future potential. Expert Rev Neurother 9(8):1133–1146, 2009 19673603

Coccaro EF, McCloskey MS, Fitzgerald DA, et al: Amygdala and orbitofrontal reactivity to social threat in individuals with impulsive aggression. Biol Psychiatry 62(2):168–178, 2007 17210136

du Toit PL, van Kradenburg J, Niehaus D, et al: Comparison of obsessive-compulsive disorder patients with and without putative obsessive-compulsive spectrum disorders using a structured clinical interview. Compr Psychiatry 45:291–300, 2005 11458303

Ettelt S, Ruhrmann S, Barnow S, et al: Impulsiveness in obsessive-compulsive disorder: results from a family study. Acta Psychiatr Scand 115(1):41–47, 2007 17201865

Fineberg NA, Chamberlain SR, Goudriaan AE, et al: New developments in human neurocognition: clinical, genetic, and brain imaging correlates of impulsivity and compulsivity. CNS Spectr 19(1):69–89, 2014 24512640

First MB, Williams JBW, Karg RS, Spitzer RL: Structured Clinical Interview for DSM-5 Disorders—Clinician Version (SCID-5-CV). Arlington, VA, American Psychiatric Association Publishing, 2016

Foa EB, Amir N, Bogert KV, et al: Inflated perception of responsibility for harm in obsessive-compulsive disorder. J Anxiety Disord 30(1):8–18, 2001

Fontenelle LF, Mendlowicz MV, Versiani M: Impulse control disorders in patients with obsessive-compulsive disorder. Psychiatry Clin Neurosci 59(1):30–37, 2005 15679537

Frankle WG, Lombardo I, New AS, et al: Brain serotonin transporter distribution in subjects with impulsive aggressivity: a positron emission study with [11C]McN 5652. Am J Psychiatry 162(5):915–923, 2005 15863793

Frick PJ, Lahey BB, Loeber R, et al: Familial risk factors to oppositional defiant disorder and conduct disorder: parental psychopathology and maternal parenting. J Consult Clin Psychol 60(1):49–55, 1992 1556285

Goodman WK, Price LH, Rasmussen SA, et al: The Yale–Brown Obsessive Compulsive Scale, II: validity. Arch Gen Psychiatry 46(11):1012–1016, 1989 2510699

Grant JE: Clinical practice: obsessive-compulsive disorder. N Engl J Med 371(7):646–653, 2014 25119610

Grant JE, Potenza MN: Compulsive aspects of impulse-control disorders. Psychiatr Clin North Am 29(2):539–551, x, 2006 16650722

Grant JE, Chamberlain SR, Odlaug BL: Clinical Guide to Obsessive Compulsive and Related Disorders. Oxford, UK, Oxford University Press, 2014

Gross-Isseroff R, Cohen R, Sasson Y, et al: Serotonergic dissection of obsessive compulsive symptoms: a challenge study with m-chlorophenylpiperazine and sumatriptan. Neuropsychobiology 50(3):200–205, 2004 15365215

Harrison BJ, Pujol J, Cardoner N, et al: Brain corticostriatal systems and the major clinical symptom dimensions of obsessive-compulsive disorder. Biol Psychiatry 73(4):321–328, 2013 23200527

Hettema JM, Neale MC, Kendler KS: A review and meta-analysis of the genetic epidemiology of anxiety disorders. Am J Psychiatry 158(10):1568–1578, 2001 11578982

Hoehn-Saric R, Barksdale VC: Impulsiveness in obsessive-compulsive patients. Br J Psychiatry 143:177–182, 1983 6616118

Hollander E, Wong CM: Obsessive-compulsive spectrum disorders. J Clin Psychiatry 56(Suppl 4):3–6, discussion 53–55, 1995 7713863

Hollander E, DeCaria C, Gully R, et al: Effects of chronic fluoxetine treatment on behavioral and neuroendocrine responses to meta-chlorophenylpiperazine in obsessive-compulsive disorder. Psychiatry Res 36(1):1–17, 1991 2017519

Korff S, Harvey BH: Animal models of obsessive-compulsive disorder: rationale to understanding psychobiology and pharmacology. Psychiatr Clin North Am 29(2):371–390, 2006 16650714

Lappalainen J, Long JC, Eggert M, et al: Linkage of antisocial alcoholism to the serotonin 5-HT1B receptor gene in 2 populations. Arch Gen Psychiatry 55(11):989–994, 1998 9819067

Lebowitz ER, Omer H, Leckman JF: Coercive and disruptive behaviors in pediatric obsessive-compulsive disorder. Depress Anxiety 28(10):899–905, 2011 21769998

Leckman JF, Zhang H, Alsobrook JP, et al: Symptom dimensions in obsessive-compulsive disorder: toward quantitative phenotypes. Am J Med Genet 105(1):28–30, 2001 11424988

Lochner C, Hemmings SMJ, Kinnear CJ, et al: Cluster analysis of obsessive-compulsive spectrum disorders in patients with obsessive-compulsive disorder: clinical and genetic correlates. Compr Psychiatry 46(1):14–19, 2005 15714189

Mannelli P, Patkar AA, Peindl K, et al: Polymorphism in the serotonin transporter gene and moderators of prolactin response to meta-chlorophenylpiperazine in African-American cocaine abusers and controls. Psychiatry Res 144(2–3):99–108, 2006 17000009

Mataix-Cols D, van den Heuvel OA: Common and distinct neural correlates of obsessive-compulsive and related disorders. Psychiatr Clin North Am 29(2):391–410, viii, 2006 16650715

Mataix-Cols D, Wooderson S, Lawrence N, et al: Distinct neural correlates of washing, checking, and hoarding symptom dimensions in obsessive-compulsive disorder. Arch Gen Psychiatry 61(6):564–576, 2004 15184236

Matsunaga H, Kiriike N, Matsui T, et al: Impulsive disorders in Japanese adult patients with obsessive-compulsive disorder. Compr Psychiatry 46(1):43–49, 2005 15714194

McCloskey MS, Phan KL, Angstadt M, et al: Amygdala hyperactivation to angry faces in intermittent explosive disorder. J Psychiatr Res 79:34–41, 2016 27145325

McElroy SL, Soutullo CA, Beckman DA, et al: DSM-IV intermittent explosive disorder: a report of 27 cases. J Clin Psychiatry 59(4):203–210, quiz 211, 1998 9590677

Moritz S, Kempke S, Luyten P, et al: Was Freud partly right on obsessive-compulsive disorder (OCD)? Investigation of latent aggression in OCD. Psychiatry Res 187(1–2):180–184, 2011 20950865

Moscovitch DA, McCabe RE, Antony MM, et al: Anger experience and expression across the anxiety disorders. Depress Anxiety 25(2):107–113, 2008 17311254

New AS, Hazlett EA, Buchsbaum MS, et al: Blunted prefrontal cortical 18fluorodeoxyglucose positron emission tomography response to meta-chlorophenylpiperazine in impulsive aggression. Arch Gen Psychiatry 59(7):621–629, 2002 12090815

New AS, Trestman RF, Mitropoulou V, et al: Low prolactin response to fen-fluramine in impulsive aggression. J Psychiatr Res 38(3):223–230, 2004 15003426

Nikolajsen KH, Nissen JB, Thomsen PH: Obsessive-compulsive disorder in children and adolescents: symptom dimensions in a naturalistic setting. Nord J Psychiatry 65(4):244–250, 2011 21062123

Öst LG, Havnen A, Hansen B, et al: Cognitive behavioral treatments of obsessive-compulsive disorder. A systematic review and meta-analysis of studies published 1993–2014. Clin Psychol Rev 40:156–169, 2015 26117062

Phan KL, Lee R, Coccaro EF: Personality predictors of antiaggressive response to fluoxetine: inverse association with neuroticism and harm avoidance. Int Clin Psychopharmacol 26(5):278–283, 2011 21795983

Pujol J, Soriano-Mas C, Alonso P, et al: Mapping structural brain alterations in obsessive-compulsive disorder. Arch Gen Psychiatry 61(7):720–730, 2004 15237084

Rachman S: Obsessions, responsibility and guilt. Behav Res Ther 31(2):149–154, 1993 8442740

Rasmussen SA, Tsuang MT: Clinical characteristics and family history in DSM-III obsessive-compulsive disorder. Am J Psychiatry 143(3):317–322, 1986 3953865

Rauch SL, Dougherty DD, Shin LM, et al: Neural correlates of factor-analyzed OCD symptom dimensions: a PET study. CNS Spectr 3(7):37–43, 1998

Sahmelikoglu Onur O, Tabo A, Aydin E, et al: Relationship between impulsivity and obsession types in obsessive-compulsive disorder. Int J Psychiatry Clin Pract 20(4):218–223, 2016 27654401

Salkovskis PM: Obsessional-compulsive problems: a cognitive-behavioural analysis. Behav Res Ther 23(5):571–583, 1985 4051930

Salkovskis PM: Cognitive-behavioural factors and the persistence of intrusive thoughts in obsessional problems. Behav Res Ther 27(6):677–682, discussion 683–684, 1989 2610662

Sanavio E: Obsessions and compulsions: the Padua Inventory. Behav Res Ther 26(2):169–177, 1988 3365207

Saudou F, Amara DA, Dierich A, et al: Enhanced aggressive behavior in mice lacking 5-HT1B receptor. Science 265(5180):1875–1878, 1994 8091214

Sheehan DV, Lecrubier Y, Sheehan KH, et al: The Mini-International Neuropsychiatric Interview (M.I.N.I.): the development and validation of a structured diagnostic psychiatric interview for DSM-IV and ICD-10. J Clin Psychiatry 59 (suppl 20):22–33, 1998 9881538

Shoval G, Zalsman G, Sher L, et al: Clinical characteristics of inpatient adolescents with severe obsessive-compulsive disorder. Depress Anxiety 23(2):62–70, 2006 16400622

Siever LJ, Buchsbaum MS, New AS, et al: d,l-Fenfluramine response in impulsive personality disorder assessed with [18F]fluorodeoxyglucose positron emission tomography. Neuropsychopharmacology 20(5):413–423, 1999 10192822

Swedo SE, Rapoport JL, Leonard H, et al: Obsessive-compulsive disorder in children and adolescents. Clinical phenomenology of 70 consecutive cases. Arch Gen Psychiatry 46(4):335–341, 1989 2930330

Taylor S: Molecular genetics of obsessive-compulsive disorder: a comprehensive meta-analysis of genetic association studies. Mol Psychiatry 18(7):799–805, 2013 22665263

van den Heuvel OA, Remijnse PL, Mataix-Cols D, et al: The major symptom dimensions of obsessive-compulsive disorder are mediated by partially distinct neural systems. Brain 132(Pt 4):853–868, 2009 18952675

Whiteside SP, Abramowitz JS: The expression of anger and its relationship to symptoms and cognitions in obsessive-compulsive disorder. Depress Anxiety 21(3):106–111, 2005 15965995

10

Anger and Aggression in Posttraumatic Stress Disorder

Jennifer R. Fanning, Ph.D.

Needs for safety, affiliation, respect, and autonomy are important for striving, fulfillment, and subjective well-being (Maslow 1943; Tay and Diener 2011). Traumatic experiences thwart these needs and challenge notions about safety, justice, and self-worth. Traumatic events involve situations that are life threatening (e.g., a violent attack), horrifying (e.g., witnessing a terrible car accident), or violations of physical integrity (e.g., a sexual assault). During such events, survival behaviors are mobilized in the form of freezing, fighting back, fleeing, or sheltering in place (Bracha 2004; Cannon 1932; Taylor et al. 2000). In the days and weeks following a traumatic event, negative effects on the individual are nearly universal: disturbed sleep, heightened arousal, emotional lability, and intrusive recollections of the event are common (Shalev 2002). Over time these sequelae may diminish as the individual returns to their pre-trauma level of functioning. For many, however, the experience of trauma sets into motion pervasive and lasting effects on self-concept, interpersonal relationships, and physiological functioning—even down to the molecular level. A common long-term effect of trauma is increased anger and aggressive behavior—problems that have their roots in the cognitive, emotional, interpersonal, and physiological effects of the trauma. In this chapter I first describe anger and aggression associated with posttraumatic stress disorder (PTSD), review psychotherapy and pharmacological approaches for treating anger associated with PTSD in adults, and discuss clinical factors that may have an impact on treatment of anger with traumatized individuals.

Phenomenology

Diagnostic Criteria

Trauma has been defined broadly as a stressful experience that overwhelms one's capacity for coping (van der Kolk 2000). When PTSD first appeared in the *Diagnostic and Statistical Manual of Mental Disorders*, in its third edition (DSM-III), trauma was described as an event that was psychologically distressing and "generally outside the range of usual human experience" (American Psychiatric Association 1980, p. 236). Unfortunately, it is now recognized that traumas are not rare events; most people (around 90%; Kilpatrick et al. 2013) will experience a traumatic event in their lifetime, and many will experience multiple traumas or prolonged exposures. The current edition, DSM-5, describes trauma as exposure to a traumatic event, defined as "actual or threatened death, serious injury, or sexual violence," which can be experienced firsthand, witnessed, or learned about happening to a loved one (American Psychiatric Association 2013, p. 271). This definition distinguishes trauma from other stressors, like job loss or divorce. ICD-10 (World Health Organization 1992, p. 344) defines trauma more broadly as "a stressful event or situation…of an exceptionally threatening or catastrophic nature, which is likely to cause pervasive distress in almost anyone."

In DSM-5, the criteria for PTSD include four clusters of symptoms that begin or worsen following a traumatic event: *intrusion* symptoms (e.g., intrusive memories, nightmares), *avoidance* (e.g., of thoughts and feelings, or of people and places, associated with the traumatic event), *negative alterations in cognitions and mood* (e.g., exaggerated negative beliefs about one's self or the world), and *arousal and reactivity* (i.e., sleep disturbance, irritability, hypervigilance). It is estimated that around 8% of the general population will develop PTSD at some point in their lifetime (Kessler et al. 1995; Kilpatrick et al. 2013).

Clinical Features

Problems with anger and aggression appear most closely related to the arousal/reactivity PTSD symptom cluster (Elbogen et al. 2010b; King and King 2004; Taft et al. 2009). The symptoms in this cluster reflect autonomic and behavior dysregulation and hyperreactivity to stimuli, and the relationship of this symptom cluster to PTSD is consistent with the role of arousal in aggressive behavior generally (Zillmann et al. 1972). Researchers have questioned whether participating in combat, a socially sanctioned form of violence, may increase the risk of anger and aggression (Beckham et al. 1997; Hiley-Young et al. 1995). However, studies that have controlled for combat exposure find little or no direct impact of combat exposure on anger and aggression (Chemtob et al. 1994; Lasko et al. 1994). Rather, the effects of combat exposure on aggression appear related to increased severity of posttraumatic stress symptoms (Taft et al. 2007b). Individuals diagnosed with PTSD have increased rates of substance use disorders (Kessler et al. 1995; Kramer et al. 2014). Substance use disorders are independently associated with aggressive behavior and have been found to exacerbate aggression in individuals with PTSD (King and King 2004). Research by Elbogen et al. (2014) attributed violence in PTSD to substance use, but other studies have found that PTSD symptoms (particularly hyperarousal) impact aggressive behavior both directly (independently) and indirectly via effects on substance use (Taft et al. 2007a). Likewise, a significant percentage of individuals with PTSD have symptoms that also meet criteria for major depressive disorder and have experienced traumatic brain injury (Breslau 2009; Stein and McAllister 2009).

Epidemiology

In 1983, the U.S. Congress commissioned a systematic study of Vietnam veterans to estimate the prevalence of PTSD, comorbid conditions, and readjustment concerns and to assess the healthcare needs of veterans, particularly those with PTSD, through the Veterans Health Administration system. The National Vietnam Veterans Readjustment Study (NVVRS; Kulka et al. 1988) was the first large-scale systematic study of PTSD in the United States. The study revealed that among veterans who developed chronic PTSD during the war, the vast majority experienced significant readjustment problems after leaving the military. From interviews with veterans and their partners, the researchers learned that male veterans who had the greatest exposure to war stress had higher rates of hostility and physical aggression compared with their civilian counterparts and compared with less trauma-exposed Vietnam era veterans. Among veterans with PTSD, 40% scored in the highest range on hostility, and 25% had committed 13 or more physically aggressive acts in the prior year alone. Women veterans demonstrated a different pattern: those with the greatest war exposure showed less physical aggression than their less-exposed female veteran counterparts.

Subsequent studies replicated the NVVRS findings. Veterans with PTSD report more anger, hostility, and aggression than veterans without PTSD (Beckham et al. 1997; Chemtob et al. 1994; Frueh et al. 1997; Lasko et al. 1994; Novaco and Chemtob 2002). The relationship between PTSD and aggression exists even when the irritability criteria from the diagnosis are excluded (Jakupcak et al. 2007; Novaco and Chemtob 2002). Increased aggression is also observed in veterans with subthreshold PTSD symptoms (Jakupcak et al. 2007). Studies show that PTSD is associated with both general aggression and intimate partner violence (IPV). IPV is physical, psychological, or sexual harm that is inflicted by a current or former partner, whereas general aggression occurs outside of intimate relationships. Taft and colleagues (2009) found that partnered and nonpartnered combat veterans seeking treatment for PTSD reported similar rates of general physical aggression (32% and 39%) in the past year. Among partnered combat veterans, 33% had engaged in physical aggression toward their partner in the previous year. PTSD is associated with aggression in civilian samples as well, among survivors of natural disaster, motor vehicle accident, violent crime, and sexual assault (Andrews et al. 2000; Ehlers et al. 1998; Feeny et al. 2000; Riggs et al. 1992). The robustness of the association between PTSD symptoms and aggression is supported by a meta-analysis of 39 studies, which demonstrated an average correlation of 0.48 between PTSD symptoms and anger and 0.29 between PTSD symptoms and aggression (Orth and Wieland 2006).

Psychobiology

How does trauma increase the risk for anger and aggression? A number of theories have been put forward. Researchers have noted that aggressive behavior among trauma-exposed individuals is often comorbid with other disinhibited behaviors, such as substance abuse, impulsivity, and antisocial behavior. Miller and colleagues observed that trauma-exposed individuals seem to develop psychopathology along internalizing or externalizing behavioral dimensions (Miller and Resick 2007; Miller et al. 2003, 2004). The symptom profile of trauma survivors, Miller and colleagues propose, is explained by broad personality dimensions as well as genetic and environmental factors (Wolf et al. 2010). There is evidence that certain specific genetic variations (e.g., *MAOA*, *FKBP5*, *ANK3*) interact with trauma exposure to increase aggression and other impulsive behaviors (Bevilacqua et al. 2012; Caspi et al. 2002; Logue et al. 2013; Waltes et al. 2016; Zannas and Binder 2014). Chemtob and colleagues have proposed that individuals with PTSD function in "survival mode" long after the traumatic event has ended (Chemtob et al. 1988, 1994; Novaco and Chemtob 2002). According to this explanation, perceived threats trigger "survival mode" behavior. Once engaged, this behavioral response precludes more extensive cognitive processing of new information; cognitions are biased toward perceiving threats, and the result is increased vigilance and reduced self-monitoring. These response tendencies become entrenched through a positive feedback loop. Similarly, social information processing theories posit that biases in how individuals perceive, interpret, and respond to social cues facilitate maladaptive behavior such as aggression (Coccaro et al. 2016; Crick and Dodge 1994; Dodge et al. 1990; Lemerise and Arsenio 2000; Taft et al. 2008).

The survival mode concept is consistent with neurobiological evidence. Individuals with PTSD show abnormal neural activity in brain regions associated with *emotional reactivity* to stimuli (amygdala and insula) and brain regions mediating *emotion regulation* (regions of prefrontal cortex [PFC], including the orbitofrontal cortex [OFC], dorsolateral PFC, dorsomedial PFC, and ventrolateral PFC). Specifically, when exposed to trauma-related stimuli and non-trauma-related threat stimuli (e.g., emotional faces), individuals with PTSD show *increased* blood-oxygen-level dependent (BOLD) activity and regional cerebral blood flow in the amygdala (Liberzon et al. 1999; Rauch et al. 1996, 2000; Shin et al. 2004, 2005) and insula (Rauch et al. 1996), and *decreased* response in the OFC (Britton et al. 2005), medial PFC (Bremner et al. 1999b; Shin et al. 2004, 2005), medial frontal gyrus (Shin et al. 2004), anterior cingulate cortex (Bremner et al. 1999a, 1999b; Britton et al. 2005; Lanius et al. 2001, 2003; Shin et al. 2004), and thalamus (Lanius et al. 2001, 2003). Studies also find positive correlations between symptom intensity and regional brain activity in the insula (flashbacks; Osuch et al. 2001), amygdala (total PTSD severity; Shin et al. 2004), PFC (inversely; Osuch et al. 2001; Shin et al. 2005), and medial frontal gyrus (inversely with total PTSD severity; Shin et al. 2004) during symptom provocation and emotion processing. Aggressive individuals also show impaired emotion regulation (Fettich et al. 2015) as well as abnormal brain structure and function of brain regions that support emotion regulation (Yang and Raine 2009).

Evidence from neuroimaging studies suggests that aggressive individuals have 1) impaired frontal lobe functioning; 2) hyperactive amygdala response to threat; and 3) abnormal connectivity between prefrontal regions and amygdala, disrupting emotion regulation (Anderson et al. 1999; Coccaro et al. 2007, 2011; Davidson et al. 2000; Grafman et al. 1996; Yang and Raine 2009). Accordingly, both PTSD and aggression have been associated with altered brain functioning, including hyperreactivity in brain regions that support threat response and negative emotionality (e.g., amygdala and insula) and hypoactivity in regions that support emotion regulation (e.g., prefrontal cortex; Coccaro et al. 2007; Etkin and Wager 2007; McCloskey et al. 2016).

Clinical Approach and Treatment

Anger and aggression are important treatment targets in PTSD. Addressing these issues has the potential to reduce harm to others and prevent negative consequences for the individual receiving treatment. Anger has been shown to predict a more negative course of PTSD

(Andrews et al. 2000; Ehlers et al. 1998; Feeny et al. 2000; Riggs et al. 1992) and has been linked to poorer treatment outcomes for patients receiving treatment for PTSD (Foa et al. 1995; Forbes et al. 2003; Riggs et al. 1992). Anger can also hinder help-seeking behavior and disrupt the development of the therapeutic relationship (Howells and Day 2003). Moreover, a substantial proportion (31%–37%) of veterans in treatment for PTSD identify anger as one of the issues they would most like to address through treatment (Rosen et al. 2013).

Pharmacological Interventions

Individually administered, manualized trauma-focused psychotherapy (such as prolonged exposure therapy or cognitive processing therapy [CPT]) is recommended as the first-line treatment of PTSD, according to recent clinical guidelines published by the U.S. Department of Veterans Affairs and Department of Defense (VA/DoD; 2017). However, when psychotherapy is unavailable or not preferred, monotherapy using a selective serotonin reputake inhibitor (SSRI) or serotonin-norepinephrine reuptake inhibitor (SNRI) is recommended. Specifically, sertraline, paroxetine, fluoxetine, and venlafaxine are recommended treatments, based on meta-analytic support for their efficacy in treating PTSD (VA/DoD 2017).

Studies of pharmacological treatment of anger in PTSD are scant. One double-blind study of sertraline in PTSD found that the drug significantly reduced rater-evaluated anger/irritability after 10 weeks of treatment, compared with placebo (Zohar et al. 2002). Monnelly and colleagues (2003) evaluated risperidone as an adjunctive treatment for irritable aggression in 15 male combat veterans with PTSD. Compared with placebo, risperidone led to a significant reduction in irritability and PTSD intrusion symptoms. However, VA/DoD guidelines recommend against treating PTSD with risperidone (as monotherapy or adjunctive therapy) because of the lack of evidence for its efficacy in PTSD and its known adverse effects and risks. Benzodiazepines have been shown to increase aggression in some patients with PTSD (see Guina et al. 2015 for a review) and may impede recovery from or worsen PTSD symptoms. Given these considerations and the risks of benzodiazepine use, which include dependency, these drugs are not recommended as monotherapy or adjunctive therapy for PTSD (VA/DoD 2017).

Psychosocial Interventions

Two trauma-informed therapeutic approaches to treating anger and aggression in PTSD are presented below, followed by a review of the literature on the efficacy of treatment of anger in PTSD.

National Center for PTSD Intervention

The National Center for PTSD (NCPTSD) offers a manual and training course for a 12-week group therapy intervention for anger (Grace et al. 2015). The course, "Managing Anger: A Treatment for Those With PTSD," is based on a manual written by Dr. Maureen Grace at the Boston division of the NCPTSD in 1999. Although the treatment was developed for groups of male veterans with PTSD, the content has been used with women, in individual therapy, with nonveteran clients, and with clients who do not have PTSD. The group focuses on psychoeducation, skill building and in-session practice of new skills, between-session practice (homework), and in-session discussion of anger patterns and troubleshooting barriers to change. The key skills practiced in group include increasing awareness of anger, assertiveness and communication training, and relaxation training.

Sessions follow a standard format, beginning with a review of the between-session assignments, during which group members are encouraged to share their work with the group. New material is introduced using handouts and psychoeducation. New skills are practiced in session using role-playing exercises. Finally, new between-session exercises are assigned.

The first session of the group is devoted to introducing and orienting clients to the group, setting expectations for the group, and discussing treatment goals. It is recommended that clinicians conduct a pretreatment assessment that includes current PTSD symptom severity, current depression severity, anger, and aggression. These assessments should be administered again posttreatment to assess treatment gains as well as the need for further treatment.

Over the course of the treatment, the group focuses on the components of anger intervention shown in Table 10–1. In addition, *time outs* are taught as a way to temporarily remove oneself from an angering situation in order to cool down and develop an effective response to the triggering event. Additional *communication skills*, such as timing important discussion, rehearsing conversations, and showing gratitude, are taught through psychoeducation and practice. At treatment end, group members and the leader share constructive feedback, discuss the material that was most helpful, and discuss ongoing goals and future treatment plans. The group concludes with a posttreatment assessment, as mentioned above.

Trauma-Informed Treatment of Intimate Partner Violence

A group therapy intervention for IPV was developed by Taft and colleagues at the Boston division of the NCPTSD. Strength at Home— Men's Program is a 12-week group psychotherapy treatment aimed at ending and preventing violence in intimate relationships (Taft et al. 2016a, 2016b). The treatment incorporates elements of cognitive-behavioral therapy (CBT) for IPV, assertiveness training, relationship-focused therapy for PTSD, and CPT for PTSD. The trauma-informed approach is considered suitable given the prevalence of trauma exposure among IPV perpetrators. The group is aimed at clients who have shown recent physically abusive, coercive, or controlling relationship behaviors, and it targets both physical and psychological IPV. Psychological IPV includes behavior that makes one's partner feel afraid, attacks her or his self-esteem, limits the partner's rights or freedoms, or punishes the person or makes her or him feel insecure.

Strength at Home groups include six to eight clients per group and two group co-leaders (Taft et al. 2016c). Sessions 1 and 2 are aimed at establishing positive group norms, including honest communication; enhancing motivation for treatment; and promoting group cohesion. The "pros and cons" of IPV are discussed. This discussion reveals that aggressive behavior is often effective in the short term for releasing stress or gaining compliance, but is detrimental in the long term. Aggression and violence are discussed as learned behaviors that can be unlearned. Other tasks in the early sessions include goal setting, discussion of healthy versus unhealthy relationship patterns, and discussion of reactions to trauma. Johnson and Lubin (2015) describe the last-mentioned as "setting the trauma-frame" of the treatment. Group members may share their traumatic experiences (though they are not required to), including past abuse experiences or military-related trauma. The discussion enhances understanding of abusive behavior patterns and facilitates emotional expression and cohesion building. The group discusses the impact of past trauma on relation-

TABLE 10–1.   Components of the National Center for PTSD anger management group treatment

Anger psychoeducation	Reviews "What is anger?" Anger is: • A normal and useful emotion • Triggered when one perceives a threat or potential loss of something important • A symptom of PTSD (hyperarousal) • Adaptive, when responded to appropriately • Made up of thoughts, feelings, and a physiological component (e.g., tension), which are interrelated
Anger awareness	Encourages clients to become more aware of their anger; this is practiced in group and in between sessions using an Anger Log. This log helps to increase awareness of anger and facilitate group discussions. Clients record the following: • Triggering situations • Physical and emotional reactions • Thoughts in the situation, and how they responded
Assertiveness training	Defines three communication styles: • Passiveness/avoidance • Aggressiveness • Assertiveness Identifies assertiveness as equally respectful of oneself and others; assertive behavior includes use of "I" statements and other ways of communicating. Often this is more effective than the other styles because it has better long-term consequences. Clients practice identifying the theee communication types using vignettes and scenarios from their own lives.

TABLE 10–1. Components of the National Center for PTSD anger management group treatment *(continued)*

Relaxation training	A variety of relaxation exercises are available, including the following: • Progressive muscle relaxation • Relaxation without tension • Diaphragmatic breathing • Cue-controlled breathing • Relaxation imagery Relaxation exercises are taught in session; they may be combined with anger-arousing imagery (either personal or from vignettes) to demonstrate the effect of relaxation on anger Clients are encouraged to use relaxation exercises outside of session, either scheduled or in response to anger triggers.

ships and beliefs about trust, self-esteem and other-esteem, and power and control. These themes are treated as "stuck points" (a concept adapted from CPT) that contribute to IPV. Recognizing and working through these stuck points is one of the primary aims of trauma-informed treatment of IPV. Finally, the concept of *communication styles* (aggressive, assertive, and passive) is introduced early in the treatment. Practice exercises are assigned to help clients more actively monitor their own anger responses.

Strength at Home sessions 3 through 6 focus on strengthening communication skills, including use of assertive communication; using "time-outs" from intense conflict situations; identifying automatic thoughts and reappraising perceived threats and insults; and managing stress through problem-focused and emotion-focused coping and relaxation skills. In session 7 the group discusses the roots of clients' communication style, noting how relationships during childhood, growing up, and in the military shaped them to rely on more aggressive, passive, or assertive communication patterns. Discussions may reveal experiences of abuse, particularly in childhood, and the ways in which families, the military, and society discourage men from communicating their feelings. Sessions 8 through 10 focus on communication skills such as active listening, assertive communication, and expressing feelings. Trauma affects communication by increasing the need for power and control (resulting in coercive behavior) or the need to avoid upsetting emotions (resulting in passive communication). Communicating feelings helps to build closeness, intimacy, and trust, which are often damaged in relationships of traumatized individuals. Trauma-exposed individuals may struggle to label their emotions. Identifying emotions and removing barriers to sharing them are a key focus of session 10. Session 11 reviews communication traps, such as generalizing, mind reading, and focusing on the negative, that undermine assertive communication. In session 12, the final session of the treatment, group members discuss their gains in treatment, their future goals, and their plans to reach those goals. Members process the end of the group. The group leaders give feedback to each member on the changes they have observed and encourage other group members to do the same. Reinforcing treatment gains is important for trauma-exposed individuals, who tend to struggle with negative self-image. Strength at Home has also been adapted as a couples therapy intervention for IPV (Taft et al. 2016c).

Efficacy of Treatment of Anger and Aggression in PTSD

Meta-analytic studies support the use of CBT interventions for managing anger and aggression in general (Beck and Fernandez 1998; DiGiuseppe and Tafrate 2003). Treatments for PTSD, such as CPT and exposure therapy, have been shown to have positive effects on anger in many (Arntz et al. 2007; Galovski et al. 2014; Stapleton et al. 2006; Taylor et al. 2003), but not all, studies (Foa et al. 1995). A small but growing body of literature has studied the efficacy of anger-focused interventions in trauma-exposed populations. Chemtob et al. (1997) examined the efficacy of a 12-session individual therapy CBT treatment for anger in Vietnam veterans with PTSD. Compared with treatment-as-usual (TAU), the intervention decreased anger reactivity to provocative stimuli and increased anger control but did not affect trait anger or reduce physiological reactivity. The treatment continued to show benefits over TAU at 18-month follow-up (Chemtob et al. 1997). Other studies have also found reductions in anger symptoms in military trauma-exposed populations (Gerlock 1994; Morland et al. 2010).

A pilot study of the Strength at Home group program with male active-duty military and military veterans showed a significant decrease from pretreatment to 6-month follow-up in both physical IPV and psychological IPV. Reductions were observed in both mild and severe IPV behaviors, with the effect sizes ranging from 1.04 to 1.57, all large effects (Taft et al. 2013). In a follow-up randomized controlled trial, Taft and colleagues compared Strength at Home with an enhanced TAU intervention in 135 male veterans. Compared with the enhanced TAU, Strength at Home was associated with greater reductions in physical and psychological IPV, based on partner reports of IPV. The Strength at Home treatment was also associated with a reduction in coercive and controlling behaviors by participants (Taft et al. 2016b). Evaluations of the Strength at Home Couples program have also demonstrated reductions in IPV in male military veterans and their partners (Taft et al. 2014, 2016a).

Mackintosh and colleagues (2014) investigated the mechanisms by which treatment reduces anger among combat veterans with PTSD. Male veteran participants ($N=109$) completed the Substance Abuse and Mental Health Services Administration Anger Management for Substance Abuse and Mental Health Clients 12-week cognitive-behavioral group therapy treatment, which teaches anger monitoring and cognitive and behavioral coping strategies, including relaxation, cognitive restructuring, and communication skills (Reilly and Shopshire 2000; Reilly et al. 2002). At the end of treatment, participants showed reductions in anger arousal, angry cognitions, and angry behaviors, and each of these reductions was associated with improvements in the ability to calm arousal, but not with improved cognitive coping or behavioral control skills. Improved calming ability was associated with better cognitive coping and behavioral control, however, suggesting that calming skills may support the acquisition of other—cognitive and behavioral—anger coping skills (Mackintosh et al. 2014). In sumary, both standard anger management approaches and trauma-informed treatments have shown positive results in addressing anger and aggression. Given the specific challenges experienced by trauma-exposed individuals, as well as the large effect sizes observed for trauma-informed anger treatments, trauma-informed interventions are particularly well suited to treating anger and aggression in this population.

Clinical Vignette

CT was a 68-year-old white male military veteran receiving treatment at his local VA medical center. CT was referred to anger management group by his primary clinician. When invited to attend the group, he readily admitted to problems with anger. He complained of feeling angry all the time and in multiple settings, including at home, in traffic, and in public. He agreed to attend the first meeting of the group.

CT joined a group of four other male and one female military veterans seeking treatment for anger. The members represented diverse military eras (Vietnam, first Iraq War, and Operation Enduring Freedom/Operation Iraqi Freedom) and service experiences (combat, stateside, and deployed Army National Guard). CT himself was a veteran of the Vietnam War. In the course of his tour, he had experienced gun battles and surprise enemy attacks and had lost several close friends and comrades. Like all the other group members except one, CT was diagnosed with chronic PTSD. He also had a history of depressive episodes and alcohol use disorder, problems that were also prevalent among the group members.

The anger management group CT attended utilized the NCPTSD group therapy treatment by Grace and colleagues, delivered over 12 weeks. The first session included an orientation to the group, discussion of confidentiality (and limits), and an assessment of anger (using the State-Trait Anger Expression Inventory–2 [STAXI-2]) and depression (using the Beck Depression Inventory–II [BDI-II]). CT's irritability was evident in the initial meeting. When the group discussed prior experiences with therapy and anger management, CT described his prior experience in a support group for veterans with PTSD negatively. CT had found the discussions of wartime trauma and atrocities overstimulating; they triggered his own traumatic memories, which would plague him for days after. Eventually he discontinued the group. CT did not want to attend a group that focused on sharing war stories. His experience led to a discussion of how traumatic experiences would be discussed in the group. The group leaders validated CT's negative past experiences of discussing trauma. They acknowledged that the group would involve some discussion of trauma, providing as a rationale the strong links between trauma and anger. They also emphasized that the goal of the group was to help the members develop new skills for coping with stress and negative emotions that would ultimately help them experience relief from their trauma. This discussion at the start of treatment helped the group members to be aware of the impact of their own stories on the other members of the group.

CT's treatment goals were to reduce his anger in a number of situations, including at home and while driving in traffic. CT was easily triggered to anger by the driving of other motorists, an experience that was common among the group members. CT would curse and yell and honk, but what bothered him the most was the way driving in traffic made him feel. He constantly felt endangered by other motorists; simply getting into his car triggered uncomfortable heightened arousal. CT also shared that he had frequent angry outbursts with his wife. He would lose his temper and yell over minor issues. Married for 35 years, CT and his wife experienced little affection in their relationship, and CT shared few of his private thoughts and feelings with her. This was not distressing to CT; he was quite comfortable with it. Instead, CT was struggling to adjust to his retirement a year earlier. With little to occupy his attention, he found himself thinking more about his past experiences and his PTSD symptoms worsened. He was isolated and had few positive, meaningful experiences in his daily life. Despite his feelings of detachment, CT's marriage was his primary relationship, and the one that was most affected by his anger. After some discussion, CT settled on the following treatment goals: 1) reduce angry feelings and outbursts while driving; and 2) improve his relationship with his wife by reducing outbursts and increasing positive communication.

CT was an active participant in the group. He engaged with the material and readily shared his own experiences with the group. Early on in the group, CT had a tendency to "yes, but" the lessons. He questioned the value of assertive communication ("The other person could just continue being a jerk!"). The group leaders acknowledged the truth in these statements. CT's comments prompted a review of early group discussions about "things we can and can't control," and about the pros and cons of anger, highlighting that the short-term rewards for anger ("winning the argument," "getting your way") are often outweighed by long-term negative consequences (isolation, lack of support). Socratic questioning and discussion helped the group to identify some long-term reasons why assertiveness is a better option than aggressiveness, even if it does not lead to the desired outcome in every situation.

During relaxation practices, the group leaders noticed that although CT participated in the exercises, he continued to show tense body posture, with his fists clenched and his jaw and shoulders tensed. In addition, when sharing events from his week during the between-session review, CT would often become quite agitated and absorbed in whatever story he was sharing. He could easily become angered all over again and begin to "litigate" the event in the group. On several occasions the group leaders had to interrupt CT to point out the way he was reexperiencing the angry event in the session and to encourage CT to notice his physiological reaction to the memory of the event. Noticing his tensed muscles during these venting episodes helped CT to recognize the need to relax to reduce his tension. After doing this, CT was able to complete his stories with much less anger intensity.

Discussion of Vignette

CT's difficulties in the group were not unusual or unexpected given the long-standing nature of his anger and his comorbid PTSD and depression diagnoses. His skills deficits were the reason he needed to be in an anger management group. CT also showed several strengths, including that he was a reliable and committed member of the group. He shared a good, albeit distant, rapport with the other group members. Because of his seniority (he was the oldest member of the group), his co-group members at times had to be encouraged by the group leaders to give CT feedback. Group processes like this highlight the importance of building group cohesion early in the treatment. For his part, CT was comfortable offering feedback and advice to the younger group members, which he did constructively, providing a good model for the group.

In spite of the early challenges, CT showed significant improvement in his anger over the course of the treatment. His STAXI-2 and BDI-II scores were lower at posttreatment. He used coping skills when driving (relaxing after getting into the car, limiting his outbursts toward other drivers, reducing his honking) and at home (taking time out and using relaxation breathing techniques while discussing plans with his wife; taking time to articulate his feelings to her; and more actively listening to her perspective). Late in the group, CT surprised everyone by announcing that he and his wife were buying a dog. This had been CT's idea, and, as he shared with the group, he committed himself to the process of selecting a breed, meeting with breeders, and finally selecting a puppy. Over the last few sessions of the group, CT shared pictures and affectionate stories about raising his new puppy. Even better, he shared the responsibility of caring for the new dog with his wife, giving them the opportunity to share positive experiences together on a regular basis. It was rewarding to see CT find an enjoyable and meaningful project that he could share with his wife, and to observe his comfort in sharing his enjoyment with the group.

Summary

Anger and aggression are common comorbidities among individuals who have been exposed to trauma and who subsequently develop PTSD. Cognitive and neurobiological models point to the role of hyperarousal symptoms, hyperresponsivity to threat, and diminished emotion regulation in trauma-related anger and aggression. Cognitive-behavioral treatments, including those that are trauma-informed, are the treatment approaches that have the most empirical support. Although there are specific challenges to working with trauma-exposed and angry clients, improvement is possible when empirically supported treatments are used and when clinicians attend to specific treatment needs of clients.

Key Clinical Points

▌ *The larger clinical picture.* Therapists working with trauma-exposed anger management clients should develop a case conceptualization based on an assessment of diagnoses, substance use, and social history. Risk assessment, a necessary component of any psychological treatment, is particularly important in work with angry and aggressive clients and trauma-exposed clients. Elbogen et al. (2010a) provide recommendations for violence risk assessment for veterans.

▌ *Treatment of court-mandated clients.* Clinicians should be aware of potential ethical issues related to having multiple roles with court-mandated clients (e.g., therapist and evaluator). Clients should be given clear information about how information about their attendance and progress will be conveyed to the mandating party as part of the treatment consent process.

▌ *Reluctance to reduce anger.* Anger may help trauma-exposed clients to feel more in control of the environment and more ready to respond to threats, and it may help them to avoid uncomfortable intimacy in relationships. The therapist should be prepared to address reluctance to change anger by promoting a secure therapeutic alliance, using motivational approaches, and actively attending to other issues such as depression, anxiety, and other symptoms of posttraumatic stress disorder (Howells and Day 2003).

▌ *Clients who are not suitable to group.* Group treatment can be an efficient and effective modality for anger management; however, clients with antisocial or psychopathic traits may disrupt group cohesion and process. Individual therapy may be a better option for such clients (Deffenbacher and McKay 2000).

▌ *Anger in the session or group.* For emotionally dysregulated clients, discussing anger may trigger venting or angry outbursts, which can derail the session agenda or elicit anger from other group members. The therapist should be prepared to intervene when this occurs. Therapists should inform clients at the outset of the group that they will interrupt "venting" that threatens to get the group off-track.

▌ *Positive reinforcement.* It is important for the therapist to notice and acknowledge constructive behaviors by the client; this is particularly important with trauma-exposed and angry clients, who experience disproportionate social isolation, stigma, and rejection.

References

American Psychiatric Association: Diagnostic and Statistical Manual of Mental Disorders, 3rd Edition. Washington, DC, American Psychiatric Association, 1980

American Psychiatric Association: Diagnostic and Statistical Manual of Mental Disorders, 5th Edition. Arlington, VA, American Psychiatric Association, 2013

Anderson SW, Bechara A, Damasio H, et al: Impairment of social and moral behavior related to early damage in human prefrontal cortex. Nat Neurosci 2(11):1032–1037, 1999 10526345

Andrews B, Brewin CR, Rose S, et al: Predicting PTSD symptoms in victims of violent crime: the role of shame, anger, and childhood abuse. J Abnorm Psychol 109(1):69–73, 2000 10740937

Arntz A, Tiesema M, Kindt M: Treatment of PTSD: a comparison of imaginal exposure with and without imagery rescripting. J Behav Ther Exp Psychiatry 38(4):345–370, 2007 18005935

Beck R, Fernandez E: Cognitive-behavioral therapy in the treatment of anger: a meta-analysis. Cognit Ther Res 22(1):63–74, 1998

Beckham JC, Feldman ME, Kirby AC, et al: Interpersonal violence and its correlates in Vietnam veterans with chronic posttraumatic stress disorder. J Clin Psychol 53(8):859–869, 1997 9403389

Bevilacqua L, Carli V, Sarchiapone M, et al: Interaction between FKBP5 and childhood trauma and risk of aggressive behavior. Arch Gen Psychiatry 69(1):62–70, 2012 22213790

Bracha HS: Freeze, flight, fight, fright, faint: adaptationist perspectives on the acute stress response spectrum. CNS Spectr 9(9):679–685, 2004 15337864

Bremner JD, Narayan M, Staib LH, et al: Neural correlates of memories of childhood sexual abuse in women with and without posttraumatic stress disorder. Am J Psychiatry 156(11):1787–1795, 1999a 10553744

Bremner JD, Staib LH, Kaloupek D, et al: Neural correlates of exposure to traumatic pictures and sound in Vietnam combat veterans with and without posttraumatic stress disorder: a positron emission tomography study. Biol Psychiatry 45(7):806–816, 1999b 10202567

Breslau N: The epidemiology of trauma, PTSD, and other posttrauma disorders. Trauma Violence Abuse 10(3):198–210, 2009 19406860

Britton JC, Phan KL, Taylor SF, et al: Corticolimbic blood flow in posttraumatic stress disorder during script-driven imagery. Biol Psychiatry 57(8):832–840, 2005 15820703

Cannon WB: The Wisdom of the Body. New York, WW Norton, 1932

Caspi A, McClay J, Moffitt TE, et al: Role of genotype in the cycle of violence in maltreated children. Science 297(5582):851–854, 2002 12161658

Chemtob C, Roitblat HL, Hamada RS, et al: A cognitive action theory of post-traumatic stress disorder. J Anxiety Disord 2(3):253–275, 1988

Chemtob CM, Hamada RS, Roitblat HL, et al: Anger, impulsivity, and anger control in combat-related posttraumatic stress disorder. J Consult Clin Psychol 62(4):827–832, 1994 7962887

Chemtob CM, Novaco RW, Hamada RS, et al: Cognitive-behavioral treatment for severe anger in posttraumatic stress disorder. J Consult Clin Psychol 65(1):184–189, 1997 9103748

Coccaro EF, McCloskey MS, Fitzgerald DA, et al: Amygdala and orbitofrontal reactivity to social threat in individuals with impulsive aggression. Biol Psychiatry 62(2):168–178, 2007 17210136

Coccaro EF, Sripada CS, Yanowitch RN, Phan KL: Corticolimbic function in impulsive aggressive behavior. Biol Psychiatry 69(12):1153–1159, 2011

Coccaro EF, Fanning JR, Keedy SK, et al: Social cognition in intermittent explosive disorder and aggression. J Psychiatr Res 83:140–150, 2016 27621104

Crick NR, Dodge KA: A review and reformulation of social information-processing mechanisms in children's social adjustment. Psychol Bull 115(1):74–101, 1994

Davidson RJ, Putnam KM, Larson CL: Dysfunction in the neural circuitry of emotion regulation—a possible prelude to violence. Science 289(5479):591–594, 2000 10915615

Deffenbacher J, McKay M: Overcoming Situational and General Anger: A Protocol for the Treatment of Anger Based on Relaxation, Cognitive Restructuring, and Coping Skills Training. Oakland, CA, New Harbinger Publications, 2000

Department of Veterans Affairs, Department of Defense: VA/DoD clinical practice guideline for the management of posttraumatic stress disorder and acute stress disorder, Version 3.0. 2017. Available at: https://www.healthquality.va.gov/guidelines/MH/ptsd/VADoDPTSDCPGFinal.pdf. Accessed April 14, 2018.

DiGiuseppe R, Tafrate RC: Anger treatment for adults: a meta-analytic review. Clin Psychol Sci Pract 10(1):70–84, 2003

Dodge KA, Bates JE, Pettit GS: Mechanisms in the cycle of violence. Science 250(4988):1678–1683, 1990 2270481

Ehlers A, Mayou RA, Bryant B: Psychological predictors of chronic posttraumatic stress disorder after motor vehicle accidents. J Abnorm Psychol 107(3):508–519, 1998 9715585

Elbogen EB, Fuller S, Johnson SC, et al: Improving risk assessment of violence among military veterans: an evidence-based approach for clinical decision-making. Clin Psychol Rev 30(6):595–607, 2010a 20627387

Elbogen EB, Wagner HR, Fuller SR, et al; Mid-Atlantic Mental Illness Research, Education, and Clinical Center Workgroup: Correlates of anger and hostility in Iraq and Afghanistan war veterans. Am J Psychiatry 167(9):1051–1058, 2010b 20551162

Elbogen EB, Johnson SC, Wagner HR, et al: Violent behaviour and posttraumatic stress disorder in US Iraq an Afghanistan veterans. Br J Psychiatry 204(5):368–375, 2014

Etkin A, Wager TD: Functional neuroimaging of anxiety: a meta-analysis of emotional processing in PTSD, social anxiety disorder, and specific phobia. Am J Psychiatry 164(10):1476–1488, 2007 17898336

Feeny NC, Zoellner LA, Foa EB: Anger, dissociation, and posttraumatic stress disorder among female assault victims. J Trauma Stress 13(1):89–100, 2000 10761176

Fettich KC, McCloskey MS, Look AE, et al: Emotion regulation deficits in intermittent explosive disorder. Aggress Behav 41(1):25–33, 2015 27539871

Foa EB, Riggs DS, Massie ED, et al: The impact of fear activation and anger on the efficacy of exposure treatment for post-traumatic stress disorder. Behav Ther 26.487–499, 1995

Forbes D, Creamer M, Hawthorne G, et al: Comorbidity as a predictor of symptom change after treatment in combat-related posttraumatic stress disorder. J Nerv Ment Dis 191(2):93–99, 2003 12586962

Frueh BC, Henning KR, Pellegrin KL, et al: Relationship between scores on anger measures and PTSD symptomatology, employment, and compensation-seeking status in combat veterans. J Clin Psychol 53(8):871–878, 1997 9403390

Galovski TE, Elwood LS, Blain LM, et al: Changes in anger relationships to responsivity to PTSD treatment. Psychol Trauma 6(1):56–64, 2014 25045416

Gerlock AA: Veterans' responses to anger management intervention. Issues Ment Health Nurs 15(4):393–408, 1994 8056569

Grace M, Niles BL, Quinn S, et al: Managing Anger: A Treatment for Those With PTSD. Boston, MA, National Center for PTSD, 2015

Grafman J, Schwab K, Warden D, et al: Frontal lobe injuries, violence, and aggression: a report of the Vietnam Head Injury Study. Neurology 46(5):1231–1238, 1996 8628458

Guina J, Rossetter SR, DeRhodes BJ, et al: Benzodiazapines for PTSD: a systematic review and meta-analysis. J Psychiatr Pract 21(4):281–303, 2015 26164054

Hiley-Young B, Blake DD, Abueg FR, et al: Warzone violence in Vietnam: an examination of premilitary, military, and postmilitary factors in PTSD in-patients. J Trauma Stress 8(1):125–141, 1995 7712051

Howells K, Day A: Readiness for anger management: clinical and theoretical issues. Clin Psychol Rev 23(2):319–337, 2003 12573674

Jakupcak M, Conybeare D, Phelps L, et al: Anger, hostility, and aggression among Iraq and Afghanistan War veterans reporting PTSD and sub-threshold PTSD. J Trauma Stress 20(6):945–954, 2007 18157891

Johnson DR, Lubin H: Principles and Techniques of Trauma-Centered Psychotherapy. Washington, DC, American Psychiatric Publishing, 2015

Kessler RC, Sonnega A, Bromet E, et al: Posttraumatic stress disorder in the National Comorbidity Survey. Arch Gen Psychiatry 52(12):1048–1060, 1995 7492257

Kilpatrick DG, Resnick HS, Milanak ME, et al: National estimates of exposure to traumatic events and PTSD prevalence using DSM-IV and DSM-5 criteria. J Trauma Stress 26(5):537–547, 2013 24151000

King LA, King DW: Male-perpetrated domestic violence: testing a series of multifactorial family models. National Institute of Justice, 2004. Available at: https://www.ncjrs.gov/pdffiles1/nij/199712.pdf. Accessed April 14, 2018.

Kramer MD, Polusny MA, Arbisi PA, et al: Comorbidity of PTSD and SUDs: toward an etiologic understanding, in Trauma and Substance Abuse: Causes, Consequences, and Treatment of Comorbid Disorders, 2nd Edition. Edited by Ouimette P, Read JP. Washington, DC, American Psychological Association, 2014, pp 53–75

Kulka RA, Schlenger WE, Fairbank JA, et al: Contractual report of findings from the National Vietnam Veterans Readjustment Study, Volume I: executive summary, description of findings, and technical appendices. November 7, 1988. Available at: https://www.ptsd.va.gov/professional/articles/article-pdf/nvvrs_vol1.pdf. Accessed April 14, 2018.

Lanius RA, Williamson PC, Densmore M, et al: Neural correlates of traumatic memories in posttraumatic stress disorder: a functional MRI investigation. Am J Psychiatry 158(11):1920–1922, 2001 11691703

Lanius RA, Williamson PC, Hopper J, et al: Recall of emotional states in posttraumatic stress disorder: an fMRI investigation. Biol Psychiatry 53(3):204–210, 2003 12559652

Lasko NB, Gurvits TV, Kuhne AA, et al: Aggression and its correlates in Vietnam veterans with and without chronic posttraumatic stress disorder. Compr Psychiatry 35(5):373–381, 1994 7995030

Lemerise EA, Arsenio WF: An integrated model of emotion processes and cognition in social information processing. Child Dev 71(1):107–118, 2000 10836564

Liberzon I, Taylor SF, Amdur R, et al: Brain activation in PTSD in response to trauma-related stimuli. Biol Psychiatry 45(7):817–826, 1999 10202568

Logue MW, Solovieff N, Leussis MP, et al: The ankyrin-3 gene is associated with posttraumatic stress disorder and externalizing comorbidity. Psychoneuroendocrinology 38(10):2249–2257, 2013 23796624

Mackintosh MA, Morland LA, Frueh BC, et al: Peeking into the black box: mechanisms of action for anger management treatment. J Anxiety Disord 28(7):687–695, 2014 25124505

Maslow AH: A theory of human motivation. Psychol Rev 50(4):370–396, 1943

McCloskey MS, Phan KL, Angstadt M, et al: Amygdala hyperactivation to angry faces in intermittent explosive disorder. J Psychiatr Res 79:34–41, 2016 27145325

Miller MW, Resick PA: Internalizing and externalizing subtypes in female sexual assault survivors: implications for the understanding of complex PTSD. Behav Ther 38(1):58–71, 2007 17292695

Miller MW, Greif JL, Smith AA: Multidimensional Personality Questionnaire profiles of veterans with traumatic combat exposure: externalizing and internalizing subtypes. Psychol Assess 15(2):205–215, 2003 12847781

Miller MW, Kaloupek DG, Dillon AL, et al: Externalizing and internalizing subtypes of combat-related PTSD: a replication and extension using the PSY-5 scales. J Abnorm Psychol 113(4):636–645, 2004 15535795

Monnelly EP, Ciraulo DA, Knapp C, et al: Low-dose risperidone as adjunctive therapy for irritable aggression in posttraumatic stress disorder. J Clin Psychopharmacol 23(2):193–196, 2003 12640221

Morland LA, Greene CJ, Rosen CS, et al: Telemedicine for anger management therapy in a rural population of combat veterans with posttraumatic stress disorder: a randomized noninferiority trial. J Clin Psychiatry 71(7):855–863, 2010 20122374

Novaco RW, Chemtob CM: Anger and combat-related posttraumatic stress disorder. J Trauma Stress 15(2):123–132, 2002 12013063

Orth U, Wieland E: Anger, hostility, and posttraumatic stress disorder in trauma-exposed adults: a meta-analysis. J Consult Clin Psychol 74(4):698–706, 2006 16881777

Osuch EA, Benson B, Geraci M, et al: Regional cerebral blood flow correlated with flashback intensity in patients with posttraumatic stress disorder. Biol Psychiatry 50(4):246–253, 2001 11522258

Rauch SL, van der Kolk B, Fisler RE, et al: A symptom provocation study of posttraumatic stress disorder using positron emission tomography and script-driven imagery. Arch Gen Psychiatry 53:380–387, 1996 8624181

Rauch SL, Whalen PJ, Shin LM, et al: Exaggerated amygdala response to masked facial stimuli in posttraumatic stress disorder: a functional MRI study. Biol Psychiatry 47(9):769–776, 2000 10812035

Reilly PM, Shopshire MS: Anger management group treatment for cocaine dependence: preliminary outcomes. Am J Drug Alcohol Abuse 26(2):161–177, 2000 10852354

Reilly PM, Shopshire MS, Durazzo TC, Campbell TA: Anger Management for Substance Abuse and Mental Health Clients: Participant Workbook. HSS Publ No (SMA) 12-4210. Rockville, MD, Center for Substance Abuse Treatment, Substance Abuse and Mental Health Services Administration, 2002

Riggs DS, Dancu CV, Gershuny BS, et al: Anger and post-traumatic stress disorder in female crime victims. J Trauma Stress 5(4):613–625, 1992

Rosen C, Adler E, Tiet Q: Presenting concerns of veterans entering treatment for posttraumatic stress disorder. J Trauma Stress 26(5):640–643, 2013 24123262

Shalev AY: Acute stress reactions in adults. Biol Psychiatry 51(7):532–543, 2002 11950455

Shin LM, Orr SP, Carson MA, et al: Regional cerebral blood flow in the amygdala and medial prefrontal cortex during traumatic imagery in male and female Vietnam veterans with PTSD. Arch Gen Psychiatry 61(2):168–176, 2004 14757593

Shin LM, Wright CI, Cannistraro PA, et al: A functional magnetic resonance imaging study of amygdala and medial prefrontal cortex responses to overtly presented fearful faces in posttraumatic stress disorder. Arch Gen Psychiatry 62(3):273–281, 2005 15753240

Stapleton JA, Taylor S, Asmundson GJ: Effects of three PTSD treatments on anger and guilt: exposure therapy, eye movement desensitization and reprocessing, and relaxation training. J Trauma Stress 19(1):19–28, 2006 16568469

Stein MB, McAllister TW: Exploring the convergence of posttraumatic stress disorder and mild traumatic brain injury. Am J Psychiatry 166(7):768–776, 2009 19448186

Taft CT, Kaloupek DG, Schumm JA, et al: Posttraumatic stress disorder symptoms, physiological reactivity, alcohol problems, and aggression among military veterans. J Abnorm Psychol 116(3):498–507, 2007a 17696706

Taft CT, Vogt DS, Marshall AD, et al: Aggression among combat veterans: relationships with combat exposure and symptoms of posttraumatic stress disorder, dysphoria, and anxiety. J Trauma Stress 20(2):135–145, 2007b 17427912

Taft CT, Schumm JA, Marshall AD, et al: Family-of-origin maltreatment, posttraumatic stress disorder symptoms, social information processing deficits, and relationship abuse perpetration. J Abnorm Psychol 117(3):637–646, 2008 18729615

Taft CT, Weatherill RP, Woodward HE, et al: Intimate partner and general aggression perpetration among combat veterans presenting to a posttraumatic stress disorder clinic. Am J Orthopsychiatry 79(4):461–468, 2009 20099937

Taft CT, Macdonald AM, Candice M, et al: "Strength at Home" group intervention for military populations engaging in intimate partner violence: pilot findings. J Fam Violence 28(3):225–231, 2013

Taft CT, Howard J, Monson CM, et al: "Strength at Home" intervention to prevent conflict and violence in military couples: pilot findings. Partn Abus 5(1):41–57, 2014

Taft CT, Creech SK, Gallagher MW, et al: Strength at Home Couples program to prevent military partner violence: a randomized controlled trial. J Consult Clin Psychol 84(11):935–945, 2016a 27599224

Taft CT, Macdonald A, Creech SK, et al: A randomized controlled clinical trial of the Strength at Home Men's Program for Partner Violence in military veterans. J Clin Psychiatry 77(9):1168–1175, 2016b 26613288

Taft CT, Murphy CM, Creech SK: Trauma-Informed Treatment and Prevention of Intimate Partner Violence. Washington, DC, American Psychological Association, 2016c

Tay L, Diener E: Needs and subjective well-being around the world. J Pers Soc Psychol 101(2):354–365, 2011 21688922

Taylor SE, Klein LC, Lewis BP, et al: Biobehavioral responses to stress in females: tend-and-befriend, not fight-or-flight. Psychol Rev 107(3):411–429, 2000 10941275

Taylor S, Thordarson DS, Maxfield L, et al: Comparative efficacy, speed, and adverse effects of three PTSD treatments: exposure therapy, EMDR, and relaxation training. J Consult Clin Psychol 71(2):330–338, 2003 12699027

van der Kolk B: Posttraumatic stress disorder and the nature of trauma. Dialogues Clin Neurosci 2(1):7–22, 2000 22034447

Waltes R, Chiocchetti AG, Freitag CM: The neurobiological basis of human aggression: A review on genetic and epigenetic mechanisms. Am J Med Genet B Neuropsychiatr Genet 171(5):650–675, 2016 26494515

Wolf EJ, Miller MW, Krueger RF, et al: Posttraumatic stress disorder and the genetic structure of comorbidity. J Abnorm Psychol 119(2):320–330, 2010 20455605

World Health Organization: International Statistical Classification of Diseases and Related Health Problems, 10th Revision. Geneva, World Health Organization, 1992

Yang Y, Raine A: Prefrontal structural and functional brain imaging findings in antisocial, violent, and psychopathic individuals: a meta-analysis. Psychiatry Res 174(2):81–88, 2009 19833485

Zannas AS, Binder EB: Gene-environment interactions at the FKBP5 locus: sensitive periods, mechanisms and pleiotropism. Genes Brain Behav 13(1):25–37, 2014 24219237

Zillmann D, Katcher AH, Milavsky B: Excitation transfer from physical exercise to subsequent aggressive behavior. J Exp Soc Psychol 8:247–259, 1972

Zohar J, Amital D, Miodownik C, et al: Double-blind placebo-controlled pilot study of sertraline in military veterans with posttraumatic stress disorder. J Clin Psychopharmacol 22(2):190–195, 2002 11910265

11

Aggression in Eating Disorders

Karen M. Jennings, Ph.D., R.N., A.P.R.N.
Lindsay P. Bodell, Ph.D.
Jennifer E. Wildes, Ph.D.

Eating disorders are serious psychiatric illnesses characterized by aberrant eating or behaviors to control weight (e.g., purging) that result in poor physical health or psychosocial functioning (American Psychiatric Association 2013). DSM-5 eating disorders include anorexia nervosa (AN), bulimia nervosa (BN), and binge-eating disorder (BED) (American Psychiatric Association 2013). The distinguishing characteristic of AN is the presence of extreme food restriction that results in a significantly low body weight. Individuals with BN are within or above a healthy weight range and experience both episodes of binge eating (i.e., eating, in a discrete period of time, an objectively large amount of food and feeling loss of control while eating) and inappropriate compensatory behaviors to prevent weight gain (e.g., vomiting, laxative use, fasting, excessive exercise). In contrast, individuals with BED engage in episodes of binge eating without recurrent compensatory behaviors. DSM-5 also includes the categories other specified feeding or eating disorder and unspecified eating or feeding disorder, which include clinically significant eating pathology that does not meet full criteria for AN, BN, or BED.

Psychiatric comorbidities are commonplace among individuals with eating disorders. As noted in other chapters in this volume, aggression and anger are associated with many psychiatric disorders (Arseneault et al. 2000; Johnson et al. 2002) and may play a role in the onset and maintenance of eating disorders (Engel et al. 2007; Fox and Power 2009; Truglia et al. 2006). Indeed, aggressive behavior toward others and self-directed aggression can increase the complexity of eating disorder clinical presentations and influence prognosis and treatment (Truglia et al. 2006). Our purpose in this chapter is to review the literature on aggression and eating disorders and provide guidance regarding the treatment of individuals with this comorbidity.

Phenomenology

Anger

Existing literature suggests that individuals with eating disorders exhibit higher levels of anger than healthy control subjects (Fassino et al. 2001; Krug et al. 2008; Miotto et al. 2008; Waller et al. 2003). For example, Krug et al. (2008) found that about 20% of adult females with AN, BN, or eating disorder not otherwise specified had moderate to high levels of "anger state" (derived from the State Anger subscale of the State-Trait Anger Expression Inventory–2 [STAXI-2]) compared with 1% of healthy controls. Similarly, individuals with eating disorders are more likely to experience "anger attacks" (i.e., the presence of irritability, overreaction to minor annoyances, autonomic arousal or behavioral outburst symptoms) than healthy controls, with approximately 33% of participants with eating disorders endorsing such symptoms (compared with 10% of healthy controls) (Fava et al. 1995). Compared with healthy control participants, individuals with BN have reported higher mean scores on both the STAXI State Anger (15.80± 6.60 vs. 12.7±4.40) and Trait Anger (23.44±5.91 vs. 19.38±5.80) subscales (Fassino et al. 2001). Furthermore, higher STAXI subscale scores have been associated with treatment dropout in adult females with BN (Fassino et al. 2003). Overall, these findings indicate that individuals with eating disorders may experience greater intensity of anger compared with healthy controls and that poor anger management may be related to treatment engagement.

Studies also have found positive associations between anger and eating disorder behaviors, including binge eating, fasting, laxative misuse, and vomiting (Engel et al. 2007; Milligan and Waller 2000; Peñas-Lledó et al. 2004; Tozzi et al. 2006), suggesting that higher levels of anger are correlated with greater severity of eating disorder symptoms. Researchers have hypothesized that individuals with eating disorders demonstrate difficulties in emotional expression and perceive anger as a threatening, uncontrollable emotion (Espeset et al. 2012; Fox and Power 2009; Ioannou and Fox 2009; Meyer et al. 2005). As such, it has been posited that eating disorder symptoms (e.g., binge eating and food restriction) may be behavioral mechanisms to avoid or suppress anger.

Aggression Toward Others

Only a few studies have evaluated aggression toward others in individuals with eating disorders, with conflicting findings (Truglia et al. 2006). Fava et al. (1995) found that among women with eating disorders who reported anger attacks, 68% endorsed physically or verbally attacking others and 46% endorsed throwing or destroying objects. Similarly, Harrison et al. (2011) found that women with AN had a greater number of "extra-aggression" responses (i.e., aggression focused on people), as measured by the Rosenzweig Picture-Frustration Study, compared with healthy control subjects. In contrast to these results, Miotto et al. (2008) found that females with AN scored lower on self-reported measures of verbal and physical aggression compared with healthy controls.

Although few studies have directly compared the prevalence of aggressive behavior in individuals with eating disorders relative to healthy control subjects, several studies using nonclinical samples have reported positive associations between disordered eating symptoms and aggression. These data suggest that individuals with eating disturbances (e.g., compensatory behaviors) are more likely to report externalizing behaviors (Marmorstein et al. 2007) and have a higher propensity to display aggressive behaviors toward others (Miotto et al. 2003; Slane et al. 2010; Thompson et al. 1999). Additionally, Thompson et al. (1999) found that adolescent girls who reported dietary restraint or binge-eating/purging were up to four times more likely to engage in robbery with a weapon, and four times more likely to engage in aggravated battery, compared with girls who did not endorse eating disorder behaviors. Furthermore, the odds of engaging in at least one aggressive behavior (i.e., group fighting, assault, robbery with a weapon, battery, violent dispute resolution, aggravated battery) were 1.6–2.1 times greater for girls who endorsed dietary restraint or binge-eating/purging, respectively. Adolescents with high eating disorder psychopathology also have demonstrated greater self-reported aggression compared with adolescents with low eating disorder psychopathology (Miotto et al. 2003). Finally, eating disorder pathology (i.e., binge eating, dietary restraint, weight preoccupation) has been correlated positively with aggressive behaviors (e.g., threatening behavior, screaming, fighting) in adult women and men (Slane et al. 2010), with stronger correlations between binge eating and aggression in men.

Self-Directed Aggression

Although beyond the scope of this chapter, associations between eating disorders and self-directed aggression (i.e., nonsuicidal self-injury [NSSI]) are worth noting. *Nonsuicidal self-injury* is defined as intentional bodily harm without the intent to die and includes behaviors such as cutting, burning, skin picking, and hair pulling (Klonsky and Muehlenkamp 2007). A recent meta-analysis found that approximately 27% of individuals with an eating disorder have a lifetime history of NSSI, with the prevalence of NSSI being higher in individuals with BN (32.7%) than in individuals with AN (21.8%) (Cucchi et al. 2016). This high comorbidity may be a result of shared risk factors, including trauma, obsessive-compulsive personality traits, impulsivity, and affective problems, that may increase likelihood of relying on NSSI or eating disorder behaviors as coping mechanisms (Klonsky and Muehlenkamp 2007; Svirko and Hawton 2007).

Overall, a relatively limited body of research has focused on associations between eating disorders and anger or aggression, with the majority of results suggesting higher prevalence of anger and aggression in individuals with eating disorders compared with healthy controls (Table 11–1). Additionally, there is some evidence to suggest that associations between facets of aggression (i.e., anger, self-directed, toward others) and eating disorder pathology are most pronounced for bulimic spectrum disorders and behaviors (e.g., binge eating).

Epidemiology

Among adults and adolescents, epidemiological studies have found a lifetime prevalence of 0.3%–0.9% for AN, 0.1%–1.6% for BN, and 0.8%–3.5% for BED (Hudson et al. 2007; Swanson et al. 2011). Eating disorders typically have their onset in adolescence or young adulthood, but cases beginning earlier and later in life have been described (American Psychiatric Association 2013). Individuals with eating disorders have a higher risk of serious medical consequences, psychosocial impairment, and death compared with the general population (American Psychiatric Association 2013; Arcelus et al. 2011; Smink et al. 2013).

Epidemiological studies suggest overlap among eating disorders, particularly bulimic spectrum disorders, and intermittent explosive disorder (IED), which is characterized by aggression that is impulsive and/or anger based (Fernández-Aranda et al. 2006, 2008; Hudson et al. 2007; Kessler et al. 2013). Approximately 2.5% and 13% of individuals with a lifetime eating disorder met criteria for lifetime IED in community and clinical samples, respectively. Moreover, at least half of individuals with comorbid IED and an eating disorder reported that onset of IED preceded onset of BN or BED (Jennings et al. 2017; Scott et al. 2016). Jennings et al. (2017) also found that individuals with eating disorders reported higher anger and aggression scores compared with healthy control subjects, and that individuals with both IED and an eating disorder had the highest levels of anger and aggression. These findings suggest that individuals with eating disorders have relatively high comorbidity with IED, which may contribute to anger and aggression in this population.

Psychobiology

Existing literature suggests that individuals with eating disorders have altered levels of endogenous hormones and disturbances in the functioning and physiology of neurotransmitters (Cotrufo et al. 2000; Culbert et al. 2015a), both of which have been shown to influence aggressive behaviors (Lucki 1998). Cotrufo et al. (2000) examined the relation between aggressiveness and endogenous hormones (i.e., tes-

TABLE 11–1.   Aggression and eating disorder behaviors in clinical and community samples

Study	Sample	Eating disorder assessment	Aggression assessment	Key findings
Clinical samples				
Cotrufo et al. 2000	33 women with BN; 22 HCs	Eating Disorder Inventory Bulimic Investigatory Test, Edinburgh	Buss-Durkee Hostility Inventory	BN < HCs, plasma levels of 17β-estradiol and prolactin BN > HCs, mean plasma levels of testosterone and cortisol ↑ plasma levels of testosterone correlated to ↑ Direct Aggression subscale scores for women with BN
Fava et al. 1995	132 women with EDs: 46 AN, 35 BN,16 AN/BN; 35 recovered; 39 HC women	Psychiatric Status Rating Scale	Anger Attacks Questionnaire	EDs> HCs met criteria for anger attacks
Fernández-Arando et al. 2008	709 women with history of EDs: 121 AN, 274 BN, 251 AN/BN, 63 EDNOS	Structured Interview for Anorexia Nervosa and Bulimic Syndromes Structured Clinical Interview for DSM-IV Axis I Disorders	A module designed by James E. Mitchell, M.D, University of North Dakota, based on DSM-IV criteria	Lifetime prevalence of IED diagnosis=0.6% ($n=4$)

TABLE 11–1. Aggression and eating disorder behaviors in clinical and community samples *(continued)*

Study	Sample	Eating disorder assessment	Aggression assessment	Key findings
Clinical samples *(continued)*				
Fernández-Arando et al. 2006	227 women with BN	Semistructured clinical interview based on DSM-IV	Structured Clinical Interview for DSM-IV Axis I Disorders	Lifetime prevalence of IED=13.2% ($n=30$)
Harrison et al. 2011	22 women with AN; 44 HC women	Eating Disorder Diagnostic Scale	Rosenzweig Picture-Frustration Study	AN > HCs, anger-focused responses AN < HCs, solution-focused responses AN sample: ↑ BMI correlated to ↑ externally directed aggression responses ↓ BMI correlated with ↑ internally directed aggression responses
Miotto et al. 2008	112 adolescent/adult females with EDs: 61 AN, 51 BN; 524 HC (adolescents)	Eating Attitudes Test Bulimic Investigatory Test Edinburgh Body Attitudes Test	Buss-Perry Aggression Questionnaire	↑ ED scores correlated to ↑ AQ scores for both groups AN < HCs, Physical Aggression and Verbal Aggression subscale scores BN > HC, Anger subscale scores

TABLE 11–1. Aggression and eating disorder behaviors in clinical and community samples *(continued)*

Study	Sample	Eating disorder assessment	Aggression assessment	Key findings
Community samples				
Arseneault et al. 2000	961 adults (women and men)	Diagnostic Interview Schedule	Court convictions for violence in the past 12 months Self-reports of violence in the past 12 months (i.e., simple assault, aggravated assault, robbery, rape, gang fighting)	No significant findings
Hudson et al. 2007	1,760 women, 1,220 men	National Comorbidity Survey	National Comorbidity Survey Replication	↑ Lifetime BED correlated to ↑ lifetime IED
Kessler et al. 2013	24,124 adults (women and men)	World Mental Health survey version of the WHO Composite International Diagnostic Interview	World Mental Health survey version of the WHO Composite International Diagnostic Interview	↑ Lifetime BN or BED correlated to: ↑ Lifetime IED ↑ Lifetime ODD ↑ Lifetime conduct disorder

TABLE 11–1. Aggression and eating disorder behaviors in clinical and community samples *(continued)*

Study	Sample	Eating disorder assessment	Aggression assessment	Key findings
Community samples *(continued)*				
Miotto et al. 2003	560 female, 258 male adolescents	Eating Attitudes Test Bulimic Investigatory Test, Edinburgh Body Attitudes Test	Buss-Perry Aggression Questionnaire	Males > females, BPAQ scores Males = females, scores ↑ than cut-off for clinically relevant EDs had ↑ AQ scores
Scott et al. 2016	88,063 adults (women and men)	World Mental Health survey version of the WHO Composite International Diagnostic Interview	World Mental Health survey version of the WHO Composite International Diagnostic Interview	Comorbidity of lifetime IED and 2.5% lifetime BED 1.7% lifetime BN 50.3% IED preceded BED 49.5% IED preceded BN Comorbidity of 12-month IED and 1.0% 12-month BED 1.2% 12-month BN
Slane et al. 2010	335 women, 206 men	Minnesota Eating Behavior Survey (MEBS) Restraint subscale of Eating Disorder Examination—Questionnaire	Aggressive Behavior subscale of the Young Adult Self-Report	Women > men, levels of aggressive behaviors ↑ Aggressive behavior correlated to ↑ weight preoccupation, ↑ binge eating, ↑ dietary restraint, and ↑ total MEBS score, for both sexes Women < men, association between aggressive behavior and binge eating

TABLE 11–1. Aggression and eating disorder behaviors in clinical and community samples *(continued)*

Study	Sample	Eating disorder assessment	Aggression assessment	Key findings
Community samples *(continued)*				
Thompson et al. 1999	3,630 female adolescents	Binge-eating/purging item: "How often do you binge-eat (eat a lot of food in a short period of time) and then make yourself throw up or use laxatives to get rid of the food you have eaten?" (Likert scale 1–4) Dietary restriction item: "Have you ever gone several months where you cut down on how much you ate and lost so much weight or became so thin that other people became worried about you?" (Yes/No)	Dichotomized violence categories based on self-reports of group fighting, aggravated battery, simple battery, robbery, assault, and violent dispute resolution in the past 12 months	Binge-eating/purging > no binge-eating/purging for each violent category: Group fighting: OR=3.2 Assault: OR=2.8 Robbery with a weapon: OR=4.0 Battery: OR=3.0 Violent resolution: OR=2.1 Aggravated battery: OR=3.9 At least one aggressive behavior: OR=2 Dietary restriction > no dietary restriction for each violence category: Group fighting: OR=2.7 Assault: OR=2.4 Robbery with a weapon: OR=3.4 Battery: OR=2.2 Violent resolution: OR=1.6 Aggravated battery: OR=4.0 At least one aggressive behavior: OR=1.6

TABLE 11–1. Aggression and eating disorder behaviors in clinical and community samples *(continued)*

Study	Sample	Eating disorder assessment	Aggression assessment	Key findings
Clinical/community samples				
Jennings et al. 2017	19,430 adolescents/adults in community sample (46.9% male) 1,642 adults in clinical research sample (56.4% male)	National Comorbidity Survey (community sample) Structured Clinical Interview for DSM diagnoses (clinical research sample)	Number of IED episodes in the past 12 months (community sample) Life History of Aggression scale; Anger subscale of BPAQ (clinical research sample)	IED > non-IED, lifetime any ED (community/clinical) IED > non-IED, lifetime BN (community) or lifetime BED (community/clinical) IED preceded any ED, BN, or BED: ≥2 years for clinical sample ≥5 years for community sample IED/ED > IED > ED > PC > HC, number of IED episodes for community sample[e] IED/ED = IED > ED = PC > HC, aggression scores for clinical sample IED/ED = IED > ED = PC > HC, Anger subscale scores for clinical sample

Note. AN=anorexia nervosa; BED=binge-eating disorder; BMI=body mass index; BN=bulimia nervosa; BPAQ=Buss-Perry Aggression Questionnaire; ED=eating disorder; EDNOS = eating disorder not otherwise specified; HC=healthy control; IED=intermittent explosive disorder; ODD=oppositional defiant disorder; OR=odds ratio; PC=psychiatric control; WHO=World Health Organization.

tosterone, 17β-estradiol, prolactin, cortisol) in 33 women with BN and 22 healthy control subjects. Results showed a significant positive correlation between testosterone plasma levels and the degree of aggressiveness in individuals with BN but not in healthy control subjects. More specifically, plasma testosterone was positively correlated with direct aggressiveness, resentment, irritability, and suspiciousness, suggesting that increased levels of testosterone may play a role in the modulation of aggression toward others and/or objects in individuals with BN (Cotrufo et al. 2000). Research also indicates that disturbances in serotonergic and dopaminergic functioning are present in women with eating disorders (Culbert et al. 2015b); thus, it is possible that shared neurobiological correlates may explain, in part, the overlap of anger or aggressive behaviors and eating disorders.

Clinical Approach and Treatment

Given associations of anger or aggression with indices of illness severity and treatment engagement in individuals with eating disorders (Fassino et al. 2003; Truglia et al. 2006), assessing these constructs may provide useful information to guide clinical decision making. Clinicians treating individuals with co-occurring anger or aggression and eating disorders should be especially attentive to the potential for self-destructive behaviors, because the presence of both an eating disorder and aggressive behavior has been linked to increased risk of suicidality and substance misuse (Thompson et al. 1999).

It also is important to consider that individuals may be more likely to seek/receive treatment for problems related to anger and aggression than for eating disorder symptoms, given the ambivalence about changing eating and weight control behaviors. Hence, it may be beneficial for providers who treat individuals with aggression (against self and others) to assess for eating disorder psychopathology. A list of efficient measures with good psychometric properties for assessing eating disorder psychopathology and aggression is provided in Table 11–2.

There are no evidence-based interventions for co-occurring aggression and eating disorders. However, the results of two randomized controlled trials conducted in the Netherlands suggest that psychomotor therapy (PMT) may have utility in the treatment of anger and aggression in patients with eating disorders (Boerhout et al. 2016,

TABLE 11–2. Self-report measures to assess eating disorder psychopathology and aggression/anger

Eating disorder psychopathology	Aggression/anger
Eating Disorder Examination Questionnaire (Fairburn et al. 2008)	Buss-Perry Aggression Questionnaire (Buss and Perry 1992)
Eating Disorder Diagnostic Scale (Stice et al. 2000)	State-Trait Anger Expression Inventory–2 (Spielberger 2010)
Eating Pathology Symptoms Inventory (Forbush et al. 2013)	

2017). PMT uses body awareness and physical activities to help individuals improve their understanding of emotions and expression skills, and may in turn, target facets of anger and aggression (Boerhout et al. 2013; Probst et al. 2010). Boerhout and colleagues randomly assigned individuals receiving outpatient (Boerhout et al. 2016) or day program (Boerhout et al. 2017) treatment for an eating disorder to either six 1-hour PMT sessions delivered by a trained psychomotor therapist or a time-and-contact control condition. Results from both studies showed statistically significant decreases in anger internalization, as measured by the Anger-In subscale score of the Self-Expression and Control Scale, from baseline to end of intervention in the PMT groups compared with the control groups. Although additional studies are needed, these findings suggest that PMT holds promise for reducing internalized anger in patients with eating disorders.

On a broader level, psychoeducation about the function of emotions, especially negative emotions, and strategies to manage and express affect may be critical components of treatment for individuals with eating disorders. Emotion regulation difficulties are well documented in this population (Lavender et al. 2015). Moreover, several scholars have theorized that eating disorder behaviors function, in part, to help patients avoid or suppress negative emotions, including anger (Espeset et al. 2012; Fox and Power 2009; Ioannou and Fox 2009; Meyer et al. 2005; Wildes et al. 2010). Thus, early identification of individuals with anger and aggression may help clinicians provide treatment interventions focused on emotion regulation and distress tolerance skills. Such treatment interventions may help individuals to accept and appropriately express feelings of anger.

Clinical Vignette

SG is a 19-year-old female who presents to outpatient treatment for binge-eating and purging behaviors. She reports eating excessive amounts of food quickly followed by self-induced vomiting several times a week over the past 6 months. She also tried laxatives for weight loss a few times as a teenager but denies current use. She has a body mass index of 22.4, has regular and normal menses, and has been taking oral birth control pills for the past 2 years. She thinks that she is "fat" and needs to lose at least 10–15 pounds, especially in her abdomen and thighs. SG reports having been a happy and "almost perfect" child, always excelling in academics with a 3.8 GPA as a college sophomore, and is an intramural soccer player. Although she has close friends and a close-knit family, she "can't truly be happy until [she] loses weight." She reports "periods of being overwhelmed." Upon further assessment, SG reports yelling at her parents and physically hitting her mom and younger brother on multiple occasions as a teenager (ages 12–14). However, she "felt horrible" and has "no idea why [she] did it." She denies a history of or current ideation, plans, or intent for suicide or self-directed aggression.

Discussion of Vignette

As a clinician, one could administer self-report measures of aggression, anger, and eating disorder psychopathology in order to gain a more thorough picture of SG's clinical presentation and to measure progress during treatment. Treatment interventions would focus on psychoeducation about the function of anger, appropriate strategies to express anger, and cognitive restructuring and problem-solving strategies to develop new schematic models for her relations with her family and friends and to help SG accept and appropriately express her anger.

Summary

Empirical evidence suggests that both self- and other-focused aggression are associated with eating disorders. Furthermore, the co-occurrence of eating disorders and aggression toward others is associated with greater risk of suicidality and substance misuse, whereas aggression toward self is related to inhibited expressions of anger and aggression toward others. Hence, clinicians should assess for the co-occurrence of eating disorders and aggressive behaviors, which may provide clinically useful information to determine the most effective treatment interventions including psychoeducation, cognitive restructuring, and problem-solving strategies.

Key Clinical Points

▌ Aggression and facets of anger may play a role in the onset and maintenance of eating disorders.

▌ Individuals with eating disorders have increased aggression toward others and greater risk of self-directed aggression, compared with the general population.

▌ Aggression increases the complexity of eating disorder clinical presentations.

▌ Emotion regulation difficulties may contribute to the link between eating disorders and aggression.

▌ Assessment of anger and aggression in the standard eating disorders interview may provide clinically useful information to determine most effective treatment interventions.

▌ Similarly, it is important to assess for eating disorder psychopathology in the standard psychiatric interview.

▌ Specific evidence-based interventions for comorbidity of aggression and eating disorders are not available.

▌ Interventions should include psychoeducation about the function of anger as well as strategies to accept, manage, and express anger.

References

American Psychiatric Association: Diagnostic and Statistical Manual of Mental Disorders, 5th Edition. Arlington, VA, American Psychiatric Association, 2013

Arcelus J, Mitchell AJ, Wales J, et al: Mortality rates in patients with anorexia nervosa and other eating disorders. A meta-analysis of 36 studies. Arch Gen Psychiatry 68(7):724–731, 2011 21727255

Arseneault L, Moffitt TE, Caspi A, et al: Mental disorders and violence in a total birth cohort: results from the Dunedin Study. Arch Gen Psychiatry 57(10):979–986, 2000 11015816

Boerhout C, van Busschbach JT, Wiersma D, et al: Psychomotor therapy and aggression regulation in eating disorders. Body Mov Dance Psychother 8(4):241–253, 2013

Boerhout C, Swart M, Van Busschbach JT, et al: Effect of aggression regulation on eating disorder pathology: RCT of a brief body and movement oriented intervention. Eur Eat Disord Rev 24(2):114–121, 2016 26679955

Boerhout C, Swart M, Voskamp M, et al: Aggression regulation in day treatment of eating disorders: two-centre RCT of a brief body and movement-oriented intervention. Eur Eat Disord Rev 25(1):52–59, 2017 27862660

Buss AH, Perry M: The aggression questionnaire. J Pers Soc Psychol 63(3):452–459, 1992 1403624

Cotrufo P, Monteleone P, d'Istria M, et al: Aggressive behavioral characteristics and endogenous hormones in women with bulimia nervosa. Neuropsychobiology 42(2):58–61, 2000 10940759

Cucchi A, Ryan D, Konstantakopoulos G, et al: Lifetime prevalence of nonsuicidal self-injury in patients with eating disorders: a systematic review and meta-analysis. Psychol Med 46(7):1345–1358, 2016 26954514

Culbert KM, Breedlove SM, Sisk CL, et al: Age differences in prenatal testosterone's protective effects on disordered eating symptoms: developmental windows of expression? Behav Neurosci 129(1):18–36, 2015a 25621790

Culbert KM, Racine SE, Klump KL: Research review: what we have learned about the causes of eating disorders—a synthesis of sociocultural, psychological, and biological research. J Child Psychol Psychiatry 56(11):1141–1164, 2015b 26095891

Engel SG, Boseck JJ, Crosby RD, et al: The relationship of momentary anger and impulsivity to bulimic behavior. Behav Res Ther 45(3):437–447, 2007 16697350

Espeset EM, Gulliksen KS, Nordbø RH, et al: The link between negative emotions and eating disorder behaviour in patients with anorexia nervosa. Eur Eat Disord Rev 20(6):451–460, 2012 22696277

Fairburn CG, Cooper Z, O'Connor M: Eating Disorders Examination (16.0D), in Cognitive Behavior Therapy and Eating Disorders. Edited by Fairburn CG. New York, Guilford, 2008, pp 265–308

Fassino S, Daga GA, Pierò A, et al: Anger and personality in eating disorders. J Psychosom Res 51(6):757–764, 2001 11750298

Fassino S, Abbate-Daga G, Pierò A, et al: Dropout from brief psychotherapy within a combination treatment in bulimia nervosa: role of personality and anger. Psychother Psychosom 72(4):203–210, 2003 12792125

Fava M, Rappe SM, West J, et al: Anger attacks in eating disorders. Psychiatry Res 56(3):205–212, 1995 7568542

Fernández-Aranda F, Jiménez-Murcia S, Alvarez-Moya EM, et al: Impulse control disorders in eating disorders: clinical and therapeutic implications. Compr Psychiatry 47(6):482–488, 2006 17067872

Fernández-Aranda F, Pinheiro AP, Thornton LM, et al: Impulse control disorders in women with eating disorders. Psychiatry Res 157(1–3):147–157, 2008 17961717

Forbush KT, Wildes JE, Pollack LO, et al: Development and validation of the Eating Pathology Symptoms Inventory (EPSI). Psychol Assess 25(3):859–878, 2013 23815116

Fox JR, Power MJ: Eating disorders and multi-level models of emotion: an integrated model. Clin Psychol Psychother 16(4):240–267, 2009 19639647

Harrison A, Genders R, Davies H, et al: Experimental measurement of the regulation of anger and aggression in women with anorexia nervosa. Clin Psychol Psychother 18(6):445–452, 2011 20859934

Hudson JI, Hiripi E, Pope HG Jr, et al: The prevalence and correlates of eating disorders in the National Comorbidity Survey Replication. Biol Psychiatry 61(3):348–358, 2007 16815322

Ioannou K, Fox JR: Perception of threat from emotions and its role in poor emotional expression within eating pathology. Clin Psychol Psychother 16(4):336–347, 2009 19639643

Jennings KM, Wildes JE, Coccaro EF: Intermittent explosive disorder and eating disorders: analysis of national comorbidity and research samples. Compr Psychiatry 75:62–67, 2017 28324677

Johnson JG, Cohen P, Kotler L, et al: Psychiatric disorders associated with risk for the development of eating disorders during adolescence and early adulthood. J Consult Clin Psychol 70(5):1119–1128, 2002 12362962

Kessler RC, Berglund PA, Chiu WT, et al: The prevalence and correlates of binge eating disorder in the World Health Organization World Mental Health Surveys. Biol Psychiatry 73(9):904–914, 2013 23290497

Klonsky ED, Muehlenkamp JJ: Self-injury: a research review for the practitioner. J Clin Psychol 63(11):1045–1056, 2007 17932985

Krug I, Bulik CM, Vall-Llovera ON, et al: Anger expression in eating disorders: clinical, psychopathological and personality correlates. Psychiatry Res 161(2):195–205, 2008 18838172

Lavender JM, Wonderlich SA, Engel SG, et al: Dimensions of emotion dysregulation in anorexia nervosa and bulimia nervosa: a conceptual review of the empirical literature. Clin Psychol Rev 40:111–122, 2015 26112760

Lucki I: The spectrum of behaviors influenced by serotonin. Biol Psychiatry 44(3):151–162, 1998 9693387

Marmorstein NR, von Ranson KM, Iacono WG, et al: Longitudinal associations between externalizing behavior and dysfunctional eating attitudes and behaviors: a community-based study. J Clin Child Adolesc Psychol 36(1):87–94, 2007 17206884

Meyer C, Leung N, Waller G, et al: Anger and bulimic psychopathology: gender differences in a nonclinical group. Int J Eat Disord 37(1):69–71, 2005 15690470

Milligan RJ, Waller G: Anger and bulimic psychopathology among nonclinical women. Int J Eat Disord 28(4):446–450, 2000 11054792

Miotto P, De Coppi M, Frezza M, et al: Eating disorders and aggressiveness among adolescents. Acta Psychiatr Scand 108(3):183–189, 2003 12890272

Miotto P, Pollini B, Restaneo A, et al: Aggressiveness, anger, and hostility in eating disorders. Compr Psychiatry 49(4):364–373, 2008 18555057

Peñas-Lledó E, Fernández JD, Waller G: Association of anger with bulimic and other impulsive behaviours among non-clinical women and men. Eur Eat Disord Rev 12(6):392–397, 2004

Probst M, Knapen J, Poot G, et al: Psychomotor therapy and psychiatry: What's in a name? Open Complement Med J 2:105–113, 2010

Scott KM, Lim CC, Hwang I, et al: The cross-national epidemiology of DSM-IV intermittent explosive disorder. Psychol Med 46(15):3161–3172, 2016 27572872

Slane JD, Burt SA, Klump KL: The road less traveled: associations between externalizing behaviors and eating pathology. Int J Eat Disord 43(2):149–160, 2010 19350646

Smink FR, van Hoeken D, Hoek HW: Epidemiology, course, and outcome of eating disorders. Curr Opin Psychiatry 26(6):543–548, 2013 24060914

Spielberger CD: State-Trait Anxiety Inventory, in The Corsini Encyclopedia of Psychology, Vol 4, 4th Edition. Edited by Weiner IB, Craighead WE. New York, Wiley, 2010

Stice E, Telch CF, Rizvi SL: Development and validation of the Eating Disorder Diagnostic Scale: a brief self-report measure of anorexia, bulimia, and binge-eating disorder. Psychol Assess 12(2):123–131, 2000 10887758

Svirko E, Hawton K: Self-injurious behavior and eating disorders: the extent and nature of the association. Suicide Life Threat Behav 37(4):409–421, 2007 17896881

Swanson SA, Crow SJ, Le Grange D, et al: Prevalence and correlates of eating disorders in adolescents: results from the National Comorbidity Survey Replication adolescent supplement. Arch Gen Psychiatry 68(7):714–723, 2011 21383252

Thompson KM, Wonderlich SA, Crosby RD, et al: The neglected link between eating disturbances and aggressive behavior in girls. J Am Acad Child Adolesc Psychiatry 38(10):1277–1284, 1999 10517061

Tozzi F, Thornton LM, Mitchell J, et al; Price Foundation Collaborative Group: Features associated with laxative abuse in individuals with eating disorders. Psychosom Med 68(3):470–477, 2006 16738081

Truglia E, Mannucci E, Lassi S, et al: Aggressiveness, anger and eating disorders: a review. Psychopathology 39(2):55–68, 2006 16391506

Waller G, Babbs M, Milligan R, et al: Anger and core beliefs in the eating disorders. Int J Eat Disord 34(1):118–124, 2003 12772176

Wildes JE, Ringham RM, Marcus MD: Emotion avoidance in patients with anorexia nervosa: initial test of a functional model. Int J Eat Disord 43(5):398–404, 2010 19670226

12

Aggression in Alcohol Use Disorder and Alcohol's Role in Aggression

David T. George, M.D.
Caroline W. Grant, B.A.

Approximately half of all homicides, assaults, rapes, or other violent interpersonal offenses are preceded by drinking (Giancola 2015; Murdoch et al. 1990). Alcohol is linked more closely with aggression than any other psychotropic substance (World Health Organization 2007). This is particularly relevant in the realm of domestic violence. Researchers have found that 60%–70% of violent men assaulted their partners after drinking alcohol (Gorney 1989). Alcohol is also closely associated with aggression outside the realm of domestic violence; for example, alcohol use disorder is the second-most prevalent psychiatric diagnosis in individuals who commit suicide (Beck and Heinz 2013).

We wish to thank Ms. Brittany Vasae Burdick for her editorial help in the preparation of this chapter.

Not everyone who drinks alcohol becomes aggressive (Bushman and Cooper 1990). Even individuals who are prone to alcohol-related violence do not become aggressive every time they drink. Why do some people become aggressive after drinking while others don't? What circumstances facilitate alcohol-related violence? What happens in the brain of an individual who is prone to alcohol-related violence?

Much research has gone into answering these questions. There are at least 15 different theoretical and empirically supported models regarding how alcohol facilitates aggression (Heinz et al. 2011). Many of these models are built on theories of cognitive disruption or theories of social learning deficits; the most recent models—namely, the "dual-process" model, the "two-channel" theory, and the "impairment of executive functioning" model—incorporate aspects of both social and cognitive processes (Heinz et al. 2011).

Phenomenology

Anger in Individuals With Alcohol Use Disorder

In our experience most of the patients seeking treatment for alcohol use disorder do not demonstrate excessive aggression. However, this is not true for two subtypes of patients: those who have reactive aggression (i.e., defensive rage) and those who have proactive aggression (i.e., predatory aggression).

Patients with reactive aggression are more likely to interpret neutral cues (e.g., facial expressions, tones of voice, perceived slights) as negative and display emotional volatility. This behavior is present when these individuals are sober and becomes accentuated under the influence of alcohol. In contrast, patients with proactive aggression typically are charming and their aggressive tendencies are less flagrant. Interestingly, in animal studies, alcohol facilitates the expression of defensive rage but suppresses instances of predatory attack (Schubert et al. 1996).

Alcohol-Induced Aggression

While great strides have been made toward understanding alcohol-induced aggression, many questions are still unanswered (Heinz et al. 2011). The greatest obstacle is a lack of a universally accepted model to describe alcohol-induced aggression.

Aggression, as discussed elsewhere in this volume, is a heterogeneous behavioral issue, yet it has often been studied as a unified concept. Laboratory paradigms have brought the field a long way, but they are limited in that they only measure certain forms of aggression. Three major laboratory paradigms have been utilized: the Taylor Aggression Paradigm (Taylor 1993), a teacher-learner task (Buss 1961), and the Point Subtraction Aggression Paradigm (Cherek 1981). These paradigms employ a competitive reaction time task, a task in which a teacher disciplines a student, and a task in which points can be taken from an opponent in exchange for money, respectively. What these paradigms fail to capture about alcohol-induced aggression is that it can occur spontaneously because of a loss of control.

Studies that describe the societal implications of alcohol-related violence often do not specify what precipitated the aggression. For example, much empirical research has used selection criteria based on a history of past aggressive behaviors, without examining the circumstances involved in the aggressive incident. This approach introduces unexamined confounding factors into many of the studies, since great variability exists in perpetrators of aggression.

Recently, there has been renewed interest in categorizing different types of aggression. By classifying different subtypes of aggressive individuals, we can avoid erroneous treatment assumptions. For example, someone who commits violence for material gain may not benefit from a therapeutic anger management program, whereas someone who struggles with low frustration tolerance may. McMurran and colleagues (2010) classified three types of alcohol-related violence. The first was violence in pursuit of nonsocial profit-based goals, which occurred in a quarter of their sample. This type of violence was often precipitated out of boredom or financial troubles. The second category of violence involved the pursuit of social dominance. This type of violence occurred in 62% of the sample and often was preceded by feelings of anger and a rush of adrenaline; remorse was uncommon. The third type of violence was characterized as a defense in response to threat. This type occurred in 14% of the sample and was precipitated by fear or anger. Unlike with the second type, excitement was not reported.

Neurobiological research has recently added to the theoretical and experimental work to explain the phenomenon of alcohol-induced aggression. This neurobiological research utilizes human, nonhuman primate, and rodent models of alcohol-induced aggression. Human research has utilized experimental paradigms with magnetic resonance imaging (MRI) and functional MRI to study various components of executive function. Individuals with damage to prefrontal cortical areas (particularly the ventral medial prefrontal cortex and the anterior cingulate cortex) exhibit an array of emotion and decision-making deficits, including, but not limited to, increased irritability, diminished guilt, shame, and empathy, and diminished abilities to plan and to learn from punishment (Koenigs 2012). Individuals who are intoxicated demonstrate similar deficits of executive functioning (Heinz et al. 2011).

Executive Function and Alcohol

Executive functioning utilizes bidirectional tracts to facilitate communication between the prefrontal cortex and the limbic areas that regulate emotion and behavior. Pihl et al. (1993) proposed a model whereby acute alcohol intoxication disrupts the activities of the prefrontal cortex and the hippocampus; these structures are essential to the executive function tasks of self-regulation and goal-directed behavior. More recent reviews point to other brain structures that are also involved in alcohol-related aggression, including the limbic, the cerebello-thalamo-cortical, and the hypothalamic-pituitary-adrenal systems (Tessner and Hill 2010). Behavioral inhibition relies on inhibitory projections from the prefrontal cortex that travel to the amygdala and other limbic areas; it is theorized that both chronic and acute alcohol exposure affect this communication. Giancola proposed that it is the acute effects of alcohol intoxication, rather than neuroadaptations from chronic exposure, that play the biggest role in facilitating alcohol-induced aggression (Giancola 2015). However, chronic ethanol exposure has been shown to significantly impair serotonergic neurotransmission within the amygdala and the prefrontal cortex (Heinz et al. 2011). This has been theorized to affect the limbic system such that threatening stimuli are processed with greater salience; therefore, serotonergic neurotransmission may be one neurobiological correlate of the alcohol myopia model (see next subsection).

Models of Alcohol Effects on Aggression

The earliest models of how alcohol may facilitate aggression include both pharmacological and expectancy theories (Chermack and Taylor 1995). The expectancy theory states that our beliefs determine how alcohol affects our behavior, rather than alcohol's psychotropic properties. Studies showing that aggression was not related to the dosage of alcohol consumed supported this theory (Lang et al. 1975). However, this theory has largely been disproved by more sophisticated experimental procedures (Bushman and Cooper 1990).

The central theme of most pharmacological models is that alcohol-induced aggression can be attributed to alcohol's effects on executive function. Executive function is a broad cognitive construct that accounts for many abilities. It encompasses but is not limited to the following: attentional control, abstract and conceptual reasoning, setting goals, envisioning the future, perspective taking, self-monitoring and social monitoring, abstract reasoning, information appraisal, information organization, set shifting, and inhibition of inappropriate responses (Heinz et al. 2011).

Many models attribute alcohol-induced violence to diminished allocation of attention and a reduction in abstract reasoning (Hull 1981; Pernanen 1976, 1991; Steele and Josephs 1990; Taylor and Leonard 1983). Steele and Josephs (1990) termed this the "alcohol myopia model," in which they state that alcohol affects executive functioning by narrowing one's perceptual field so that only the most salient cues in the environment are perceived and processed. This narrowed scope of attention (i.e., the alcohol myopia) can be conceptualized as hitting the "zoom" function on a camera such that only a small portion of the larger scene is in focus (Heinz et al. 2011). This means that when some intoxicated individuals encounter a threatening stimulus, they have less access to environmental cues and cognitive resources that inhibit them from responding.

This narrowed scope of attention becomes increasingly dangerous when the most salient cues in the environment are threatening. Beck and Heinz (2013) proposed one scenario where alcohol myopia can lead to violence: if someone bumps into you at a bar and you interpret it as an attack, other interpretations (i.e., it was inadvertent, there are long-term consequences of retaliating) are less salient in the moment; therefore, you are less restrained and may respond aggressively to the perceived attack (Beck and Heinz 2013). Unfortunately, individuals who are intoxicated are more likely to perceive neutral cues as threatening (Bartholow and Heinz 2006). This has been termed "hostile perception bias," and it occurs because alcohol disrupts threat-related processing (Giancola et al. 2002).

Another aspect of executive function that is central to models of alcohol-induced aggression is inhibition. The disinhibition hypothesis was an early theory that proposed that the pharmacological properties of alcohol disrupt brain centers that maintain inhibitory control over behavior (Cherek 1981). While this hypothesis serves as a good building block, it is not sufficient to explain why disinhibited individuals act aggressively (as opposed to acting in other disinhibited ways), and it must be combined with other social models to more accurately describe alcohol-induced aggression. A recent review by Giancola (2015) states that a combination of models, rather than any single model or executive function component, is necessary to provide a theoretical framework for alcohol-induced aggression.

Comorbidity

Alcohol use disorders are comorbid with many disorders that are also associated with increased aggression. These include mood, anxiety, trauma-related, other substance use, and personality disorders, among others (see relevant chapters in this volume). Psychopathic personality is especially notable in this regard because there is a high incidence of alcohol and drug abuse among psychopaths and because there appear to be significant differences in the way alcohol affects these individuals (Alterman and Cacciola 1991; Cao et al. 2010). Specifically, Cope et al. (2014) imaged incarcerated psychopaths with substance abuse histories to see the effect of psychopathy on neurobiological craving while viewing drug-related pictures and neutral pictures and reported inverse correlations between psychopathy and activation of many brain structures previously cited to be involved with psychopathy and craving. These included inverse correlations with 1) anterior cingulate, which is purported to be involved with cognitive control and conflict processing; 2) amygdala, which is typically activated by salient cues; and 3) nucleus accumbens, which is critical for the motivation to seek substances. Unfortunately, there was not any specific mention regarding the effects of alcohol versus other substances. However, taken collectively, the results suggest that psychopaths process substance abuse cues differently. This is consistent with observations by Cope and colleagues (2014) that psychopaths experience minimal withdrawal while incarcerated.

Psychobiology

Behavioral and Molecular Genetics

In considering the genetics of aggression, we will limit our discussion to an evolving literature identifying genetic differences between reactive aggression occurring in response to a perceived threat and proactive aggression that is driven by reward or the desire to control (Waltes et al. 2016). Twin studies provide strong evidence for a gene × environmental interaction such that reactive aggression has more contributions from family adversity, maltreatment, and so forth, whereas proactive aggression is associated with higher levels of heritability (Tuvblad and Baker 2011; Waltes et al. 2016). Genetic studies focusing on catecholamines show that the short allele of *SLC6A4* (5-HTTLPR) is associated with increased impulsive aggression in children (Beitchman et al. 2006; Davidge et al. 2004). Individuals with a history of adverse childhood trauma and L alleles of the monoamine oxidase A gene (*MAOA* L) are at increased risk of adult proactive aggression (Caspi et al. 2002; Reif et al. 2007). Changes in *MAOA* L–induced dopamine activity could contribute to reward-driven aggression and potentially alcohol consumption. It is anticipated that epigenetics is going to be increasingly important as we consider the gene × environmental interaction associated with aggression and alcohol use disorder.

Neurobiology

Nonhuman primates raised in stressful environments have decreased central serotonin metabolism that is associated with increased impulsiveness, aggression, and alcohol consumption (Higley et al. 1996). Subsequent work suggests that these alterations in serotonin metabolism are specific to one allele of the serotonin transporter gene, namely, 5-HTTLPR (Lesch et al. 1996). Only monkeys with the short allele in this study had reduced serotonin metabolism, which correlated with both increased aggression and greater alcohol consumption.

Individuals with low serotonin metabolism perceive alcohol's effects differently from others. Specifically, these individuals do not perceive the sedative effects of alcohol as strongly as their counterparts (Heinz et al. 2011). Low sedation predisposes individuals to engage in excessive drinking, because sedation serves as a signal to alert them that they have had too much to drink. Without this signal, the individual is predisposed to excessive drinking and, therefore, greater disinhibition.

Other findings support that abnormalities in serotonin function can facilitate alcohol-induced aggression. For example, low levels of the serotonin metabolite 5-hydroxyindoleacetic acid are found in the cerebrospinal fluid of individuals with early-onset alcoholism, anxiety, and impulsive aggression (Cloninger 1987; Kruesi et al. 1990). Furthermore, fluoxetine, which binds to the serotonin transporter to block transport function, has been shown to reduce anger and physical aggression in perpetrators of domestic violence with alcohol dependence (George et al. 2011).

Clinical Neuroscience

Conceptually, the symptoms and behaviors associated with acts of domestic violence can be subdivided into assessment and response components. Perpetrators have an increased sensitivity to environmental stimuli that is associated with an escalating sense of anxiety and/or fear (George et al. 2006). The response behaviors are characterized by a compulsive need for the perpetrator to "defend" himself that typically leads to verbal and/or physical aggression. The perpetrator's assessment of danger typically occurs independent of an actual physical threat posed by his or her spouse or significant other.

External stimuli, which serve to alert the animal or individual to threat, are received by the thalamus. The information is then transmitted to both the amygdala and the cortex, which together serve to evaluate the threat and initiate an appropriate response (Phelps and LeDoux 2005). The thalamic input to the amygdala allows an individual to process the threat quickly. Conditioned fear responses arise in the amygdala and can result in the activation of autonomic, behavioral, and hormonal responses (Davis et al. 1994).

In contrast to the amygdala, the polysynaptic processing of the cortex is slower but results in a more detailed evaluation of environmental stimuli. The medial and orbital areas of the prefrontal cortex provide affective and cognitive input to the sensory information (Bechara et al. 2000; Elliott et al. 2000; Ongür and Price 2000). The pathways between the orbital cortex and the amygdala integrate environmental stimuli with fear responses (Schoenbaum et al. 1998). The presence of threatening stimuli causes the amygdala to decrease the firing rate of the medial prefrontal cortex neurons (Garcia et al. 1999). Lesions to the medial prefrontal cortex impair the ability to extinguish conditioned fear responses (Morgan and LeDoux 1995; Morgan et al. 1993).

Other brain structures are critical to the processing of fear as well. In humans, the periaqueductal gray (PAG) located in the midbrain only measures approximately 14×5 mm but is critical for survival. It consists of four columns: the dorsomedial PAG (dmPAG), the dorsolateral PAG (dlPAG), the lateral PAG (lPAG) and the ventrolateral PAG (vlPAG). Pain is also registered here. The PAG has reciprocal connections to the spinal cord, prefrontal cortex, insula, hypothalamus, hippocampus, and amygdala (Coulombe et al. 2016; Linnman et al. 2012; Menant et al. 2016). The dmPAG and dlPAG innervate the sympathetic nervous system, while the vlPAG innervates the parasympathetic nervous system (Bandler et al. 2000). The strategic location of the PAG, with its connections to the thalamus (Li et al. 2014), hypothalamus (Hadjipavlou et al. 2006), and amygdala, (Johansen et al. 2010), serves to integrate emotions and behaviors (i.e., anger with fight, fear with flight, and depression with shutdown) with the autonomic, endocrine, and immune systems. The PAG's connections to the heart, lungs, gastrointestinal tract, and bladder are a critical mind-body connection for survival (Holstege 2014).

Normally, when an individual is faced with a perceived threat, cognitive processes evaluate the degree and nature of the threat in the cortex and send this information to the PAG, which then elicits a response that is commensurate with the threat (Mobbs et al. 2007). In the case of overwhelming threat, connections from the amygdala to the PAG facilitate a rapid emotional and behavioral response that occurs outside of the person's conscious awareness (Rizvi et al. 1991). Psychopathology can arise when the top-down control of the amygdala is impaired; such impairment can occur because of early life stressors and emotional trauma (Caspi et al. 2010; Fonzo et al. 2010), changes in serotonin function (Graeff and Del-Ben 2008), alcohol or drug insult (Koob and Volkow 2016), or genetic predisposition (Pezawas et al. 2005). This results in the PAG being activated inappropriately.

To explore the etiology of the heightened fear and aggressive responses evidenced by perpetrators of domestic violence, we performed fluorodeoxyglucose–positron emission tomography (FDG-PET) scans on perpetrators with alcoholism and compared them with scans from nonviolent individuals with alcohol use disorder and healthy control subjects (George et al. 2004). Results showed that perpetrators had significantly lower right hypothalamic activity. The clinical relevance of this finding is elucidated by animal studies showing that the hypothalamus, in conjunction with the PAG, is critical for the circuitry that mediates fear-induced aggression (Siegel et al. 1999).

Perpetrators also showed decreased connections between various cortical structures and the amygdala. These differences theoretically compromise the ability of the perpetrators to modulate the rapid but imprecise evaluation of environmental stimuli by the amygdala. Without cortical inhibition of the amygdala, the PAG can be activated (Gross and Canteras 2012). This provides an explanation for the perpetrators' previously described hypersensitivity to environmental stimuli; they are predisposed to conditioned fear responses, which manifest as fight behaviors (i.e., a "need" to defend themselves).

Clinical Approach and Treatment

Assessment of Aggression in Alcohol Use Disorder

In our domestic violence research, we found the Modified Overt Aggression Scale (MOAS; Coccaro et al. 1991) to be effective as a surrogate marker for anger and physical aggression. The Global Anger and Aggression (GAA) subscale score is composed of 1) subjective anger, measuring feelings of anger and annoyance, and 2) overt anger, measuring argumentativeness, shouting, loss of temper, and physical aggression. Aggression can be quantified by numerous other measures, such as the Barratt Impulsiveness Scale, Life History of Aggression, and Buss-Durkee Hostility Inventory. Alcohol use can be tracked with the Timeline Followback (Sobell and Sobell 1992).

Treatment of Aggression in Alcohol Use Disorder

Descriptive studies show that individuals with high trait anger are the most likely to exhibit alcohol-associated aggression (Parrott and Giancola 2004). Traditionally, these individuals have been treated with psychoeducation and cognitive-based therapies. However, a meta-analysis examining the results of court-mandated treatment programs for perpetrators of domestic violence showed that these programs are largely ineffective in reducing the likelihood of future violence (Feder and Wilson 2005).

Therefore, to test the potential benefit of a pharmacological intervention, we performed a 12-week double-blind, randomized, placebo-controlled study employing fluoxetine (at a dosage of up to 40 mg/day), in addition to alcohol treatment and cognitive-behavioral therapies. The GAA subscale of the MOAS was used as an outcome measure (George et al. 2011). The perpetrators who received fluoxetine showed a greater reduction in global subjective anger and global overt aggression compared with the perpetrators who received placebo. Clinical interviews with the perpetrators at the end of the study substantiated that those taking fluoxetine were less reactive to environmental stimuli and "had more time to think" before reacting. The Irritability subscale score changes were not found to be correlated with either anxiety or depression.

Clinical Vignette

AW was a 48-year-old married male with a master's degree in engineering. He reported that he had had regular childhood fights with his brothers that were so intense that his mother had to physically separate them. His father had been a strict disciplinarian who regularly beat him and his siblings. His mother also occasionally had swatted him with a stick. As an adult, he was easily frustrated with his boss, who was a "micromanager," and on occasion he lost control or overreacted to what he perceived as disparaging remarks by his boss. On his way home from work, AW frequently stopped off at the local watering hole to unwind. His wife hated his drinking because he became irritable and more unpredictable. Once home, the slightest thing, such as the dinner being a few minutes late, dirty dishes in the sink, or kids asking questions about homework, could set him off into a litany of curse words and caustic remarks. This escalated to approximately two times per week when it also progressed to pushing, shoving, punching, and hair pulling. These actions were typically followed by remorse.

Discussion of Vignette

AW's patterns of domestic aggression are not unique. Subsequent interviews with other perpetrators and their spouses provide additional information (Bitler et al. 1994; George et al. 2006). Like AW, many were exposed to violence growing up. Almost universally the perpetrators felt disrespected or belittled. These feelings were often triggered by a look, a tone of voice, or a body posture. In AW's case, his boss's micromanaging was perceived as demeaning, and it fueled feelings of incompetency. Individuals who become violent with drinking often identified feeling trapped immediately before "losing control" and becoming violent. Somatic changes typically preceded or accompanied the aggression and included increased motor activity, palpitations, shaking, sweating, and hyperventilation. At the height of activation, individuals became totally focused on the victim, and any influence of reason or sense of consequences disappeared. For some perpetrators, violence ended when they saw blood, or when they experienced a sense of release or fatigue. Following the aggressive outburst, most reported feeling extreme guilt that soon morphed into rationalization: "If you had not done that, I would not have gone off." Although loss of control was a common theme, it played a complex role in this regard. While individuals reported losing touch with reality, thereby signaling a loss of control, they also appeared to exert total control over the victim. Perplexingly, this loss of control rarely occurred outside of their home environment. In AW's case, he would show some signs of inappropriate hostility toward his boss, but it never morphed into the more extreme aggression demonstrated at home. Overall, alcohol was an inconsistent variable that made the individuals' behavior more unpredictable.

Summary

The literature provides strong evidence that alcohol can facilitate reactive aggression: thus, alcohol treatment is essential for this patient population. To better understand the interaction between alcohol and aggression, we have, in this chapter, focused on the PAG. The PAG is a midbrain structure with reciprocal connections to the spinal cord, prefrontal cortex, insula, hypothalamus, hippocampus, and amygdala. It serves as the final common pathway integrating the autonomic, endocrine, and immune systems to respond to threat and promote survival. Stimulation of specific regions of the PAG gives rise to defensive rage and predatory aggression. These forms of aggression can occur appropriately in response to a bona fide threat or, pathologically, secondarily to poor inhibitory control. Animal studies suggest that alcohol functions to facilitate defensive rage but appears to inhibit predatory aggression (Schubert et al. 1996). Since the PAG receives input from cortical as well as subcortical structures, it is likely that alcohol could also be impacting aggression at multiple sites.

Key Clinical Points

▮ Alcohol use is closely associated with violent crimes, yet most individuals with alcohol use disorder do not demonstrate excessive aggression.

▮ Individuals with alcohol use disorder may be comorbid with reactive or proactive aggression.

▮ Intoxication facilitates defensive rage while suppressing predatory aggression.

▮ Activity of the periaqueductal gray in the midbrain is closely linked to both reactive and proactive aggression.

▮ Short- and long-term alcohol-induced disruptions in cortical and limbic brain activity may result in diminished executive function and increased emotional liability, both of which can facilitate aggression.

▮ Fluoxetine combined with alcohol treatment and cognitive-behavioral therapy reduces reactive aggression.

References

Alterman AI, Cacciola JS: The antisocial personality disorder diagnosis in substance abusers: problems and issues. J Nerv Ment Dis 179(7):401–409, 1991 1869868

Bandler R, Keay KA, Floyd N, et al: Central circuits mediating patterned autonomic activity during active vs. passive emotional coping. Brain Res Bull 53(1):95–104, 2000 11033213

Bartholow BD, Heinz A: Alcohol and aggression without consumption. Alcohol cues, aggressive thoughts, and hostile perception bias. Psychol Sci 17(1):30–37, 2006 16371141

Bechara A, Damasio H, Damasio AR: Emotion, decision making and the orbitofrontal cortex. Cereb Cortex 10(3):295–307, 2000 10731224

Beck A, Heinz A: Alcohol-related aggression—social and neurobiological factors. Dtsch Arztebl Int 110(42):711–715, 2013 24223671

Beitchman JH, Baldassarra L, Mik H, et al: Serotonin transporter polymorphisms and persistent, pervasive childhood aggression. Am J Psychiatry 163(6):1103–1105, 2006 16741214

Bitler DA, Linnoila M, George DT: Psychosocial and diagnostic characteristics of individuals initiating domestic violence. J Nerv Ment Dis 182(10):583–585, 1994 7931207

Bushman BJ, Cooper HM: Effects of alcohol on human aggression: an integrative research review. Psychol Bull 107(3):341–354, 1990 2140902

Buss AH: The Psychology of Aggression. New York, Wiley, 1961

Cao JL, Covington HE 3rd, Friedman AK, et al: Mesolimbic dopamine neurons in the brain reward circuit mediate susceptibility to social defeat and antidepressant action. J Neurosci 30(49):16453–16458, 2010 21147984

Caspi A, McClay J, Moffitt TE, et al: Role of genotype in the cycle of violence in maltreated children. Science 297(5582):851–854, 2002 12161658

Caspi A, Hariri AR, Holmes A, et al: Genetic sensitivity to the environment: the case of the serotonin transporter gene and its implications for studying complex diseases and traits. Am J Psychiatry 167(5):509–527, 2010 20231323

Cherek DR: Effects of smoking different doses of nicotine on human aggressive behavior. Psychopharmacology (Berl) 75(4):339–345, 1981 6803276

Chermack ST, Taylor SP: Alcohol and human physical aggression: pharmacological versus expectancy effects. J Stud Alcohol 56(4):449–456, 1995 7674681

Cloninger CR: Neurogenetic adaptive mechanisms in alcoholism. Science 236(4800):410–416, 1987 2882604

Coccaro EF, Harvey PD, Kupsaw-Lawrence E, et al: Development of neuropharmacologically based behavioral assessments of impulsive aggressive behavior. J Neuropsychiatry Clin Neurosci 3(2):S44–S51, 1991 1821222

Cope LM, Vincent GM, Jobelius JL, et al: Psychopathic traits modulate brain responses to drug cues in incarcerated offenders. Front Hum Neurosci 8:87, 2014 24605095

Coulombe MA, Erpelding N, Kucyi A, et al: Intrinsic functional connectivity of periaqueductal gray subregions in humans. Hum Brain Mapp 37(4):1514–1530, 2016 26821847

Davidge KM, Atkinson L, Douglas L, et al: Association of the serotonin transporter and 5HT1Dbeta receptor genes with extreme, persistent and pervasive aggressive behaviour in children. Psychiatr Genet 14(3):143–146, 2004 15318027

Davis M, Rainnie D, Cassell M: Neurotransmission in the rat amygdala related to fear and anxiety. Trends Neurosci 17(5):208–214, 1994 7520203

Elliott R, Dolan RJ, Frith CD: Dissociable functions in the medial and lateral orbitofrontal cortex: evidence from human neuroimaging studies. Cereb Cortex 10(3):308–317, 2000 10731225

Feder L, Wilson DB: A meta-analytic review of court-mandated batterer intervention programs: can courts affect abusers' behavior? J Exp Criminol 1:239–262, 2005

Fonzo GA, Simmons AN, Thorp SR, et al: Exaggerated and disconnected insular-amygdalar blood oxygenation level-dependent response to threat-related emotional faces in women with intimate-partner violence post-traumatic stress disorder. Biol Psychiatry 68(5):433–441, 2010 20573339

Garcia R, Vouimba RM, Baudry M, et al: The amygdala modulates prefrontal cortex activity relative to conditioned fear. Nature 402(6759):294–296, 1999 10580500

George DT, Rawlings RR, Williams WA, et al: A select group of perpetrators of domestic violence: evidence of decreased metabolism in the right hypothalamus and reduced relationships between cortical/subcortical brain structures in position emission tomography. Psychiatry Res 130(1):11–25, 2004 14972365

George DT, Phillips MJ, Doty L, et al: A model linking biology, behavior and psychiatric diagnoses in perpetrators of domestic violence. Med Hypotheses 67(2):345–353, 2006 16580153

George DT, Phillips MJ, Lifshitz M, et al: Fluoxetine treatment of alcoholic perpetrators of domestic violence: a 12-week, double-blind, randomized, placebo-controlled intervention study. J Clin Psychiatry 72(1):60–65, 2011 20673556

Giancola PR: Development and evaluation of theories of alcohol-related violence: covering a 40-year span. Subst Use Misuse 50(8–9):1182–1187, 2015 26361926

Giancola PR, Helton EL, Osborne AB, et al: The effects of alcohol and provocation on aggressive behavior in men and women. J Stud Alcohol 63(1):64–73, 2002 11925061

Gorney B: Domestic violence and chemical dependency: dual problems, dual interventions. J Psychoactive Drugs 21(2):229–238, 1989 2668487

Graeff FG, Del-Ben CM: Neurobiology of panic disorder: from animal models to brain neuroimaging. Neurosci Biobehav Rev 32(7):1326–1335, 2008 18573531

Gross CT, Canteras NS: The many paths to fear. Nat Rev Neurosci 13(9):651–658, 2012 22850830

Hadjipavlou G, Dunckley P, Behrens TE, et al: Determining anatomical connectivities between cortical and brainstem pain processing regions in humans: a diffusion tensor imaging study in healthy controls. Pain 123(1–2):169–178, 2006 16616418

Heinz AJ, Beck A, Meyer-Lindenberg A, et al: Cognitive and neurobiological mechanisms of alcohol-related aggression. Nat Rev Neurosci 12(7):400–413, 2011 21633380

Higley JD, Suomi SJ, Linnoila M: A nonhuman primate model of type II alcoholism? Part 2. Diminished social competence and excessive aggression correlates with low cerebrospinal fluid 5-hydroxyindoleacetic acid concentrations. Alcohol Clin Exp Res 20(4):643–650, 1996 8800379

Holstege G: The periaqueductal gray controls brainstem emotional motor systems including respiration. Prog Brain Res 209:379–405, 2014 24746059

Hull JG: A self-awareness model of the causes and effects of alcohol consumption. J Abnorm Psychol 90(6):586–600, 1981 7320328

Johansen JP, Tarpley JW, LeDoux JE, et al: Neural substrates for expectation-modulated fear learning in the amygdala and periaqueductal gray. Nat Neurosci 13(8):979–986, 2010 20601946

Koenigs M: The role of prefrontal cortex in psychopathy. Rev Neurosci 23(3):253–262, 2012 22752782

Koob GF, Volkow ND: Neurobiology of addiction: a neurocircuitry analysis. Lancet Psychiatry 3(8):760–773, 2016 27475769

Kruesi MJ, Rapoport JL, Hamburger S, et al: Cerebrospinal fluid monoamine metabolites, aggression, and impulsivity in disruptive behavior disorders of children and adolescents. Arch Gen Psychiatry 47(5):419–426, 1990 1691910

Lang AR, Goeckner DJ, Adesso VJ, et al: Effects of alcohol on aggression in male social drinkers. J Abnorm Psychol 84(5):508–518, 1975 1194512

Lesch KP, Bengel D, Heils A, et al: Association of anxiety-related traits with a polymorphism in the serotonin transporter gene regulatory region. Science 274(5292):1527–1531, 1996 8929413

Li S, Shi Y, Kirouac GJ: The hypothalamus and periaqueductal gray are the sources of dopamine fibers in the paraventricular nucleus of the thalamus in the rat. Front Neuroanat 8:136, 2014 25477789

Linnman C, Moulton EA, Barmettler G, et al: Neuroimaging of the periaqueductal gray: state of the field. Neuroimage 60(1):505–522, 2012 22197740

McMurran M, Jinks M, Howells K, et al: Alcohol-related violence defined by ultimate goals: a qualitative analysis of the features of three different types of violence by intoxicated young male offenders. Aggress Behav 36(1):67–79, 2010 19890905

Menant O, Andersson F, Zelena D, et al: The benefits of magnetic resonance imaging methods to extend the knowledge of the anatomical organisation of the periaqueductal gray in mammals. J Chem Neuroanat 77:110–120, 2016 27344962

Mobbs D, Petrovic P, Marchant JL, et al: When fear is near: threat imminence elicits prefrontal-periaqueductal gray shifts in humans. Science 317(5841):1079–1083, 2007 17717184

Morgan MA, LeDoux JE: Differential contribution of dorsal and ventral medial prefrontal cortex to the acquisition and extinction of conditioned fear in rats. Behav Neurosci 109(4):681–688, 1995 7576212

Morgan MA, Romanski LM, LeDoux JE: Extinction of emotional learning: contribution of medial prefrontal cortex. Neurosci Lett 163(1):109–113, 1993 8295722

Murdoch D, Pihl RO, Ross D: Alcohol and crimes of violence: present issues. Int J Addict 25(9):1065–1081, 1990 2090635

Ongür D, Price JL: The organization of networks within the orbital and medial prefrontal cortex of rats, monkeys and humans. Cereb Cortex 10(3):206–219, 2000 10731217

Parrott DJ, Giancola PR: A further examination of the relation between trait anger and alcohol-related aggression: the role of anger control. Alcohol Clin Exp Res 28(6):855–864, 2004 15201628

Pernanen K: Alcohol and Crimes of Violence. New York, Plenum, 1976

Pernanen K: Alcohol in Human Violence. New York, Guilford, 1991

Pezawas L, Meyer-Lindenberg A, Drabant EM, et al: 5-HTTLPR polymorphism impacts human cingulate-amygdala interactions: a genetic susceptibility mechanism for depression. Nat Neurosci 8(6):828–834, 2005 15880108

Phelps EA, LeDoux JE: Contributions of the amygdala to emotion processing: from animal models to human behavior. Neuron 48(2):175–187, 2005 16242399

Pihl RO, Peterson JB, Lau MA: A biosocial model of the alcohol-aggression relationship. J Stud Alcohol Suppl 11:128–139, 1993 8410954

Reif A, Rösler M, Freitag CM, et al: Nature and nurture predispose to violent behavior: serotonergic genes and adverse childhood environment. Neuropsychopharmacology 32(11):2375–2383, 2007 17342170

Rizvi TA, Ennis M, Behbehani MM, et al: Connections between the central nucleus of the amygdala and the midbrain periaqueductal gray: topography and reciprocity. J Comp Neurol 303(1):121–131, 1991 1706363

Schoenbaum G, Chiba AA, Gallagher M: Orbitofrontal cortex and basolateral amygdala encode expected outcomes during learning. Nat Neurosci 1(2):155–159, 1998 10195132

Schubert K, Shaikh MB, Han Y, et al: Differential effects of ethanol on feline rage and predatory attack behavior: an underlying neural mechanism. Alcohol Clin Exp Res 20(5):882–889, 1996 8865964

Siegel A, Roeling TA, Gregg TR, et al: Neuropharmacology of brain-stimulation-evoked aggression. Neurosci Biobehav Rev 23(3):359–389, 1999 9989425

Sobell LC, Sobell MB: Timeline follow-back: a technique for assessing self-reported ethanol consumption, in Measuring Alcohol Consumption: Psychosocial and Biochemical Methods. Edited by Allen J, Litten R. Totowa, NJ, Humana Press, 1992, pp 41–72

Steele CM, Josephs RA: Alcohol myopia. Its prized and dangerous effects. Am Psychol 45(8):921–933, 1990 2221564

Taylor SP: Experimental investigation of alcohol-induced aggression in humans. Alcohol Health Res World 17:108–112, 1993

Taylor SP, Leonard KE: Alcohol and Human Aggression. New York, Academic Press, 1983

Tessner KD, Hill SY: Neural circuitry associated with risk for alcohol use disorders. Neuropsychol Rev 20(1):1–20, 2010 19685291

Tuvblad C, Baker LA: Human aggression across the lifespan: genetic propensities and environmental moderators. Adv Genet 75:171–214, 2011 22078481

Waltes R, Chiocchetti AG, Freitag CM: The neurobiological basis of human aggression: A review on genetic and epigenetic mechanisms. Am J Med Genet B Neuropsychiatr Genet 171(5):650–675, 2016 26494515

World Health Organization: WHO Expert Committee on Problems Related to Alcohol Consumption. Second Report. Geneva, World Health Organization, 2007

13

Aggression in Substance Use Disorders

Rachel L. Gunn, Ph.D.
Kyle R. Gerst, M.Sc.
Daniel J. Fridberg, Ph.D.

Considerable literature suggests that substance use and misuse are associated with aggressive behavior (e.g., Beck et al. 2014; Boles and Miotto 2003; Hoaken and Stewart 2003). Specifically, individuals with a substance use disorder (SUD) are at an increased risk of being the perpetrator or victim of interpersonal violence, including intimate partner violence (Boles and Miotto 2003; Chermack et al. 2008; Low et al. 2016; Moore et al. 2008; Teten et al. 2009). Among family members supporting an individual with substance misuse, approximately 70% report family aggression and/or violence related to the substance use (McCann et al. 2017). Therefore, understanding the association between substance misuse and aggression has considerable importance in terms of both clinical practice and public health.

Although there is substantial evidence demonstrating a link between aggressive behavior and SUD, the mechanisms underlying this association are complex. Whereas multiple studies have documented the association between acute alcohol intoxication and aggressive or violent behavior (Duke et al. 2011; Pihl and Sutton 2009), relatively less work has focused on potential associations between misuse of other substances and aggression. In this chapter, we review the existing literature on the associations between substance misuse (excluding alcohol) and aggression. Specifically, we provide an overview of the psychological and neurobiological factors believed to account for these complex associations. We also discuss clinical approaches to treating patients with SUD and aggression to guide practitioners in better understanding and treating these problems. Of note, for the purposes of this review, we use the term *aggression* to refer to the broad class of hostile or violent verbal or physical behavior directed toward another individual. In contrast, we use the term *violence* to refer specifically to the subset of aggressive behaviors that result in physical harm (e.g., assault) (Anderson and Bushman 2002).

Phenomenology

Direct Links Between Substance Misuse and Aggression

Researchers have devised theoretical models to account for the co-occurrence of SUD and aggression. Regarding the associations between SUD and violent behavior specifically, Goldstein (1985) proposed three types of violence associated with substance misuse (see also Boles and Miotto 2003): psychopharmacological violence, systemic violence, and economic compulsive violence. *Psychopharmacological violence* results from acute or long-term effects of substance intoxication on the cognitive functions associated with behavioral control (e.g., impulsive disinhibition) and is most readily associated with stimulant (e.g., cocaine and amphetamines), phencyclidine (PCP), and benzodiazepine misuse. In contrast, Goldstein (1985) proposed that acute intoxication from use of other drugs, such as heroin or tranquilizers, may attenuate aggressive or violent behavior because of the sedating effects of those substances. *Systemic violence* is characterized by patterns of aggression or violent behavior that result from interactions within the system of illicit drug distribution and is most commonly associated with amphetamine and cocaine use. According to this theory, involvement in drug distribution as either a dealer or a user puts one at greater risk for being a victim or perpetrator of violence. Examples of systemic violence include violence resulting from rivalry between drug dealers, as a way of enforcing hierarchy within a drug distribution organization, or as a means of collecting payment from users. Last, *economic compulsive violence* is characterized by violence perpetrated by individuals with a SUD on others in order to acquire substances and is most commonly associated with heroin and cocaine because of their high economic value (Goldstein 1985). In sum, this model highlights the associations between substance misuse and violent aggression and has informed later laboratory studies examining causal associations between chronic or acute substance use and aggressive behavior.

Although significant scientific literature has investigated the association between alcohol use and aggression in the laboratory (see Tomlinson et al. 2016 for review), significantly less work has examined the putative causal association between illicit substance intoxication and aggressive behavior. The theory accounting for this association suggests that acute intoxication causes disinhibited behavior generally, including hostile, violent aggression (Boles and Miotto 2003; Hoaken and Stewart 2003). While a few laboratory studies have found evidence for a link between acute intoxication and aggressive behavior, results are inconsistent and vary across substances. Many laboratory studies involve use of laboratory behavioral paradigms such as the Taylor Aggression Paradigm (TAP; Taylor 1967). In the TAP, the participant competes in a reaction time task against a fictional "opponent" who "provokes" the participant by delivering the highest-level (i.e., most painful) finger shocks to the participant on those trials in which the participant's response time is deemed to be slower than that of the "opponent." Unbeknownst to the participant, the shocks delivered by the "opponent" are manipulated by the experimenter to lead the participant to believe that their opponent is delivering the most painful shock available. Aggression is measured in this task by the intensity of the shock the participant delivers in response on trials they "win"; higher shocks reflect more aggressive behavior. The TAP and similar protocols have been used frequently and shown to successfully elicit aggressive responding in laboratory studies (see, e.g., Giancola et al. 1998).

Among studies of the effects of stimulant intoxication on aggression, only one placebo-controlled study has demonstrated a dose-related effect of cocaine on aggressive behavior on the TAP in humans (Licata et al. 1993). In this study, 30 male undergraduate students received either a high dose (2 mg) or low dose (1 mg) of orally administered cocaine, or placebo. Participants in the high-dose condition exhibited more aggressive responding on the TAP relative to those in the low-dose and placebo groups (Licata et al. 1993). Studies examining the association between methamphetamine administration and aggressive behavior have produced mixed results in mice (Crowley 1972; Miczek and O'Donnell 1978), nonhuman primates (Smith and Byrd 1984, 1985), and humans (Cherek et al. 1986, 1987, 1990). In humans, Cherek and colleagues (1986) found increased aggressive responding on a variant of the TAP in subjects administered doses of 5 and 10 mg D-amphetamine, relative to a 20-mg dose and placebo. Of note, these results were not replicated in follow-up studies by the same group (Cherek et al. 1987, 1990), and research in children with attention-deficit/hyperactivity disorder has shown that D-amphetamine can effectively reduce aggressive behavior in that group (Connor and Steingard 1996).

Regarding opiates, limited evidence suggests that morphine (Berman et al. 1993) and codeine (Spiga et al. 1990) acutely increase aggressive responding on variants of the TAP. However, studies in mice have found contradictory findings, with morphine administration reducing aggressive behavior (Espert et al. 1993; Haney and Miczek 1989). Last, there is no evidence to date to suggest that cannabis intoxication increases aggression, and some studies have reported decreased aggressive behavior following administration of liquid tetrahydrocannabinol, the primary psychoactive constituent of cannabis (Myerscough and Taylor 1985; Taylor et al. 1976).

Overall, laboratory studies do not suggest a robust causal association between acute use of stimulants, opioids, or cannabis and aggressive behavior. More recent work has proposed that the high co-occurrence between substance misuse and aggression may reflect shared psychological mechanisms rather than a direct causal association per se.

Models of Co-occurring Substance Use Disorders and Aggressive Behavior

Before we discuss the putative common etiological factors underlying SUD and co-occurring aggression, it is first important to review the distinct types of aggression described in the literature. Aggression research distinguishes between instrumental aggression and hostile aggression. *Instrumental aggression* refers to aggressive behavior that derives from premeditated and goal-directed action. In contrast, *hostile aggression* refers to aggressive behavior that is reactive and emotion driven (Anderson and Bushman 2002; Polman et al. 2007). This type of impulsive aggression is characterized by rash action without consideration of future consequences, and parallels the impulsive behavior characteristic of SUD, such as the decision to use substances for their short-term hedonic effects despite negative long-term consequences (Bechara 2005). A shared mechanism of poor impulse control may link SUD and aggressive behavior and has been the primary focus of research in this field (Brady et al. 1998).

A parallel classification can be drawn in considering proactive versus reactive aggression. *Proactive aggression* is goal oriented, premeditated, and motivated by an external stimulus (e.g., gaining control over another individual), while *reactive aggression* occurs in response to behavior that is perceived as threatening (Barratt et al. 1997; Cornell et al. 1996; Dodge and Coie 1987). Proactive aggression as it relates to antisocial personality traits is implicated in models of externalizing psychopathology that suggest similar etiology with SUD (Krueger et al. 2002). Research showing that proactive aggression in childhood predicts adult substance misuse reflects this notion (Moffitt 1993). Comparatively, reactive aggression may relate to substance misuse via poor self-control (i.e., difficulty inhibiting impulsive behavior) (Caspi et al. 1996; Finn et al. 2000, 2002).

There is little research further examining causal factors contributing to the high co-occurrence of aggressive behavior and SUD specifically. One study by Fite and colleagues (2007) sought to explain the unique risk pathways between proactive and reactive aggression and substance misuse via social variables in a longitudinal study of an aggressive adolescent population. They found that both types of aggression were indirectly associated with substance misuse. Proactive aggression was indirectly associated with substance misuse through peer delinquency, where reactive aggression exhibited the same mediational pathway, but only among individuals who experienced high levels of peer rejection (Fite et al. 2007). These findings suggest that although both types of aggression are associated with substance misuse, their pathways are unique and strongly related to social (i.e., peer delinquency) variables. Future research should examine other mediating variables that further explain the association between aggression and SUD.

Models of externalizing psychopathology suggest the co-occurrence of SUD and aggression may reflect shared genetic and/or environmental factors (Krueger et al. 2007). Impulsivity or behavioral disinhibition is one factor common to multiple forms of externalizing psychopathology that may confer risk for both substance misuse and aggression. Impulsivity has long been identified as a risk factor for substance misuse and SUD (see de Wit 2009 for review). Additionally, impulsivity has been found to be an important personality trait predicting aggression across multiple diverse samples (Derefinko et al. 2011; Lynam and Miller 2004; Miller et al. 2003). Therefore, comorbid aggression and SUD may represent a shared deficit in impulse control, or a tendency to focus on the potential immediate (i.e., more salient) benefit of the aggressive behavior rather than on the long-term consequences of that behavior (e.g., injury or legal consequences). Models of externalizing psychopathology, which encompasses both antisocial personality and substance use disorders, suggest impulsivity as a core underlying mechanism of these frequently co-occurring problems (see Bogg and Finn 2010; Krueger and Markon 2006).

Other studies have examined the temporal association between comorbid SUD and impulsive aggression. In two well-powered studies, Coccaro and colleagues (2016, 2017) observed that individuals with a prior history of intermittent explosive disorder (IED), a psychiatric disorder characterized by frequent episodes of impulsive aggressive behavior (American Psychiatric Association 2013), showed significantly higher rates of SUD later in life, relative to individuals without a history of IED. Results from this study suggest that aggressive behavior precedes and may be a risk factor for the development of future SUD. Additionally, some evidence suggests that polydrug users report more aggressive behavior than do monodrug users (Steele and Peralta 2017). Thus, the number of substances used (i.e, polydrug versus monodrug) may be an important consideration in the development and implementation of prevention, intervention, and treatment approaches for aggression in the context of substance misuse.

Psychobiology

Studies in both humans and animals suggest that aggressive behavior and substance misuse may reflect common neurobiological factors. The serotonergic and dopaminergic systems have been implicated in the reinforcing effects of substances of abuse and the development of addiction (Nordahl et al. 2003; Volkow et al. 1999, 2004), as well as in the modulation of impulsive aggressive behavior (Berman et al. 1997; Coccaro et al. 1997; Siegel and Schubert 1995; Yanowitch and Coccaro 2011). For example, there is a consistent association between serotonergic hypofunction and impulsive forms of aggression in both human and nonhuman samples (Coccaro et al. 2009; Ferrari et al. 2003; Ferris et al. 1999; Higley et al. 1992; Kyes et al. 1995; Miczek et al. 1994; Westergaard et al. 2003). In contrast, it is increased dopamine activity in the nucleus accumbens (NAc) that is associated with increased impulsive aggression in rats (van Erp and Miczek 2000), with administration of a dopamine receptor antagonist into the NAc significantly reducing aggressive responding compared with administration outside of boundaries of the NAc (Couppis and Kennedy 2008). The authors interpreted these findings to suggest that dopaminergic activity in the NAc is involved in the rewarding properties of aggression.

There is considerable evidence that genetic factors contribute to both impulsive aggression and risk for substance misuse as well. Berggård and colleagues (2003) found associations between low levels of a polymorphism of the serotonin receptor gene *5-HT2A* (–1438 GG) and violent criminal behavior. Similar associations were found in separate studies of two other serotonin-related gene polymorphisms and aggression-related outcomes: violent suicide (Courtet et al. 2001), and anger-related traits and aggression (Manuck et al. 1999; Rujescu et al. 2002). Genetic factors may also play a key role in substance-induced effects via alterations of pharmacodynamics and pharmacokinetics of the substance (Kreek et al. 2005). Furthermore, using established models of drug addiction, Golden and colleagues (2017) observed "addiction-like" aggressive behavior in a subpopulation of CD-1 mice, including high motivation to seek aggressive encounters despite consequences, and increased rates of recidivism (i.e., relapse to aggression-seeking behavior). Taken together, these studies suggest that reward pathways similar to those implicated in the development of SUD are implicated in the expression of aggressive behavior as well. This similarity further points to common etiological factors underlying comorbid SUD and aggression.

Clinical Approach and Treatment

Several studies suggest that patients with SUD self-report high rates of violence, as both perpetrators and victims (Macdonald et al. 2003, 2008). Associated psychosocial consequences (e.g., complex legal or interpersonal difficulties) pose a unique set of challenges for clinicians and complicate treatment delivery. Patients who report impulsive aggression contributing to psychosocial problems should be evaluated for IED. Recent data showing that IED precedes SUD in 80% of comorbid cases suggest that early intervention for IED may aid in preventing the development of SUD (Coccaro et al. 2016, 2017).

To date, there is minimal literature regarding the treatment of comorbid impulsive aggression and SUD, and no randomized controlled trials for the treatment of comorbid IED and SUD have been conducted as of the time of this writing. However, several studies have demonstrated support for the efficacy and effectiveness of treatment for IED and SUD independently, which can assist treatment planning (e.g., McCloskey et al. 2008; McHugh et al. 2010. Additionally, as with treating all comorbidities, it is important to consider the severity of presenting problems when making treatment decisions. For example, if a patient presents with a severe SUD resulting in difficulty arriving sober for treatment sessions or with serious withdrawal symptoms requiring inpatient detoxification, treatment for IED symptoms is unlikely to be effective before the SUD is effectively treated. It is imperative that clinicians collaboratively discuss presenting problems with patients to identify those symptoms causing the most distress before choosing an integrative treatment approach.

Psychopharmacological Treatment

There are no currently approved psychopharmacological treatments for patients with comorbid IED and SUD. However, clinical trials have demonstrated the efficacy of psychopharmacological agents to treat IED and SUD independently. Double-blind, placebo-controlled trials have shown that fluoxetine 20–40 mg/day reduces various forms of impulsive aggression relative to placebo in patients with symptoms meeting diagnostic criteria for IED (Coccaro et al. 2009), personality disorder (Silva et al. 2010), and alcohol use disorder (George et al. 2011). Divalproex at 500 mg twice daily, with the dosage increased by 250 mg after 3–7 days, has also been found to reduce impulsive aggression in patients with IED and comorbid Cluster B personality traits (Hollander et al. 2003). Regarding SUD, there is robust evidence for the efficacy of agonist replacement therapies, such as methadone and buprenorphine for heroin and other opiates, as well as nicotine for tobacco (Gonzalez et al. 2004; O'Malley and Kosten 2006). Additionally, drugs that inhibit a substance's reinforcing effects via the dopamine system, such as disulfiram for cocaine use disorder, have shown promise (Carroll et al. 2004; Schottenfeld et al. 2014).

There is some minimal evidence for integrative psychopharmacology for comorbid aggression and SUD. For instance, anticonvulsant and selective serotonin reuptake inhibitors have shown promise in the independent treatment of both impulsive and aggressive behaviors and SUD, compared with placebo (Brady et al. 1998). Additionally, given that the mood instability that is associated with withdrawal can be a significant contributor to the acute aggressive episodes associated with SUD (Boles and Miotto 2003), there is some evidence that opiate replacement therapies have also been effective in attenuating aggression via reduction in withdrawal symptoms among individuals with opioid use disorder (Doran et al. 2012). Additional research is needed to identify effective pharmacotherapy for the comorbid SUD and aggression.

Psychotherapy

Research evidence has supported integrative treatment models for SUD and comorbid psychiatric conditions (Mueser et al. 2006). Much of the empirical support for this approach comes from studies of persons with severe mental illness, and additional research on psychotherapeutic treatment for SUD and other common comorbid disorders, such as IED, is needed. Indeed, there have been no randomized controlled trials of behavioral therapies for comorbid SUD and impulsive aggression as of this writing. However, there are well-established psychotherapeutic interventions for both diagnoses that may be useful in guiding treatment planning for patients with both disorders.

Several meta-analyses have suggested cognitive-behavioral therapy (CBT) can be helpful in treating impulsive aggression as it occurs in the context of diverse psychiatric conditions (Beck and Fernandez 1998; Del Vecchio and O'Leary 2004; DiGiuseppe and Tafrate 2003; Edmondson and Conger 1996). Although treatment of anger and aggression could be considered conceptually similar, there is less research support for protocols aimed at reducing aggression specifically, especially in the context of IED. In a randomized controlled trial, CBT was found to reduce aggression, anger, hostile thinking, and depressive symptoms in individuals with IED, relative to wait-list control subjects. These effects were maintained at 3-month follow-up and did not differ based on whether treatment was delivered via group or individually (McCloskey et al. 2008). There is also significant evidence for the use of CBT for SUD (McHugh et al. 2010). Furthermore, there are other evidence-based treatments for SUD with good empirical support, including 12-step facilitation, motivational interviewing, and contingency management (Carroll and Rounsaville 2006). Note, however, that these interventions are intended to treat SUD and may not address aggression specifically.

Regarding current established integrative treatments for SUD and aggression, the Substance Abuse and Mental Health Services Administration has developed a protocol to address co-occurring substance misuse and excessive or inappropriate anger (Reilly and Shopshire 2002). Although the efficacy and effectiveness of this protocol have not been evaluated within the context of a randomized control trial, its format and content resemble those of evidence-based CBT approaches, and it may be delivered in a group or individual setting. In addition, some work has adapted motivational enhancement therapy, originally developed to treat SUD, to target aggression in persons with SUD. One study examining the efficacy of motivational enhancement among domestic violence offenders (approximately 50% of whom had clinical presentation that met criteria for SUD) found that it was effective in increasing readiness to change substance misuse in this group (Easton et al. 2000). This study provides initial evidence for the feasibility of motivational enhancement strategies among populations with SUD and history of violent aggression. A review of evidence-based treatments for SUD and aggression among adolescents confirms that these standard treatments—motivational enhancement, contingency management, and CBT—are all promising models of treating this comorbidity (Doran et al. 2012). Mindfulness-based treatments for SUD and aggression are another area of potential development. One study suggests that trait mindfulness is negatively associated with aggression among SUD treatment-seeking individuals (Shorey et al. 2015). These data suggest that mindfulness-based interventions may be an effective area for intervention in reducing aggression among individuals seeking treatment for SUD.

Clinical Vignette

DN was a 64-year-old white male who presented to a hospital-based outpatient substance use clinic. His chief complaint was "anger and frustration in relationships and having cravings." DN had a psychiatric history significant for cocaine use disorder and alcohol use disorder, both in remission, and antisocial personality features. He had grown up witnessing significant domestic violence perpetrated against his mother by his father. At the time of treatment, he was on parole for armed robbery and assault, for which he had served a reduced sentence of 15 years. DN completed 2 years of group psychotherapy for SUD at the clinic and then enrolled in a group treatment for anger management. During the course of the treatment protocol, he became engaged in a series of verbal altercations with patients and clinic staff, at which point staff transferred him to an individual provider for treatment of anger and ongoing relapse prevention. The initial treatment plan included CBT for SUD and anger (Reilly and Shopshire 2002). DN reported abstinence from cocaine and alcohol since being released from prison. His initial treatment goals were maintaining abstinence from cocaine and alcohol and managing anger to prevent verbal and physical aggression in the personal and professional relationships in his life.

Early assessment and case conceptualization revealed that DN suffered significantly from impulse-control problems that likely contributed to his history of SUD and violent aggression. For example, DN's temper and verbal expression of anger quickly escalated when the clinician set boundaries in session regarding appropriate topics for discussion. Developing and maintaining rapport was a challenge as well, as DN's antisocial personality features contributed to frequently externalizing blame for his problems and attempting to control the session by discussing topics previously agreed to be outside the focus of treatment. His difficulty regulating his anger also became readily apparent in discussion of the interpersonal experiences in his life. For example, he had significant difficulty interacting with his parole officer, who he believed was actively seeking reasons to place DN back in custody. His rigidity made it difficult to challenge this cognitive belief and focus on improving his relationships. Challenging statements by the clinician were met with significant opposition and at least one rapport rupture. DN's aggressive behavior in session posed an additional challenge for the clinician. He would often pace around the office, shout, and occasionally express his anger by pounding his fist on the desk, which the clinician found threatening.

DN was able to make progress over 10 sessions with increased rapport and more careful and subtle challenging of his assumptions and beliefs by the clinician. The use of several shared themes between behavioral treatment for SUD and anger treatment helped to create a synchronous treatment plan for both presenting problems. For example, DN benefited from learning and understanding the function of environmental and emotional stimuli (i.e., "triggers") that elicited urges to act out aggressively or use substances, using behavioral coping strategies to manage urges to engage in those behaviors, and cognitive restructuring of anger and substance-related thoughts. DN agreed to weekly practice exercises focused on improving his ability to cope effectively with urges to act aggressively or use substances, and noted that this was helpful in reducing the frequency and intensity of those urges as well as the incidence of aggressive outbursts. DN and the clinician worked together to develop a relapse prevention plan for both anger and substance use that involved anticipating situations that might increase anxiety (which DN identified as a significant trigger for his aggression and substance use), practicing self-care (e.g., exercise) regularly, and filling free time with positive social interactions.

By the end of treatment, DN was able to identify major triggers for aggression and substance use as well as strategies to cope effectively with those stimuli without engaging in problem behaviors. He discussed the frustration, anger, and helplessness he felt as a child while observing the physical abuse of his mother by his father. DN stated his belief that he used substances to "numb" and distract himself from these unpleasant memories and subsequent anger. He benefited greatly from cognitive restructuring focused on challenging his maladaptive beliefs about the utility of using substances to manage negative emotional states, including anger, and from behavioral strategies to manage anger, including diaphragmatic breathing, guided relaxation, and regular cardiovascular exercise. At termination, DN reported reduced anger and aggression, reduced anxiety, improved sleep, reduced cravings, and improved interpersonal relationships, including the initiation of a romantic relationship.

Discussion of Vignette

This case vignette illustrates several important principles to consider when treating individuals with comorbid aggression and SUD. First, setting clear boundaries is important to ensure a safe environment for both clinician and patient. Second, understanding common etiological factors underlying both aggression and substance misuse can increase effectiveness of treatment and streamline care for the patient. Last, implementing tailored behavioral and cognitive skills training can be helpful for reducing aggressive behavior and preventing relapse to substance use (e.g. using deep breathing to manage both cravings and anger caused by known triggers).

Summary

Treating patients with comorbid aggression and SUD presents significant challenges, and aggression is associated with poor treatment outcomes among patients with SUD (Crowley et al. 1998a, 1998b). As reviewed in this chapter, research examining the comorbidity of SUD and aggression points to shared factors that contribute to the development of both problems, including an impulsive or disinhibited personality type. These findings suggest that each of these problems may benefit from a similar treatment approach, but evidence-based treatments for comorbid SUD and aggression are not well established as of this writing, and more research is needed.

Key Clinical Points

▮ When treating patients with comorbid aggression and substance use disorder (SUD), clinicians should remain mindful of risk factors and safety precautions standard for treating any patient, including but not limited to:

　▮ Implementing workplace safeguards (e.g., panic buttons, having other staff present in the office when seeing patients).

▌ Evaluating patients with SUD for potential withdrawal symptoms. Patients who present to treatment with a history of dependence on substances with the potential for a fatal withdrawal syndrome (e.g., benzodiazepines, alcohol) should be evaluated by a medical professional to determine the need for detoxification prior to treatment.

▌ Cognitive-behavioral therapy holds promise as a treatment for comorbid aggression and SUD, but more research on the effectiveness of this approach in this population is needed.

▌ As with all patients with complex presentations, treatment planning for patients with comorbid aggression and SUD should consider the degree of impairment for each set of problems on the patient's functioning and quality of life in order to collaboratively determine treatment goals and plan.

References

American Psychiatric Association: Diagnostic and Statistical Manual of Mental Disorders, 5th Edition. Arlington, VA, American Psychiatric Association, 2013

Anderson CA, Bushman BJ: Human aggression. Annu Rev Psychol 53:27–51, 2002 11752478

Barratt ES, Stanford MS, Kent TA, et al: Neuropsychological and cognitive psychophysiological substrates of impulsive aggression. Biol Psychiatry 41(10):1045–1061, 1997 9129785

Bechara A: Decision making, impulse control and loss of willpower to resist drugs: a neurocognitive perspective. Nat Neurosci 8(11):1458–1463, 2005 16251988

Beck A, Heinz AJ, Heinz A: Translational clinical neuroscience perspectives on the cognitive and neurobiological mechanisms underlying alcohol-related aggression. Curr Top Behav Neurosci 17:443–474, 2014 24338662

Beck R, Fernandez E: Cognitive-behavioral therapy in the treatment of anger: a meta-analysis. Cognit Ther Res 22(1):63–74, 1998

Berggård C, Damberg M, Longato-Stadler E, et al: The serotonin 2A –1438 G/A receptor polymorphism in a group of Swedish male criminals. Neurosci Lett 347(3):196–198, 2003

Berman M, Taylor S, Marged B: Morphine and human aggression. Addict Behav 18(3):263–268, 1993 8342439

Berman M, Kavoussi RJ, Coccaro EF: Neurotransmitter correlates of human aggression, in Handbook of Antisocial Behaviour. Edited by Stoff DM, Breiling J, Maser JD. Hoboken, NJ, Wiley, 1997, pp 305–313

Bogg T, Finn PR: A self-regulatory model of behavioral disinhibition in late adolescence: integrating personality traits, externalizing psychopathology, and cognitive capacity. J Pers 78(2):441–470, 2010 20433626

Boles SM, Miotto K: Substance abuse and violence: a review of the literature. Aggress Violent Behav 8(2):155–174, 2003

Brady KT, Myrick H, McElroy S: The relationship between substance use disorders, impulse control disorders, and pathological aggression. Am J Addict 7(3):221–230, 1998 9702290

Carroll KM, Rounsaville BJ: Behavioral therapies: the glass would be half full if only we had a glass, in Rethinking Substance Abuse: What the Science Shows, and What We Should Do About It. Edited by Miller WR, Carroll KM. New York, Guilford, 2006, pp 223–239

Carroll KM, Fenton LR, Ball SA, et al: Efficacy of disulfiram and cognitive behavior therapy in cocaine-dependent outpatients: a randomized placebo-controlled trial. Arch Gen Psychiatry 61(3):264–272, 2004 14993114

Caspi A, Moffitt TE, Newman DL, et al: Behavioral observations at age 3 years predict adult psychiatric disorders. Longitudinal evidence from a birth cohort. Arch Gen Psychiatry 53(11):1033–1039, 1996 8911226

Cherek DR, Steinberg JL, Kelly TH, et al: Effects of d-amphetamine on human aggressive behavior. Psychopharmacology (Berl) 88(3):381–386, 1986 3083459

Cherek DR, Steinberg JL, Kelly TH, et al: Effects of d-amphetamine on aggressive responding of normal male subjects. Psychiatry Res 21(3):257–265, 1987 3628610

Cherek DR, Steinberg JL, Kelly TH, et al: Effects of acute administration of diazepam and d-amphetamine on aggressive and escape responding of normal male subjects. Psychopharmacology (Berl) 100(2):173–181, 1990 2305007

Chermack ST, Murray RL, Walton MA, et al: Partner aggression among men and women in substance use disorder treatment: correlates of psychological and physical aggression and injury. Drug Alcohol Depend 98(1–2):35–44, 2008 18554825

Coccaro EF, Kavoussi RJ, Trestman RL, et al: Serotonin function in human subjects: intercorrelations among central 5-HT indices and aggressiveness. Psychiatry Res 73(1–2):1–14, 1997 9463834

Coccaro EF, Lee RJ, Kavoussi RJ: A double-blind, randomized, placebo-controlled trial of fluoxetine in patients with intermittent explosive disorder. J Clin Psychiatry 70(5):653–662, 2009 19389333

Coccaro EF, Fridberg DJ, Fanning JR, et al: Substance use disorders: relationship with intermittent explosive disorder and with aggression, anger, and impulsivity. J Psychiatr Res 81:127–132, 2016 27442963

Coccaro EF, Fanning JR, Lee R: Intermittent explosive disorder and substance use disorder: analysis of the National Comorbidity Study Replication Sample. J Clin Psychiatry 78(6):697–702, 2017 28252880

Connor DF, Steingard RJ: A clinical approach to the pharmacotherapy of aggression in children and adolescents. Ann N Y Acad Sci 794:290–307, 1996 8853610

Cornell DG, Warren J, Hawk G, et al: Psychopathy in instrumental and reactive violent offenders. J Consult Clin Psychol 64(4):783–790, 1996 8803369

Couppis MH, Kennedy CH: The rewarding effect of aggression is reduced by nucleus accumbens dopamine receptor antagonism in mice. Psychopharmacology (Berl) 197(3):449–456, 2008 18193405

Courtet P, Baud P, Abbar M, et al: Association between violent suicidal behavior and the low activity allele of the serotonin transporter gene. Mol Psychiatry 6(3):338–341, 2001 11326306

Crowley TJ: Dose-dependent facilitation or supression of rat fighting by methamphetamine, phenobarbital, or imipramine. Psychopharmacology (Berl) 27(3):213–222, 1972 4674515

Crowley TJ, Macdonald MJ, Whitmore EA, et al: Cannabis dependence, withdrawal, and reinforcing effects among adolescents with conduct symptoms and substance use disorders. Drug Alcohol Depend 50(1):27–37, 1998a 9589270

Crowley TJ, Mikulich SK, MacDonald M, et al: Substance-dependent, conduct-disordered adolescent males: severity of diagnosis predicts 2-year outcome. Drug Alcohol Depend 49(3):225–237, 1998b 9571387

de Wit H: Impulsivity as a determinant and consequence of drug use: a review of underlying processes. Addict Biol 14(1):22–31, 2009 18855805

Del Vecchio T, O'Leary KD: Effectiveness of anger treatments for specific anger problems: a meta-analytic review. Clin Psychol Rev 24(1):15–34, 2004 14992805

Derefinko K, DeWall CN, Metze AV, et al: Do different facets of impulsivity predict different types of aggression? Aggress Behav 37(3):223–233, 2011 21259270

DiGiuseppe R, Tafrate RC: Anger treatment for adults: a meta-analytic review. Clin Psychol Sci Pract 10(1):70–84, 2003

Dodge KA, Coie JD: Social-information-processing factors in reactive and proactive aggression in children's peer groups. J Pers Soc Psychol 53(6):1146–1158, 1987 3694454

Doran N, Luczak SE, Bekman N, et al: Adolescent substance use and aggression: a review. Crim Justice Behav 39(6):748–769, 2012

Duke AA, Giancola PR, Morris DH, et al: Alcohol dose and aggression: another reason why drinking more is a bad idea. J Stud Alcohol Drugs 72(1):34–43, 2011

Easton C, Swan S, Sinha R: Motivation to change substance use among offenders of domestic violence. J Subst Abuse Treat 19(1):1–5, 2000 10867294

Edmondson CB, Conger JC: A review of treatment efficacy for individuals with anger problems: conceptual, assessment, and methodological issues. Clin Psychol Rev 16(3):251–275, 1996

Espert R, Navarro JF, Salvador A, et al: Effects of morphine hydrochloride on social encounters between male mice. Agg Behav 19(5):377–383, 1993

Ferrari PF, van Erp AMM, Tornatzky W, et al: Accumbal dopamine and serotonin in anticipation of the next aggressive episode in rats. Eur J Neurosci 17(2):371–378, 2003 12542674

Ferris CF, Stolberg T, Delville Y: Serotonin regulation of aggressive behavior in male golden hamsters (Mesocricetus auratus). Behav Neurosci 113(4):804–815, 1999 10495088

Finn PR, Sharkansky EJ, Brandt KM, et al: The effects of familial risk, personality, and expectancies on alcohol use and abuse. J Abnorm Psychol 109(1):122–133, 2000 10740943

Finn PR, Mazas CA, Justus AN, et al: Early onset alcoholism with conduct disorder: go/no go learning deficits, working memory capacity, and personality. Alcohol Clin Exp Res 26(2):186–206, 2002 11964558

Fite PJ, Colder CR, Lochman JE, et al: Pathways from proactive and reactive aggression to substance use. Psychol Addict Behav 21(3):355–364, 2007 17874886

George DT, Phillips MJ, Lifshitz M, et al: Fluoxetine treatment of alcoholic perpetrators of domestic violence: a 12-week, double-blind, randomized, placebo-controlled intervention study. J Clin Psychiatry 72(1):60–65, 2011 20673556

Giancola PR, Chermack ST, Dingell JD: Construct validity of laboratory aggression paradigms: a response to Tedeschi and Quigley (1996). Aggress Violent Behav 3(3):237–253, 1998

Golden SA, Heins C, Venniro M, et al: Compulsive addiction-like aggressive behavior in mice. Biol Psychiatry 82(4):239–248, 2017

Goldstein PJ: The drugs/violence nexus: a tripartite conceptual framework. J Drug Issues 15(4):493–506, 1985

Gonzalez G, Oliveto A, Kosten TR: Combating opiate dependence: a comparison among the available pharmacological options. Expert Opin Pharmacother 5(4):713–725, 2004 15102558

Haney M, Miczek KA: Morphine effects on maternal aggression, pup care and analgesia in mice. Psychopharmacology (Berl) 98(1):68–74, 1989 2498961

Higley JD, Mehlman PT, Taub DM, et al: Cerebrospinal fluid monoamine and adrenal correlates of aggression in free-ranging rhesus monkeys. Arch Gen Psychiatry 49(6):436–441, 1992 1376105

Hoaken PNS, Stewart SH: Drugs of abuse and the elicitation of human aggressive behavior. Addict Behav 28(9):1533–1554, 2003 14656544

Hollander E, Tracy KA, Swann AC, et al: Divalproex in the treatment of impulsive aggression: efficacy in Cluster B personality disorders. Neuropsychopharmacology 28(6):1186–1197, 2003 12700713

Kreek MJ, Nielsen DA, Butelman ER, et al: Genetic influences on impulsivity, risk taking, stress responsivity and vulnerability to drug abuse and addiction. Nat Neurosci 8(11):1450–1457, 2005 16251987

Krueger RF, Markon KE: Reinterpreting comorbidity: a model-based approach to understanding and classifying psychopathology. Annu Rev Clin Psychol 2:111–133, 2006 17716066

Krueger RF, Hicks BM, Patrick CJ, et al: Etiologic connections among substance dependence, antisocial behavior, and personality: modeling the externalizing spectrum. J Abnorm Psychol 111(3):411–424, 2002 12150417

Krueger RF, Markon KE, Patrick CJ, et al: Linking antisocial behavior, substance use, and personality: an integrative quantitative model of the adult externalizing spectrum. J Abnorm Psychol 116(4):645–666, 2007 18020714

Kyes RC, Botchin MB, Kaplan JR, et al: Aggression and brain serotonergic responsivity: response to slides in male macaques. Physiol Behav 57(2):205–208, 1995 7716193

Licata A, Taylor S, Berman M, et al: Effects of cocaine on human aggression. Pharmacol Biochem Behav 45(3):549–552, 1993 8332615

Low S, Tiberio SS, Shortt JW, et al: Associations of couples' intimate partner violence in young adulthood and substance use: a dyadic approach. Psychol Violence 7(1):120, 2016

Lynam DR, Miller JD: Personality pathways to impulsive behavior and their relations to deviance: results from three samples. J Quant Criminol 20(4):319–341, 2004

Macdonald S, Anglin-Bodrug K, Mann RE, et al: Injury risk associated with cannabis and cocaine use. Drug Alcohol Depend 72(2):99–115, 2003 14636965

Macdonald S, Erickson P, Wells S, et al: Predicting violence among cocaine, cannabis, and alcohol treatment clients. Addict Behav 33(1):201–205, 2008 17689875

Manuck SB, Flory JD, Ferrell RE, et al: Aggression and anger-related traits associated with a polymorphism of the tryptophan hydroxylase gene. Biol Psychiatry 45(5):603–614, 1999 10088047

McCann TV, Lubman DI, Boardman G, et al: Affected family members' experience of, and coping with, aggression and violence within the context of problematic substance use: a qualitative study. BMC Psychiatry 17(1):209, 2017 28578666

McCloskey MS, Noblett KL, Deffenbacher JL, et al: Cognitive-behavioral therapy for intermittent explosive disorder: a pilot randomized clinical trial. J Consult Clin Psychol 76(5):876–886, 2008 18837604

McHugh RK, Hearon BA, Otto MW: Cognitive behavioral therapy for substance use disorders. Psychiatr Clin North Am 33(3):511–525, 2010 20599130

Miczek KA, O'Donnell JM: Intruder-evoked aggression in isolated and non-isolated mice: effects of psychomotor stimulants and L-dopa. Psychopharmacology (Berl) 57(1):47–55, 1978 26933

Miczek KA, DeBold JF, van Erp AM: Neuropharmacological characteristics of individual differences in alcohol effects on aggression in rodents and primates. Behav Pharmacol 5(4 and 5):407–421, 1994 11224293

Miller J, Flory K, Lynam D, et al: A test of the four-factor model of impulsivity-related traits. Pers Ind Diff 34(8):1403–1418, 2003

Moffitt TE: Adolescence-limited and life-course-persistent antisocial behavior: a developmental taxonomy. Psychol Rev 100(4):674–701, 1993 8255953

Moore TM, Stuart GL, Meehan JC, et al: Drug abuse and aggression between intimate partners: a meta-analytic review. Clin Psychol Rev 28(2):247–274, 2008 17604891

Mueser KT, Drake RE, Turner W, et al: Comorbid substance use disorders and psychiatric disorders, in Rethinking Substance Abuse: What the Science Shows and What We Should Do About It. Edited by Miller WR, Carroll KM. New York, Guilford, 2006, pp 115–133

Myerscough R, Taylor S: The effects of marijuana on human physical aggression. J Pers Soc Psychol 49(6):1541–1546, 1985 3003332

Nordahl TE, Salo R, Leamon M: Neuropsychological effects of chronic methamphetamine use on neurotransmitters and cognition: a review. J Neuropsychiatry Clin Neurosci 15(3):317–325, 2003 12928507

O'Malley SS, Kosten TR: Pharmacotherapy of addictive disorders, in Rethinking Substance Abuse: What the Science Shows and What We Should Do About It. Edited by Miller WR, Carroll KM. New York, Guilford, 2006, pp 241–256

Pihl RO, Sutton R: Drugs and aggression readily mix: so what now? Subst Use Misuse 44(9–10):1188–1203, 2009 19938914

Polman H, Orobio de Castro B, Koops W, et al: A meta-analysis of the distinction between reactive and proactive aggression in children and adolescents. J Abnorm Child Psychol 35(4):522–535, 2007 17340178

Reilly PM, Shopshire MS: Anger Management for Substance Abuse and Mental Health Clients: A Cognitive Behavioral Therapy Manual (HHS Publ No SMA-02-3661). Rockville, MD, Substance Abuse and Mental Health Services Administration, 2002. Available at: http://www.centerwatch.com/ drug-information/fda-approved-drugs/year/ 2009. Accessed April 17, 2018.

Rujescu D, Giegling I, Bondy B, et al: Association of anger-related traits with SNPs in the TPH gene. Mol Psychiatry 7(9):1023–1029, 2002 12399958

Schottenfeld RS, Chawarski MC, Cubells JF, et al: Randomized clinical trial of disulfiram for cocaine dependence or abuse during buprenorphine treatment. Drug Alcohol Depend 136:36–42, 2014 24462581

Shorey RC, Brasfield H, Anderson S, et al: The relation between trait mindfulness and early maladaptive schemas in men seeking substance use treatment. Mindfulness (N Y) 6(2):348–355, 2015 26085852

Siegel A, Schubert K: Neurotransmitters regulating feline aggressive behavior. Rev Neurosci 6(1):47–61, 1995 7633640

Silva H, Iturra P, Solari A, et al: Fluoxetine response in impulsive-aggressive behavior and serotonin transporter polymorphism in personality disorder. Psychiatr Genet 20(1):25–30, 2010 20010449

Smith EO, Byrd LD: Contrasting effects of d-amphetamine on affiliation and aggression in monkeys. Pharmacol Biochem Behav 20(2):255–260, 1984 6538973

Smith EO, Byrd LD: d-Amphetamine induced changes in social interaction patterns. Pharmacol Biochem Behav 22(1):135–139, 1985 4038801

Spiga R, Cherek DR, Roache JD, et al: The effects of codeine on human aggressive responding. Int Clin Psychopharmacol 5(3):195–204, 1990 2230064

Steele JL, Peralta RL: Are polydrug users more physically and verbally aggressive? An assessment of aggression among mono- versus polydrug users in a university sample. J Interpers Viol June 1, 2017 [Epub ahead of print] 29294803

Taylor SP: Aggressive behavior and physiological arousal as a function of provocation and the tendency to inhibit aggression. J Pers 35(2):297–310, 1967 6059850

Taylor S, Vardaris RM, Rawtich AB, et al: The effects of alcohol and delta-9-tetrahydrocannabinol on human physical aggression. Agg Behav 2(2):153–161, 1976

Teten AL, Schumacher JA, Bailey SD, et al: Male-to-female sexual aggression among Iraq, Afghanistan, and Vietnam veterans: co-occurring substance abuse and intimate partner aggression. J Trauma Stress 22(4):307–311, 2009 19588515

Tomlinson MF, Brown M, Hoaken PNS: Recreational drug use and human aggressive behavior: a comprehensive review since 2003. Agg Viol Behav 27:9–29, 2016

van Erp AM, Miczek KA: Aggressive behavior, increased accumbal dopamine, and decreased cortical serotonin in rats. J Neurosci 20(24):9320–9325, 2000 11125011

Volkow ND, Wang GJ, Fowler JS, et al: Prediction of reinforcing responses to psychostimulants in humans by brain dopamine D2 receptor levels. Am J Psychiatry 156(9):1440–1443, 1999 10484959

Volkow ND, Fowler JS, Wang G-J, et al: Dopamine in drug abuse and addiction: results from imaging studies and treatment implications. Mol Psychiatry 9(6):557–569, 2004 15098002

Westergaard GC, Suomi SJ, Chavanne TJ, et al: Physiological correlates of aggression and impulsivity in free-ranging female primates. Neuropsychopharmacology 28(6):1045–1055, 2003 12700686

Yanowitch R, Coccaro EF: The neurochemistry of human aggression. Adv Genet 75:151–169, 2011 22078480

14

Aggression in Personality Disorders

Royce J. Lee, M.D.

Aggression in the context of personality disorder has been the focus of empirical and theoretical attention since the inception of personality disorder as a diagnostic/theoretical construct. In this chapter, I summarize how this knowledge has been translated into clinical approaches to aggressive behavior in personality disorder. These approaches will be operationalized in a clinical vignette to illustrate clinical issues that arise when treating aggression in the context of a personality disorder.

Aggression in the context of personality disorder represents a serious societal and public health problem. In the largest meta-analysis of forensic samples to date, data from nearly 23,000 prisoners, about a quarter of whom were violent offenders, showed that 65% of men and 42% of females had a personality disorder. The personality disorders most frequently encountered tended to be those most closely associated with aggression: antisocial personality disorder (AsPD), borderline personality disorder (BPD), narcissistic personality disorder (NPD), and paranoid personality disorder (PPD) (Blackburn and

Coid 1999). Outside of the forensic setting, in clinical settings such as inpatient psychiatric hospitals, personality disorder remains the strongest prospective risk factor for committing acts of interpersonal violence, to a greater degree than other psychiatric disorders (Tardiff et al. 1997).

Aggression is encountered across the diagnostic spectrum of personality disorders (Dunne et al. 2017). Because of this complexity, issues with nosology are of paramount importance. The field is transitioning from a categorical to a dimensional classification system (Oldham 2017). In the United States, the transition from DSM-IV to DSM-5 can be summarized as movement away from a categorical system of three personality disorder clusters and 10 disorders toward a dimensional system of overall severity and severity of five dimensional traits (Negative Affectivity, Detachment, Antagonism, Disinhibition, and Psychoticism). In Europe, the transition from ICD-10 to ICD-11 (Reed et al. 2016) is toward a dimensional trait system of five trait domains (Negative Affectivity, Detachment, Dissociality, Disinhibition, and Anankastia). In this transition point, categorical and dimensional systems both have merit and champions.

The relationship of impulsive aggression to personality disorder raises important issues relevant to both categorical and dimensional approaches to nosology. DSM-5 intermittent explosive disorder (IED) permits the comorbidity of IED and personality disorder (American Psychiatric Association 2013); its expression is taxonic, supporting the validity of a categorical approach (Ahmed et al. 2010). Counterintuitively, impulsive aggressive behavior is dimensional in the population, as are its biological correlates (Coccaro et al. 1989). The categorical nature of the clinical diagnosis and the dimensional nature of behavior in the population can be reconciled by the fact that there may be a threshold at which problems become a problem for the individual or society. In summary, there is a paradoxical movement toward a dimensional nosology of personality disorder just as a categorical diagnosis of IED has been created.

Dimensional, personality measure correlates of aggression have been examined. Aggression encompasses premeditated and reactive aggression (Bondü and Richter 2016); these two subforms are correlated ($r=0.7$; Vitaro and Brendgen 2005). A meta-analytic review of the relationship between laboratory measures of aggression and personality dimensions found that irritability, impulsivity, neuroticism, and narcissism were associated with reactive aggression. Antagonism was associated with unprovoked aggression (Bettencourt et al. 2006). Anger predicted provoked aggression, but not neutral, aggression.

The pragmatic approach is to use the diagnostic tools available. Presently, the diagnosis of DSM-5 IED can be given along with a personality disorder diagnosis. AsPD and BPD are the two disorders that are more frequently found in individuals with IED. Even so, the presence of either of these disorders is associated with approximately 50% of the variance in aggressive behavior that IED accounts for (Coccaro 2012). This is particularly important because the diagnostic criteria for and psychological models of these disorders are based on high levels of innate aggression, raising the possibility that the IED diagnosis is superfluous. But this is not the case. The level of aggression found when IED co-occurs with AsPD or BPD is not additive, but mostly determined by IED. Thus, the IED diagnosis provides powerful predictive information about severity of aggression (Coccaro 2012) and should be used in the clinic when diagnostic criteria are met.

The transition to dimensional personality disorder diagnostic schemes will raise new issues with respect to the diagnostic classification of aggression, because of the multicollinearity of aggression and personality dimensions. Neuroscience-based classification systems, such as the National Institute of Mental Health's Research Domain Criteria (Carcone and Ruocco 2017; Insel et al. 2010), are being developed that may provide the ability to biologically validate behavioral trait dimensions. Such approaches could provide a solution to some of the current nosological problems the field faces.

Phenomenology

The presence of aggression in personality disorders is highlighted by the fact that anger and aggression are included as a specific diagnostic criterion for both BPD and AsPD. Other personality disorders have diagnostic features that likely increase the proneness for anger and aggression (e.g., holding grudges in those with PPD). Diagnostic and psychological data from a sample of 1,500 Chicago adults evaluated with semistructured interviews at the Clinical Neurosciences and Psychopharmacology Research Unit at the University of Chicago can help to elucidate the relationship between aggression and specific personality disorders. Aggressive behavior was measured with the Life History of Aggression (LHA). We found that AsPD, BPD, NPD, obsessive-compulsive personality disorder (OCPD), and PPD were positively, and significantly, related to LHA Aggression. Not surprisingly, each of these personality disorders was found to exhibit significant comorbidity with IED. Thus, even personality disorders without anger and aggression as diagnostic features are associated with high life histories of actual aggressive behavior. Finally, these data suggest possible triggers for impulsive aggressive behavior in those with different personality disorders—for example, threat to reaching an objective (AsPD), threat of abandonment (BPD), threat of disrespect (NPD), threat to sense of order (OCPD), and existential social threat (PPD).

Borderline Personality Disorder

Because the diagnostic construct of BPD derived from the clinical observations of psychodynamic therapists, it is useful to review its early history. The first descriptions of borderline psychopathology were in fact dimensional, proposing a third form of psychopathology of intermediate severity between mood (neurotic) and psychotic disorders (Stern 1938). In a startlingly prescient description of this new class of psychopathology, in 1938 Stern described nine characteristics that would eventually transform into modern diagnostic criteria: narcissism, stress sensitivity, interpersonal hypersensitivity, rigidity, feelings of inferiority, masochism, an externalizing and outward focus, regression and dependency, and proneness to micropsychotic episodes. Shortly thereafter, borderline psychopathology was described in psychoanalytic, metapsychological terms, leading to the development of a metapsychological developmental model of the self. These theories posited a high level of aggressive drives. Freud proposed that primitive drives shape early life development as a "death" drive that opposes the libidinal drive for pleasure, closely related to what might be considered today as trait aggression (Freud 1920/1955). Otto Kernberg (1967) incorporated these drives with object relations theory. He hypothesized that the high intensity, and possibly constitutional nature, of aggressive drives in the borderline patient lead to defensive splitting of "self-objects," or working models of the self and early relationships.

Empirical data have confirmed the importance of aggression in BPD. The majority of patients with BPD have had aggressive outbursts in the past year, usually in close relationships (Newhill et al. 2009). Mancke and others proposed four biobehavioral dimensions to underlie aggressive behavior in BPD: 1) affective dysregulation (neuroticism), 2) impulsivity (disinhibition), 3) threat hypersensitivity (hostility), and 4) empathic functioning (Mancke et al. 2015). It is known that angry ruminations are a precursor to angry responding in BPD (Baer and Sauer 2011). In adolescent females with BPD, perceived rejection triggers anger, which then leads to "hot" aggression (Scott et al. 2017). This effect has some specificity for BPD traits, as young women with antisocial traits do not show the same angry reactions to perceived rejection. In BPD, levels of aggression decline over the lifespan but can persist in the face of concurrent substance abuse and adversity (Zanarini et al. 2017).

Antisocial Personality Disorder

AsPD encompasses behavioral and biological heterogeneity. Psychopathy represents the severe end of a wide spectrum of irresponsible, destructive, and aggressive behavior (Coid and Ullrich 2010). This spectrum encompasses both hot (impulsive) and cold (premeditated) aggression. Analysis of populations with AsPD detects two dimensions of psychopathy: the first (Hare Psychopathy Checklist—Revised [PCL-R] Factor 1) is associated with narcissism, instrumental aggression, and low fear, while the second (PCL-R Factor 2) is related to reactive aggression, substance abuse problems, and suicidal behavior and can be characterized by impulsive responsivity (Bezdjian et al. 2011; Fite et al. 2009). A recent modification to this classification includes three, rather than two, factors: meanness, disinhibition, and a third factor related to low fear, boldness (Patrick 2014). External factors such as alcohol consumption can potently interact with AsPD, leading to aggression and violence (Moeller and Dougherty 2001). Unusually cruel behavior, such as that seen in sexual violence or serial killing, is at the extreme end of the spectrum of the psychopathy continuum. DSM-III-R described a pattern of antisocial behavior characterized by sadistic and controlling behavior, not including rule-breaking behavior characteristic of AsPD (Myers et al. 2006). This population has a unique constellation of personality traits, characterized by Personality Inventory for DSM-5 Suspiciousness, Cognitive and Perceptual Dysregulation, and Grandiosity, and a lack of Eccentricity (Russell and King 2017). Neurobiological studies to date point to deficits in limbic and cortical activation in relation to callousness (Michalska et al. 2016; Patrick 2014), frontal disinhibition and diminished working memory updating in impulsivity (Pasion et al. 2017), and abnormal recruitment of temporoparietal circuits mediating cognitive empathy in sadism (Harenski et al. 2012).

Narcissistic Personality Disorder

Early metapsychological models of NPD differentiated it from BPD while acknowledging the shared characteristic of interpersonal hypersensitivity and ensuing relationship difficulties. Kernberg hypothesized that "oral rage" may be an early life factor and assumed that constitutional aggression played a developmental role. But he also observed that in comparison to patients with BPD, impulse control was not as severe a problem. When aggression was overt, it was brief and elicited in moments of frustration (Kernberg 1970) secondary to challenges to their unrealistic image of their own self-worth. This subtle differentiation has not been fully explicated in theoretical work. Empirical research on narcissism has consistently found it to be a risk factor for aggression. More severe, pathological forms of narcissism, such as lack of empathy and self-aggrandizement, overlap with AsPD and psychopathy (Geberth and Turco 1997; Gunderson and Ronningstam 2001). Pathological narcissism is more closely associated with aggression (Beasley and Stoltenberg 1992), even after adjustment for comorbid AsPD (Coid 2002). The type of narcissism present may also predict subtypes of aggressive behavior. In a study of laboratory aggression, grandiose narcissism, closely related to traits of callousness, predicted both reactive and premeditated aggression, while vulnerable narcissism, related to neuroticism and interpersonal hypersensitivity, did not (Lobbestael et al. 2014). Likewise, more severe forms of physical aggression appear to have a stronger relationship with narcissism (Lambe et al. 2018).

Obsessive-Compulsive Personality Disorder

OCPD has not received as much scientific attention as AsPD and BPD, but impulsive aggression is often seen in this personality disorder.

While none of the OCPD diagnostic criteria directly relate to impulsive aggressive behavior, the rigidity and perfectionism stemming from the anxiety that without great effort "things will go out of control" set up those with OCPD to react with an impulsive aggressive outburst when their "sense of order" is violated.

Paranoid Personality Disorder

PPD has not received as much scientific attention as AsPD and BPD, but in fact it is commonly encountered in the clinical and forensic settings (Lee 2017). It is one of the only personality disorder diagnoses uniquely related to aggression after AsPD and BPD are controlled for (Berman et al. 1998), contributing unique variance to history of aggression not accounted for by other personality disorder symptoms. It is closely associated with the risk factors of childhood trauma (Lee 2017) and chronic social stress (Raza et al. 2014). PPD has not been the focus of intense psychoanalytic attention, but psychodynamic and cognitive-behavioral models of the disorder are coherent, focusing on shame aversion, externalizing, and hostility (Lee 2017). Its neurobiology is poorly understood. It is probably more closely related genetically to delusional disorder than to schizophrenia and is less closely related to schizophrenia than to schizotypal personality disorder (Lee 2017). Given its relationship to trauma and social stress, it is not surprisingly associated with biomarkers of chronic stress activation, such as cerebrospinal fluid levels of corticotropin-releasing hormone (Lee et al. 2005). Treatment approaches for PPD have not been well articulated in the literature and there have been no randomized controlled trials (RCTs) for it. Interpersonal sensitivity and hostility, defining features of the disorder, are strongly related to a hostile attribution bias that is shared with impulsive aggression (Chen et al. 2012; Coccaro et al. 2016; Dodge and Crick 1990). Future research should examine the degree to which this can be modified in psychotherapy.

Psychobiology

Neurobiology and Neuroimaging

Given the role of serotonergic dysfunction in impulsive aggression (Coccaro et al. 1989), there have been efforts to identify abnormalities in serotonergic signaling in BPD. Ligand positron emission tomography studies have identified serotonergic abnormalities in the prefrontal cortex of patients with BPD (Kolla et al. 2016; Soloff et al. 2014). A meta-analysis of volumetric magnetic resonance imaging (MRI) brain imaging studies in BPD implicates the superior and middle temporal lobes, including the arcuate fasciculus, and supplementary motor area. Differences were also seen over the lifespan, with BPD patients starting out with a smaller volume of the left superior parietal gyrus, with the volume normalizing with age, and then having a smaller right amygdala over time with advancing age. These results suggest subtle but widespread gray matter abnormalities associated with BPD. The longitudinal pattern of parietal lobe changes parallels the longitudinal course of BPD, with normalization in advancing age (Gunderson et al. 2011). Meta-analysis of functional MRI studies in BPD shows that during processing of negatively valenced emotional stimuli, BPD is associated with greater limbic, posterior cingulate, and middle temporal lobe metabolic activity but blunting of lingual and superior parietal regions (Schulze et al. 2016). These results point to network dysfunction spanning limbic and associative functions of the brain. Examining aggression in BPD, work as of this writing points to regional brain dysfunction in frontal executive, limbic, and association circuits (Herpertz et al. 2017; New et al. 2009; Soloff et al. 2017). An important causal factor in the widespread network dysfunction that is found to be associated with both aggression and BPD may be the white matter connections between distant brain regions. Indeed, we have found an area of decreased white matter integrity in the area of the superior longitudinal fasciculus common to both BPD subjects with IED and those without IED (Lee 2017). The regions supported by the superior longitudinal fasciculus are thought to play an important role in visual working memory, language, and social cognition.

The neurobiological findings, thus far, in BPD and aggression in the context of BPD point toward abnormalities in widely distributed brain networks that encompass a range of mental functions. These findings are reinforced by the curiously broad range of subtle neuropsychological findings in the disorder (Ruocco 2005). They also provide a biological explanation for the complexity of the nosological issues raised by BPD. Future neuroscience-based work, perhaps using the Research Domain Criteria framework, may help to solve the problems of nosological theory.

Molecular Genetics

Two small genomewide association studies have provided preliminary evidence for genes encoding proteins associated with BPD (dihydropyrimidine dehydrogenase [*DPYD*]; involved in pyrimidine metabolism and oxidative stress), Plakophilin 4 ([*PKP4*]; for cell-cell adhesion), and serine incorporator 5 ([*SERINC5*]; involved in membrane lipids and myelination). These gene products, if altered, could cause widespread network dysfunction (Cond et al. 2017; Witt et al. 2017). Interestingly, the most recent genomewide association study of BPD concluded that it was closely related genetically to mood and psychotic disorders (Witt et al. 2017), confirming an early dimensional theory of the borderline personality (Stern 1938).

Clinical Approach and Treatment

Psychopharmacological Treatment

Borderline Personality Disorder

Antipsychotics have been tested in the treatment of BPD, in part because of hypothesized relationships between BPD and psychotic disorders. Meta-analysis reveals that as a class, antipsychotics can be helpful for anger in BPD (standardized mean difference [SMD]=-0.31, 95% confidence interval [CI] =-0.63 to -0.003) (National Collaborating Centre for Mental Health 2009). One of the first antipsychotic drugs tested, haloperidol, has been found to reduce anger intensity (SMD=-0.46, 95% CI=-0.84 to -0.09; Lieb et al. 2010) but increase global BPD severity (SMD=0.3, 95% CI=-0.22 to 0.82; Soloff et al. 1993). Given this finding, the usefulness of haloperidol is limited. Newer antipsychotics likewise show effects of uncertain benefit. The atypical antipsychotic olanzapine has a beneficial but small sized effect on anger (*N*=661; mean change standard deviation=-0.27, 95% CI=-0.43 to -0.12; Stoffers et al. 2010). However, these beneficial effects are undone by negative effects on metabolic status and negative effects on suicidality (SMD=0.15; 95% CI=-0.36 to 0.65) and self-injury (relative risk=1.20, 95% CI=0.50 to 2.88). The closely related molecule quetiapine has also been found to reduce aggression. Interestingly, the effect size is slightly higher for low-dose (150 mg/day) compared with higher-dose (300 mg/day) treatment (effect size=-0.82 for low dose) and -0.76 for higher dose) (Black et al. 2014).

Antidepressant medications have been tested for the treatment of impulsive aggression. Impulsive aggression in adults with personality disorder is reduced by fluoxetine, at dosages of 20–40 mg/day (Coccaro et al. 2009). Meta-analysis of selective serotonin reuptake inhibitors (SSRI) trials for the treatment of anger and aggression found a moderate to large effect (SMD=-0.55, 95% CI=-0.17 to -0.92) (Coccaro and Kavoussi 1997; Rinne et al. 2002; Salzman et al. 1995; Simpson et al. 2004). The monoamine oxidase inhibitors phenelzine and tranylcypromine have been found in small controlled trials to reduce anger, hostility, and violent behavioral dyscontrol (Cowdry and Gardner 1988; Soloff et al. 1993). Given the higher risk to benefit ratio of monoamine oxidase inhibitors, these medications should only be used when other interventions have failed. Tricyclic antidepressants (TCAs) are generally avoided in this population because of evidence of clinical deterioration while these drugs are being taken and their dangerousness in overdose (Soloff et al. 1986).

The anticonvulsant mood stabilizers also have some evidence of efficacy. Valproate has been found to reduce anger in three studies (SMD=-1.83, 95% CI=-3.17 to -0.48) (Kendall et al. 2010). A single study has found preliminary evidence for reduced anger after treatment with lamotrigine relative to placebo (SMD=-1.69, 95% CI=-2.62 to -0.75) (Tritt et al. 2005). Most of the evidence for anticonvulsant mood stabilizer use comes from single, relatively small studies, and this decreases the reliability of the findings. Benzodiazepine medications are to be avoided, given evidence for worsening of aggression in BPD (Cowdry and Gardner 1988).

Other Personality Disorders With Aggressive Features

There are no double-blind, placebo-controlled trials of agents to treat aggression in specific individuals with AsPD, NPD, OCPD, or PPD, though the few studies on the psychopharmacology of impulsive aggression have included individuals with these personality disorders. That said, we have not found any difference in the anti-aggressive response to agents, such as fluoxetine, as a function of any of the five personality disorders with aggressive features.

Psychotherapeutic Approaches

Borderline Personality Disorder

While BPD was once thought of as being resistant to treatment or even "uncurable," several psychotherapeutic techniques have been shown to be effective in RCTs. Dialectical behavior therapy (DBT) is able to reduce suicide attempt rates in BPD and anger ($n = 46$; two RCTs; SMD = –0.83, 95% CI = –1.43 to –0.22) (Kliem et al. 2010). Transference-focused therapy (TFP) has been found to effective reduce anger and interpersonal problems in BPD (Choi-Kain et al. 2017). General psychiatric management (GPM), which combines a structured supportive therapy with an algorithm of medication and case management, has also been found to reduce anger in BPD, to a degree comparable to DBT (McMain et al. 2012). These findings suggest that anger can be treated with evidence-based psychotherapy. Further research using validated measures of aggressive behavior is needed to know if the reductions in anger result in decreased frequency and/or intensity of interpersonal aggression.

Antisocial Personality Disorder

Although, as with BPD, claims of "untreatableness" have been attached to AsPD, there have been efforts to develop new approaches. In one study, in which a preventative approach was used, psychoanalytic psychotherapy was found to be effective in preventing or delaying the onset of aggressive behavior in individuals with ASPD, compared with wait-list, in adolescents with severe conduct disorder (Weitkamp et al. 2017). Mentalization-based therapy, targeting cognitive empathy, was found to be more effective than an intensity-matched comparison condition in the treatment of interpersonal problems in adults with comorbid BPD and AsPD (Bateman and Krawitz 2013). However, even treatments that have been previously identified to be effective for externalizing behavior have been less effective in individuals with high levels of psychopathic traits (Manders et al. 2013). Therefore, innovative approaches have been developed, such as cognitive skills training, which has been shown to reduce violence and aggression in prisoners with psychotic (Cullen et al. 2012) and personality disorders (Young et al. 2013). Treatment guidelines have been scarce in this area, with the exception of National Institute for Health and Care Excellence guidelines (National Collaborating Centre for Mental Health

2010) for the treatment of AsPD. These guidelines direct clinicians to target impulsivity with cognitive-behavioral interventions and do not recommend pharmacotherapy, given the paucity of evidence supporting its use. Targeting the treatment of impulsive aggression is a priority when appropriate, given the lack of strong treatment recommendations for other AsPD symptoms.

Clinical Vignette

HK is a 42-year-old unmarried, professional, medically healthy male who was seen in the outpatient clinic, having requested "expert" medication management of his previously diagnosed bipolar affective disorder. He was taking nortriptyline 150 mg per day, carbamazepine 400 mg twice a day, alprazolam 1 mg three times a day, and fluoxetine 20 mg per day. HK complained of volatile temper, irritability, depression, and insomnia. He came seeking treatment for a treatment-refractory mood disorder. On examination, he exhibited prominent irritability, professed to passive suicidal ideation, and focused on an interpersonal conflict that had resulted in him daydreaming about murdering a female acquaintance. Exploration of these thoughts revealed that his ruminations had not led him to plan a homicidal act; his fear of the consequences had strongly deterred him (e.g., "I just want her to acknowledge me"). Over the course of several diagnostic interview sessions, it became clear that there was no history of mania, but there was a recurrent pattern of volatile outbursts in the face of perceived rejection and/or challenge to his self-esteem. There also was a prominent history of childhood abuse and neglect. He had a history of several suicide attempts and psychiatric hospitalizations, the first of which was at the age of 21. Although he had not recently been hospitalized, he continued to have a history of volatility and unstable relationships through his 20s, 30s, and now his 40s.

HK's presentation met diagnostic criteria for BPD and NPD, as well as IED. The recommended treatment plan included weaning him off of the ineffective and possibly deleterious TCA and benzodiazepine drugs while retaining his mood stabilizer and SSRI antidepressant. He underwent a sequence of TFP for 3 years, followed by a year of DBT, and then GPM (which he continued to participate in). For the past 10 years, he has remained out of the hospital and has had reduced intensity of affective outbursts, but he has continued to struggle with interpersonal relationships. He acknowledges the problem of interpersonal sensitivity and is able to perceive his role in conflicts at work and his personal life. The criteria for NPD are no longer met, and he has only subthreshold IED symptoms; he reports reduced severity of BPD symptoms. He remains active and well respected in his volunteer advocacy work. There have been several challenges to the therapeutic relationship, but he prides himself on his ability to discuss them and overcome his inclination to end the therapeutic relationship. He retains a reality-based view of the relationship as a collaborative one, in which the primary challenges are the implementation of reasonable therapeutic choices to target his problems, rather than a quest to find the perfect therapist. The treatment remains focused on continuing psychotherapy to target his interpersonal hypersensitivity.

Discussion of Vignette

This vignette reflects a realistic view of what occurs in a complex case. Although there are no U.S. Food and Drug Administration–approved treatments for personality disorder, by adhering to the evidence base a clinician can avoid iatrogenically harming, or reduce the risk of such harm to, the patient. In this case, the TCA and benzodiazepine medications were likely deleterious and were discontinued safely. The SSRI appears to be helpful in preventing depression and reducing anger outburst frequency. Most of the therapy is directed toward his problems with interpersonal sensitivity and shows an effect size consistent with that predicted by the empirical literature: symptoms, more than function, show the larger response. Although his symptoms are only subthreshold for making a diagnosis of posttraumatic stress disorder, he is able to talk about the connections between his volatility and the chronic verbal abuse he received as a child.

Summary

Aggression is a significant correlate of personality disorder, even when anger, aggression, or impulsivity is not part of the diagnostic criteria for the specific personality disorder. Overall, AsPD, BPD, NPD, OCPD, and PPD are associated with high levels of aggression. The association of aggression with OCPD and PDD was initially unexpected and deserves further study. The results of this analysis reinforce the relevance of these specific personality disorders to aggression. New insights about BPD in the clinic, with regard to neurobiology and treatment response, have led to recommendations regarding the use of medications and evidence-based psychotherapies.

Key Clinical Points

▌ Treatment guidelines encompassing therapy, medications, and case management have been developed for borderline personality disorder: the National Institute for Health and Care Excellence Borderline Personality Disorder: Treatment and Management guidelines (National Collaborating Centre for Mental Health 2009) and, in the context of stepped, or resource-limited care, general psychiatric management (Choi-Kain et al. 2016). Both of these guidelines were developed with an understanding of the research literature of these interacting conditions.

▌ Psychopharmacological interventions are off-label, without specific approval by regulatory agencies such as the U.S. Food and Drug Administration. Therefore, prescribing must involve informed consent for the off-label use. Documentation of this in the chart is advised.

▌ Personality disorders associated with aggression, even if biologically related to mood and psychotic disorders, are separate conditions, requiring specific and targeted interventions (Gunderson et al. 2011).

▌ Although psychotherapy can be enormously helpful, evidence indicates that not every therapy helps in every domain of impaired function (Choi-Kain et al. 2017).

▌ Psychoeducation is an important goal in its own right. By understanding their diagnosis and the proposed treatment, patients transform into active participants in treatment and are better prepared for the ups and downs that can occur.

▌ Experience in research populations using semistructured interviews reveals that most patients with one personality disorder have multiple comorbid personality disorders.

References

Ahmed AO, Green BA, McCloskey MS, et al: Latent structure of intermittent explosive disorder in an epidemiological sample. J Psychiatr Res 44(10):663–672, 2010 20064645

American Psychiatric Association: Diagnostic and Statistical Manual of Mental Disorders, 5th Edition. Arlington, VA, American Psychiatric Association, 2013

Baer RA, Sauer SE: Relationships between depressive rumination, anger rumination, and borderline personality features. Pers Disord 2(2):142–150, 2011 22448733

Bateman AW, Krawitz R: Borderline Personality Disorder: An Evidence-Based Guide for Generalist Mental Health Professionals. Oxford, UK, Oxford University Press, 2013

Beasley R, Stoltenberg CD: Personality characteristics of male spouse abusers. Prof Psychol Res Pr 23(4):310–317, 1992

Berman ME, Fallon AE, Coccaro EF: The relationship between personality psychopathology and aggressive behavior in research volunteers. J Abnorm Psychol 107(4):651–658, 1998 9830252

Bettencourt BA, Talley A, Benjamin AJ, et al: Personality and aggressive behavior under provoking and neutral conditions: a meta-analytic review. Psychol Bull 132(5):751–777, 2006 16910753

Bezdjian S, Tuvblad C, Raine A, et al: The genetic and environmental covariation among psychopathic personality traits, and reactive and proactive aggression in childhood. Child Dev 82(4):1267–1281, 2011 21557742

Black DW, Zanarini MC, Romine A, et al: Comparison of low and moderate dosages of extended-release quetiapine in borderline personality disorder: a randomized, double-blind, placebo-controlled trial. Am J Psychiatry 171(11):1174–1182, 2014 24968985

Blackburn R, Coid JW: Empirical clusters of DSM-III personality disorders in violent offenders. J Pers Disord 13(1):18–34, 1999 10228924

Bondü R, Richter P: Interrelations of justice, rejection, provocation, and moral disgust sensitivity and their links with the hostile attribution bias, trait anger, and aggression. Front Psychol 7(5):795, 2016 27303351

Carcone D, Ruocco AC: Six years of research on the National Institute of Mental Health's Research Domain Criteria (RDoC) initiative: a systematic review. Front Cell Neurosci 11:46, 2017 28316565

Chen P, Coccaro EF, Lee R, et al: Moderating effects of childhood maltreatment on associations between social information processing and adult aggression. Psychol Med 42(6):1293–1304, 2012 22008562

Choi-Kain LW, Albert EB, Gunderson JG: Evidence-based treatments for borderline personality disorder: Implementation, integration, and stepped care. Harv Rev Psychiatry 24(5):342–356, 2016 27603742

Choi-Kain LW, Finch EF, Masland SR, et al: What works in the treatment of borderline personality disorder. Curr Behav Neurosci Rep 4(1):21–30, 2017 28331780

Coccaro EF: Intermittent explosive disorder as a disorder of impulsive aggression for DSM-5. Am J Psychiatry 169(6):577–588, 2012 22535310

Coccaro EF, Kavoussi RJ: Fluoxetine and impulsive aggressive behavior in personality-disordered subjects. Arch Gen Psychiatry 54(12):1081–1088, 1997 9400343

Coccaro EF, Siever LJ, Klar HM, et al: Serotonergic studies in patients with affective and personality disorders. Correlates with suicidal and impulsive aggressive behavior. Arch Gen Psychiatry 46(7):587–599, 1989 2735812

Coccaro EF, Lee RJ, Kavoussi RJ: A double-blind, randomized, placebo-controlled trial of fluoxetine in patients with intermittent explosive disorder. J Clin Psychiatry 70(5):653–662, 2009 19389333

Coccaro EF, Fanning JR, Keedy SK, et al: Social cognition in intermittent explosive disorder and aggression. J Psychiatr Res 83:140–150, 2016 27621104

Coid J, Ullrich S: Antisocial personality disorder is on a continuum with psychopathy. Compr Psychiatry 51(4):426–433, 2010 20579518

Coid JW: Personality disorders in prisoners and their motivation for dangerous and disruptive behaviour. Crim Behav Ment Health 12(3):209–226, 2002 12830313

Cond LC, Amin N, Hottenga J-J, et al: The first genome-wide association meta-analysis of borderline personality disorder features. Eur Neuropsychopharmacol 27(S3):S504–S505, 2017

Cowdry RW, Gardner DL: Pharmacotherapy of borderline personality disorder: alprazolam, carbamazepine, trifluoperazine, and tranylcypromine. Arch Gen Psychiatry 45(2):111–119, 1988 3276280

Cullen AE, Clarke AY, Kuipers E, et al: A multisite randomized trial of a cognitive skills program for male mentally disordered offenders: violence and antisocial behavior outcomes. J Consult Clin Psychol 80(6):1114–1120, 2012 23025249

Dodge KA, Crick NR: Social information-processing bases of aggressive behavior in children. Pers Soc Psychol Bull 16(1):8–22, 1990

Dunne AL, Gilbert F, Daffern M: Investigating the relationship between DSM-5 personality disorder domains and facts and aggression in an offender population using the personality inventory for the DSM-5. J Pers Disord 31:1–26, 2017 28972816

Fite PJ, Stoppelbein L, Greening L: Proactive and reactive aggression in a child psychiatric inpatient population: relations to psychopathic characteristics. Crim Justice Behav 36(5):481–493, 2009

Freud S: Beyond the pleasure principle (1920), in The Standard Edition of the Complete Psychological Works of Sigmund Freud, Vol 18. Translated and edited by Strachey J. London, Hogarth Press, 1955, pp 1–64

Geberth VJ, Turco RN: Antisocial personality disorder, sexual sadism, malignant narcissism, and serial murder. J Forensic Sci 42(1):49–60, 1997 8988574

Gunderson JG, Ronningstam E: Differentiating narcissistic and antisocial personality disorders. J Pers Disord 15(2):103–109, 2001 11345846

Gunderson JG, Stout RL, McGlashan TH, et al: Ten-year course of borderline personality disorder: psychopathology and function from the Collaborative Longitudinal Personality Disorders study. Arch Gen Psychiatry 68(8):827–837, 2011 21464343

Harenski CL, Thornton DM, Harenski KA, et al: Increased frontotemporal activation during pain observation in sexual sadism: preliminary findings. Arch Gen Psychiatry 69(3):283–292, 2012 22393220

Herpertz SC, Nagy K, Ueltzhöffer K, et al: Brain mechanisms underlying reactive aggression in borderline personality disorder—sex matters. Biol Psychiatry 82(4):257–266, 2017 28388995

Insel T, Cuthbert B, Garvey M, et al: Research Domain Criteria (RDoC): toward a new classification framework for research on mental disorders. Am J Psychiatry 167(7):748–751, 2010 20595427

Kendall T, Burbeck R, Bateman A: Pharmacotherapy for borderline personality disorder: NICE guideline. Br J Psychiatry 196(2):158–159, 2010 20118465

Kernberg O: Borderline personality organization. J Am Psychoanal Assoc 15(3):641–685, 1967 4861171

Kernberg OF: Factors in the psychoanalytic treatment of narcissistic personalities. J Am Psychoanal Assoc 18(1):51–85, 1970 5451020

Kliem S, Kröger C, Kosfelder J: Dialectical behavior therapy for borderline personality disorder: a meta-analysis using mixed-effects modeling. J Consult Clin Psychol 78(6):936–951, 2010 21114345

Kolla NJ, Chiuccariello L, Wilson AA, et al: Elevated monoamine oxidase–A distribution volume in borderline personality disorder is associated with severity across mood symptoms, suicidality, and cognition. Biol Psychiatry 79(2):117–126, 2016 25698585

Lambe S, Hamilton-Giachritsis C, Garner E, et al: The role of narcissism in aggression and violence: a systematic review. Trauma Violence Abuse 19(2):209–230, 2018 27222500

Lee R: Mistrustful and misunderstood: a review of paranoid personality disorder. Curr Behav Neurosci Rep 4(2):151–165, 2017 29399432

Lee R, Geracioti TD Jr, Kasckow JW, et al: Childhood trauma and personality disorder: positive correlation with adult CSF corticotropin-releasing factor concentrations. Am J Psychiatry 162(5):995–997, 2005 15863804

Lieb K, Völlm B, Rücker G, et al: Pharmacotherapy for borderline personality disorder: Cochrane systematic review of randomised trials. Br J Psychiatry 196(1):4–12, 2010 20044651

Lobbestael J, Baumeister RF, Fiebig T, et al: The role of grandiose and vulnerable narcissism in self-reported and laboratory aggression and testosterone reactivity. Pers Ind Diff 69:22–27, 2014

Mancke F, Herpertz SC, Bertsch K: Aggression in borderline personality disorder: A multidimensional model. Pers Disord 6(3):278–291, 2015 26191822

Manders WA, Dekovic M, Asscher JJ, et al: Psychopathy as predictor and moderator of multisystemic therapy outcomes among adolescents treated for antisocial behavior. J Abnorm Child Psychol 41(7):1121–1132, 2013 23756854

McMain SF, Guimond T, Streiner DL, et al: Dialectical behavior therapy compared with general psychiatric management for borderline personality disorder: clinical outcomes and functioning over a 2-year follow-up. Am J Psychiatry 169(6):650–661, 2012 22581157

Michalska KJ, Zeffiro TA, Decety J: Brain response to viewing others being harmed in children with conduct disorder symptoms. J Child Psychol Psychiatry 57(4):510–519, 2016 26472591

Moeller FG, Dougherty DM: Antisocial personality disorder, alcohol, and aggression. Alcohol Res Health 25(1):5–11, 2001 11496966

Myers WC, Burket RC, Husted DS: Sadistic personality disorder and comorbid mental illness in adolescent psychiatric inpatients. J Am Acad Psychiatry Law 34(1):61–71, 2006 16585236

National Collaborating Centre for Mental Health: Borderline Personality Disorder: Treatment and Management. NICE Clinical Guideline 78. Leicester, UK, British Psychological Society, 2009

National Collaborating Centre for Mental Health: Antisocial Personality Disorder: Treatment, Management and Prevention. Leicester, UK, British Psychological Society, 2010

New AS, Hazlett EA, Newmark RE, et al: Laboratory induced aggression: a positron emission tomography study of aggressive individuals with borderline personality disorder. Biol Psychiatry 66(12):1107–1114, 2009 19748078

Newhill CE, Eack SM, Mulvey EP: Violent behavior in borderline personality. J Pers Disord 23(6):541–554, 2009 20001173

Oldham JM: DSM models of personality disorders. Curr Opin Psychol 21:86–88, 2017 29065382

Pasion R, Fernandes C, Pereira MR, et al: Antisocial behaviour and psychopathy: uncovering the externalizing link in the P3 modulation. Neurosci Biobehav Rev March 22, 2017 [Epub ahead of print] 28342766

Patrick CJ: Physiological correlates of psychopathy, antisocial personality disorder, habitual aggression, and violence. Curr Top Behav Neurosci 21:197–227, 2014 25129139

Raza GT, DeMarce JM, Lash SJ, et al: Paranoid personality disorder in the United States: the role of race, illicit drug use, and income. J Ethn Subst Abuse 13(3):247–257, 2014 25176118

Reed GM, First MB, Elena Medina-Mora M, et al: Draft diagnostic guidelines for ICD-11 mental and behavioural disorders available for review and comment. World Psychiatry 15(2):112–113, 2016 27265692

Rinne T, van den Brink W, Wouters L, et al: SSRI treatment of borderline personality disorder: a randomized, placebo-controlled clinical trial for female patients with borderline personality disorder. Am J Psychiatry 159(12):2048–2054, 2002 12450955

Ruocco AC: The neuropsychology of borderline personality disorder: a meta-analysis and review. Psychiatry Res 137(3):191–202, 2005 16297985

Russell TD, King AR: Distrustful, conventional, entitled, and dysregulated: PID-5 personality facets predict hostile masculinity and sexual violence in community men. J Interpers Violence January 1, 2017 [Epub ahead of print] 29294638

Salzman C, Wolfson AN, Schatzberg A, et al: Effect of fluoxetine on anger in symptomatic volunteers with borderline personality disorder. J Clin Psychopharmacol 15(1):23–29, 1995 7714224

Schulze L, Schmahl C, Niedtfeld I: Neural correlates of disturbed emotion processing in borderline personality disorder: a multimodal meta-analysis. Biol Psychiatry 79(2):97–106, 2016 25935068

Scott LN, Wright AGC, Beeney JE, et al: Borderline personality disorder symptoms and aggression: a within-person process model. J Abnorm Psychol 126(4):429–440, 2017 28383936

Simpson EB, Yen S, Costello E, et al: Combined dialectical behavior therapy and fluoxetine in the treatment of borderline personality disorder. J Clin Psychiatry 65(3):379–385, 2004 15096078

Soloff PH, George A, Nathan RS, et al: Paradoxical effects of amitriptyline on borderline patients. Am J Psychiatry 143(12):1603–1605, 1986 3538914

Soloff PH, Cornelius J, George A, et al: Efficacy of phenelzine and haloperidol in borderline personality disorder. Arch Gen Psychiatry 50(5):377–385, 1993 8489326

Soloff PH, Chiappetta L, Mason NS, et al: Effects of serotonin-2A receptor binding and gender on personality traits and suicidal behavior in borderline personality disorder. Psychiatry Res 222(3):140–148, 2014 24751216

Soloff PH, Abraham K, Burgess A, et al: Impulsivity and aggression mediate regional brain responses in borderline personality disorder: an fMRI study. Psychiatry Res 260:76–85, 2017 28039797

Stern A: Psychoanalytic investigation of and therapy in the border line group of neuroses. Psychoanalytic Quarterly 7(4), 1938

Stoffers J, Völlm BA, Rücker G, et al: Pharmacological interventions for borderline personality disorder. Cochrane Database Syst Rev (6):CD005653, 2010 20556762

Tardiff K, Marzuk PM, Leon AC, et al: A prospective study of violence by psychiatric patients after hospital discharge. Psychiatr Serv 48(5):678–681, 1997 9144823

Tritt K, Nickel C, Lahmann C, et al: Lamotrigine treatment of aggression in female borderline-patients: a randomized, double-blind, placebo-controlled study. J Psychopharmacol 19(3):287–291, 2005 15888514

Vitaro F, Brendgen M: Proactive and reactive aggression: a developmental perspective, in Developmental Origins of Aggression. Edited by Tremblay RE, Hartup WW, Archer J. New York, Guilford, 2005, pp 178–201

Weitkamp K, Daniels JK, Romer G, et al: Psychoanalytic psychotherapy for children and adolescents with severe externalizing psychopathology: an effectiveness trial. Z Psychosom Med Psychother 63(3):251–266, 2017 28974184

Witt SH, Streit F, Jungkunz M, et al; Bipolar Disorders Working Group of the Psychiatric Genomics Consortium; Major Depressive Disorder Working Group of the Psychiatric Genomics Consortium; Schizophrenia Working Group of the Psychiatric Genomics Consortium: Genome-wide association study of borderline personality disorder reveals genetic overlap with bipolar disorder, major depression and schizophrenia. Transl Psychiatry 7(6):e1155, 2017 28632202

Young S, Hopkin G, Perkins D, et al: A controlled trial of a cognitive skills program for personality-disordered offenders. J Atten Disord 17(7):598–607, 2013 22308561

Zanarini MC, Temes CM, Ivey AM, et al: The 10-year course of adult aggression toward others in patients with borderline personality disorder and Axis II comparison subjects. Psychiatry Res 252:134–138, 2017 28264784

Legal and Forensic Aspects of Aggression

Michael Greenage, D.O.
Robert L. Trestman, Ph.D., M.D.

When aggression is looked at in the context of mental illness, forensic and legal issues relate largely to risk assessment and the prediction of violence. The risk assessment of violence plays out legally in a number of ways, including sentencing and parole issues, as well as involuntary civil commitment. Despite much evidence to the contrary, the fact that the legal system anticipates that psychiatrists and psychologists can reliably and consistently assess violence has had a profound impact on our civil and criminal justice systems. The nature of this impact has shaped these systems and affects individual patients and the clinicians involved in their assessment or treatment.

In this chapter, we examine some of the complex issues relating to legal and forensic aspects of aggression and risk assessment. We begin with a discussion about forensic implications of aggression classifications and then turn to the implications of assessment within a legal and forensic framework. *Tarasoff* and derivative rulings are subsequently examined, as are several legal precedents relating to risk assessment and the tools commonly used. We conclude the chapter with a few key clinical points to take away for everyday use.

Overview of Aggression From Forensic and Legal Perspectives

Broadly, and from a forensic point of view, aggression can be thought as having two, relatively orthogonal facets: impulsive/affective aggression and predatory/psychopathic aggression (McDermott and Holoyda 2014). Impulsive/affective aggression is often reactive in nature and results from an inability to control one's response to a provocation. As such, impulsive/affective aggression may speak to the presence of a mental illness, such as intermittent explosive disorder (IED), a personality disorder, or other disorders discussed in this volume. In contrast, predatory/psychopathic aggression is typically characterized as planned or instrumental, such that the aggressor is initiating a series of events (typically one in which the aggression is believed to bring about a tangible benefit) rather than simply responding to the actions of others. As such, predatory/psychopathic aggression can be characterized as "purposeful, controlled, and unemotional" (Quanbeck et al. 2007), and is seen as an indicator of social deviancy or even potentially sociopathy. Thus, it is not surprising that impulsive/affective aggression is more prevalent on inpatient psychiatric wards and that predatory/psychopathic aggression is more common in correctional facilities.

A third type of aggression has been described as well, which arises as a result of psychosis (see Chapter 5, "Aggression in Primary Psychotic Disorders," in this volume). A popular framework for considering psychosis and the potential for aggression is the concept of *threat/control override* (TCO). The work, originally conceptualized by Link and Stueve (1994), posited that one explanation for violence occurring in some psychotic patients and not others was related to TCO, a set of personality traits relating to psychosis. Individuals with a TCO disturbance perceive either a threat that could inflict harm on them or a threat that controls the individual's behaviors. Several studies have suggested that the emotional reactions to positive symptoms, anger especially, are more related to aggressive behaviors than are the emotional reactions to control symptoms (Nederlof et al. 2011; Stompe et al. 2004).

On a day-to-day basis, dealing with aggressive patients on an inpatient psychiatric unit is commonplace. The experience of assessing the risk these patients pose is vastly different from formal forensic assessments or expert testimony. It should be emphasized that from a legal/forensic point of view, many of the risk assessment tools require trained users and are validated for specific populations. Quanbeck et al. (2007) looked at categorizing aggression in a state hospital using a three-armed schema of impulsive, predatory, and psychotic types. They found that 54% of aggressive patients were impulsive and that, notably, impulsive aggression most often targeted staff rather than other patients. One possible explanation for this finding is that anger appears to be a driving element of the TCO. Accordingly, because staff set limits and are in positions of authority, this power differential could be influencing the focus of the aggressive behavior of psychotic patients.

Although not a precise delineation, predatory aggression may most often be found within the criminal or correctional justice systems, whereas psychotic aggression is more likely to be found in traditional mental health settings. Impulsive/affective aggression may be encountered in either setting depending on circumstances. If the psychotic aggressive patient is found in the justice system, and aggression is the cause of the instant offense, an insanity defense or psychosis as mitigation at sentencing may be a consideration. Such issues are not within the traditional mental health arena. Though it is not uncommon to have a mental health professional provide insight into the potential role of psychosis as it relates to an offense, *insanity* is a legal, rather than a psychiatric, construct, and as such any mitigation of an offense is determined by a court of law.

It should also be noted that no typology is perfect. A patient's behavior may well fit into more than one box and, indeed, may cross over into different categories depending on the details. Patients can exhibit aggressive behavior both out of anger and in an attempt to secure some tangible gain. An example of this would be an abuser committing acts of aggression against his or her spouse both as a result of frustration and as a means of asserting control. Patients can also show both psychotic and predatory aggression. A good example of this is Theodore Kaczynski, the so-called Unabomber, who was diagnosed with paranoid schizophrenia and convicted of multiple predatory homicides and attempted homicides. This characterization is also salient in the selection of violence risk assessment tools, as each risk assessment tool is optimized for subsets of behavioral types.

Approach to the Evaluation of Aggression in a Forensic Context

Risk assessment itself has two broad types: unstructured and structured. In actual clinical practice, only a very small number of clinicians utilize structured risk assessment tools. Elbogen et al. (2002) demonstrated that of 134 clinicians surveyed who do use such assessments, most indicated a clear preference for directly observable "behavioral and dynamic" variables over more actuarial "research variables" from the Violence Risk Appraisal Guide (VRAG) and Historical Clinical Risk Management–20 (HCR-20) tools. This finding is in contrast to the court's view of risk assessment, which often considers the use of structured risk assessment tools as a prerequisite for admissibility. There is good reason for this. For example, after examining 136 empirical studies comparing actuarial with clinical prediction, Grove and Meehl (1996) came to the overwhelming conclusion that actuarial tools were superior. Notably these authors went on to state, "We know of no social science controversy for which the empirical studies are so numerous, varied, and consistent as this one" (p. 322). It should be highlighted that Virginia adopted a requirement of a named structured assessment tool in the civil commitment of sexually violent individuals in 1993.

There are a multitude of violence risk assessment tools available, notably the revised Hare Psychopathy Checklist—Revised (PCL-R), the Classification of Violence Risk (COVR), and the HCR-20, among others. A meta-analysis of nine different risk assessment instruments demonstrated that those tools were able to reliably separate (95% confidence interval) risk of violence in high-risk versus low-risk groups (Singh et al. 2013). Such actuarial tools have a clarity and lack of bias that lend themselves to the courtroom.

Assessments Targeting Impulsive/Affective Aggression

The HCR-20, a risk assessment tool developed by Webster et al. and first published in 1997 that has had several revisions since then, is a

20-item list that looks at historical, clinical, and risk management factors (Webster et al. 1997a, 1997b). Of note, the Clinical subscale of HCR-20 showed a strong relationship with long-term impulsive aggression. The HCR-20 has been utilized and validated in multiple settings with a variety of populations, including incarcerated offenders (Belfrage et al. 2000) and civilly committed psychiatric inpatients (Nicholls et al. 2004).

When a violence risk assessment is being conducted, it is important to distinguish aspects of impulsivity from aggression. One common tool for doing so is the Barratt Impulsiveness Scale (BIS). Developed in 1959, this 30-item questionnaire is one of the most commonly used assessments of impulsivity. Swogger et al. (2015) reported that a tendency toward premeditated aggression was predictive of violent recidivism. Further, they argued that impulsive aggression did not predict violent recidivism. Most interestingly, these authors found that impulsive and premeditated aggression often coexist. Stanford et al. (2009) reviewed the literature on the BIS-11 across multiple domains and generally concluded that the BIS-11 might be considered "a standard point of reference" for assessment of impulsivity.

Assessments for Predatory Aggression

Predatory aggression, a substantial issue within the justice system, can be assessed with several different instruments. The PCL-R, a 90- to 120-minute interview developed by Robert Hare, has been used extensively to predict the risk for criminal re-offense and the probability of rehabilitation (Hare 2003). The PCL-R has 20 items that assess different aspects of psychopathy. Hare describes four "facets" in the PCL-R: interpersonal traits, affective deficits, characteristics of lifestyle, and socially deviant behaviors. These facets span two "factors." Factor 1 facets suggest a primary psychopathology that is causing the undesirable behavior. Factor 2 facets suggest that the behaviors are consequential to a primary issue, such as poor impulse control or trouble regulating emotions. Notably, affective aspects present are not characterized, and thus for assessing affectively driven aggression, this tool may not be optimal. The PCL-R is commonly used in the criminal justice system to predict risks of failure in the context of parole and probation.

Another actuarial tool, the VRAG, published in 1993 (Quinsey et al. 1998), uses 12 factors, including the PCL-R, to predict the likelihood of aggression and recidivism at time of parole among mentally disordered and criminal inmates. The 12 items assessed are 1) living with both biological parents to age 16, 2) a history of maladjustment in elementary school, 3) alcohol problems, 4) marital status at the time of the index offense, 5) nonviolent criminal history before the index offense, 6) failure of a prior conditional release, 7) age at the time of the index offense, 8) the extent of injury of the index victim, 9) whether the victim of the index offense was female, 10) presence of a personality disorder, 11) a diagnosis of schizophrenia, and 12) PCL-R score. None of these tools have a high positive predictive value individually. They are best used in combination together with clinical judgment; this has indeed become the standard of care.

The Static-99 is a frequently used assessment of violence. Developed by Hanson and Thornton, it is used with male sex offenders at the time of release into the community to assess future risk of sexual violence (Hanson and Thornton 2000). The Static-99 includes 10 items: 1) age at time of release, 2) having ever lived with a lover for at least 2 years, 3) past convictions for nonsexual violence, 4) current conviction (index) for nonsexual violence, 5) past sexual offenses, 6) past sentencing, 7) past convictions for noncontact sexual offenses, 8) past victims being unrelated, 9) past victims being stranger, and 10) past victims being male. The Static-99 is widely applied as a risk assessment tool, with more than 60 replications in a variety of settings, and has demonstrated moderate predictive value (Helmus et al. 2009).

Limitations of Current Assessments of Violence Risk

Each violence risk assessment instrument has strengths and limitations. For all instruments administered by clinicians (or trained professionals), fidelity to the validated procedure and population is critical but often lacking in real-world settings (Singh et al. 2011). The VRAG is interesting in its limitation because it is a purely actuarial tool; that is, it does not allow for any clinical review of the results produced. Additionally, it was developed for male offenders, and its extrapolation to other populations should be considered cautiously. McDermott et al. (2008) reported that when they examined data collected about aggressive patients in an inpatient setting, only Factor 3 of the PCL-R (i.e., lifestyle characteristics) was higher in aggressive patients. This makes sense given that many inpatients have unstable circumstances. Complicating this, the clinical environment itself may contribute to increases in the rate of certain types of aggression. Daffern et al. (2004) posited that living in close quarters contributes to elevations in certain rating scales of aggression and that this is not captured by pure psychopathy.

Additionally, the time course of the prediction is important when one is considering which instrument to use. Inpatient community psychiatric facilities are typically most concerned with near-future violence (i.e., days or weeks), whereas a correctional facility may be interested in risk for violence in the ensuing months or years when probation of a sexual offender is being considered.

In a recent paper, Large and Nielssen (2017) identified a key issue with actuarial risk assessment that also reasonably applies to structured clinical judgment risk assessments. They considered the question of usefulness once risk has been stratified; that is, is it reasonable to intervene by treating all those at high risk for violence (true and false positives)? This treatment ideology must also justify not treating individuals in the low-risk category, even though they are known to contribute to some of the total amount of violence. Additionally, there is concern that rates of violence scored on various structured risk assessment tools show marked variance and as such should be used cautiously when interventions based on those assessments are being considered.

In addition, one must consider the results from the MacArthur Violence Risk Assessment Study (Monahan et al. 2005). From 1992 to 1995, 951 patients from various inpatient units were followed every 10 weeks after discharge. This group was compared with a community group of people, randomly chosen, living in Pittsburgh. Broadly, the study concluded that mentally ill patients were no more dangerous than the general population. Torrey et al. (2008), reassessing those findings 10 years later, argued several points about the initial conclusions. Of note, they pointed out that the sample population did not include any patients in forensic hospitals, jails, or prisons. The majority of risk assessment studies are conducted within the criminal justice system, and using these risk assessment tools within the context of the general population may not produce meaningful results. A related criticism by Torrey et al. was related to the association of treatment adherence and reduction in violence. Torrey et al. pointed out that one possible explanation is that patients who are amenable to treatment compliance are those less likely to be violent and that the intervention itself may not explain the result. This is something that should be considered when mandated outpatient therapy is ordered, if part of the expectation is a reduction in aggression.

Duty to Warn

One thing common to all forms of risk assessment is that it has the potential to bring into play a mental health professional's duty to warn other of potential harm. At its core, the drivers necessitating violence risk assessment are intended to give objective weight to decisions relating to disposition, whether that be release from a hospital, at sentencing, or at a parole hearing. The duty to warn has become a complex and sophisticated concern that has become more codified over the last several decades.

One of the most difficult and consequential aspects of caring for the mentally ill who are deemed dangerous is the legality tied up in that issue. The legacy of the 1976 *Tarasoff* ruling and the impact of this ruling on decision making, violence risk assessment, and liability are still very much felt today.

In brief, the case of *Tarasoff v. Regents of the University of California* (1976) changed how the law views risk, and subsequently how practitioners manage risk. Prior to the *Tarasoff* ruling, much was made of the predictive acumen of the day as it related to confinement. Interestingly, in the *Tarasoff* brief, the psychiatrists and psychologists made it a point to talk about their inability to reliably predict violence and argued that they were therefore not liable for mismanaging the care of patient Poddar.

Perhaps the most salient point to come out of the *Tarasoff* case was the idea that while under common law "one person owed no duty to control the conduct of another" (Harper and Kime 1934), an exception was made because of the existence of a special relationship, that of the treating physician or therapist to a patient who needs to be "controlled." Within the purview of California's section 315 of the Restatement Second of Torts (*Tarasoff*), although the psychologist in the *Tarasoff* case had no special relationship with the victim, the duty owed to her came from the relationship of the therapist and the patient; in other words, a third party. The California Supreme Court also discussed ways to discharge that duty: by warning the victims, contacting law enforcement, or "protecting" the potential victims.

The *Tarasoff* ruling had echoes in every state. Most states have not taken the *Tarasoff* ruling verbatim, but rather have taken pieces of it and tried to place limits on those various pieces (Lake 1994). One of those pieces is that of the issue of an identifiable potential victim. Again, in California, in the case of *Thompson v. County of Alameda* (1980), a man had threatened an unidentified victim in a neighborhood, and when a child was killed, a suit was brought; ultimately, the California Supreme Court ruled that because the potential victim was a public group of potential victims, there was no duty to warn (California Government Code Section: 820.2, 1963). In the case of *Lipari v. Sears Roebuck, Co.* (1980), a federal court upheld just the opposite. In that case, the court looked at the fact that a practitioner could have reasonably foreseen that a group was at risk to become potential victims, even if those victims were not specifically and individually identifiable.

In similar fashion, the question of identifying a potential victim is another sequela of the ruling that has manifested in courtrooms. In the case of *Shaw v. Glickman* (1980), a man released from a psychiatric hospital shot the lover of his wife. The man who was shot brought suit and argued that the psychiatric team had a duty to warn him of both the patient's violent tendencies and his release from the hospital. The shooter had never voiced to the treatment team his intentions, and so the Maryland appellate court ruled there was no duty to warn because no threats had been voiced. Further, it would have been a violation of the patient's confidentiality to warn the victim and discuss anything related to his mental health.

Clearly, one of the more practical issues arising from a duty to warn is the sheer volume of reporting that would occur if every threat or potential threat were called to potential victims or law enforcement. Given the various interpretations in case law, most states have taken care to try and place parameters around what constitutes risk and obligation. For example, many states have statutes that define concepts such as "imminent risk" and the "likelihood" that the threat could be carried out. Threatening to kill a specific person "one day" or "a thousand years from now" can generally be thought of as either not imminent or not believable. Means, their availability, and their believability are also practical considerations in many states. If a patient threatens to build a nuclear bomb but has no access to fissionable material, such a threat may be considered unbelievable, or at least unlikely. A patient who speaks about using his rifle at home to kill his neighbor when he gets out of the hospital and who is known to have a weapon at home and a history of known contention with his neighbor presents a very different risk. Further complicating issues, many states (e.g., Texas among others) reject the *Tarasoff* ruling outright, stating that psychiatrists and psychologists "may" warn or "are not required" to warn (Soulier et al. 2010).

So, what are we to do? There is no clear algorithmic consensus about when to warn. An interesting problem that arises as a consequence is the notion of whether formal informed consent exists regarding our potential obligation to satisfy a duty to care. What happens when a practitioner violates confidentiality to warn but the threat is later determined not to be sufficient to have demanded disclosure? For example, suppose that as part of an evaluation of any patient, the practitioner discusses with the patient the fact that confidentiality is not absolute and explains what limits exist specifically upon it. What happens to rapport and trust? Could a situation be created whereby patients no longer disclose those threats? This is an ongoing concern, since an evaluation of any patient is expected to discuss disclosure and the limitations thereof.

The other mechanism practitioners have for protecting people from violent patients is to confine those patients. Many physicians working in acute care settings report direct experiences with violent mentally ill patients (Bourget et al. 2002). This is in stark contrast with the fact that the majority of mentally ill patients are not violent. One way to reconcile these ideas is to look at how civil commitment pushes only those at the highest risk of violence into the acute care settings. Indeed, several studies looking at factors of aggression in acute care settings found that a multitude of factors that relate mostly to the environment (Katz and Kirkland 1990), such as milieu, patient density, and amount and structure of activities, have more in common with violence than simply having a mental illness. The question that then arises is: Are practitioners committing dangerous people because they are mentally ill, or are practitioners committing mentally ill people who are dangerous? Of note, in Swanson's (1994) study using data from the Epidemiologic Catchment Area Study, the increase in attributable risk for violence due to the presence of a mental disorder was only 4.3%.

The Daubert Standard: Scientific Evidence in Court Cases

Clinical assessment of risk has repercussions for a patient clinically as well as legally. A brief review of *Daubert v. Merrell Dow Pharmaceuticals* (1993) provides a constructive framework for examining both of these ideas. In *Daubert*, the plaintiff alleged that a product made by Merrell Dow resulted in certain birth defects. Merrell Dow argued that epidemiology was the standard of review for birth defects and that no studies existed demonstrating them. The plaintiff brought several research experts who argued a different way of analyzing the data, and their testimony was rejected. The U.S. Supreme Court, in its ruling, created a legal standard of the courts being the arbiters of the admissibility of scientific evidence. Put another way, the decision brought into question why a court should believe an expert's testimony. Even with this fallout, many courts still give heavy weight to an expert's testimony. To date, many jurisdictions do not demand high standards of scientific support for expert testimony, and still rely on the opinion of the testifying psychiatrist as derived from the Frye "general acceptance" test (Calhoun 2008).

Another legal aspect of violence assessment is its relationship to the insanity defense. It is important to recognize that *insanity defense* is a legal term, not a clinical one, and does not in any way suggest a clinical diagnosis. Moreover, there are different definitions of insanity, in its legal usage, varying from state to state. Common language is "did not possess a will sufficient," "unable to appreciate the nature of," or "lacked capacity to appreciate." It is important to note that the presence of a psychiatric disorder is itself insufficient grounds for an insanity defense. It is also important to note that competency to stand trial is not synonymous with being found insane at the time of an offense.

Clinical Vignette

A useful lens through which to view the legal issues surrounding violence assessment and its ramifications is the 2007 Virginia Tech shooting:

> On April 16, 2007, Seung-Hui Cho shot and killed 32 people and injured nearly as many more. At the time of the shooting, Virginia had a standard of involuntary civil commitment that was far narrower than that of many other states. Prior to 2007 and the review that followed the shooting, "imminent danger" was the standard used to identify when an individual is a candidate for involuntary civil commitment.
>
> In this case, Cho had been identified by a prescreener at the Virginia Tech Police Department as being in imminent danger. He was brought to a nearby hospital and assessed by an independent examiner to not be at imminent risk. The treating psychiatrist also reported that Cho was not an imminent risk. At the initial hearing to determine if Cho should be hospitalized against his wishes, the special justice did find Cho to be an imminent danger but deemed that outpatient treatment was the least restrictive alternative to involuntary inpatient hospitalization.

Discussion of Vignette

This tragic event led to a series of legislative debates and proposals that were presented to the Virginia governor, Tim Kaine. Following the review of the then current standards, the governor signed legislation that broadened the scope for involuntary civil commitment from "imminent danger" to "a substantial likelihood" and "significant risk" "in the near future" (VA. Civ. Code § 37.2–81).

Prior to the changes to the scope of involuntary civil commitment laws in Virginia, it was in some respects harder to commit an individual, but there was also a marked difference in Virginia's gun laws relative to federal gun laws. Virginia had placed itself in a position that protecting the potentially violent mentally ill was harder compared with other states, while having a gun policy that made it easier to acquire firearms. The importance of the relationships and ramifications of mental health laws as they relate to the potential for violence to other political and legal issues cannot be stressed enough.

Taking a closer look at involuntary civil commitment, one obvious intent of these laws, however enacted, is to treat mentally ill individuals who may not themselves be able to identify their need of treatment. That said, the other use of involuntary civil commitment is an extension into "duty to protect." Due process is guaranteed under the Fourteenth Amendment for anyone undergoing involuntary civil commitment. Likewise, someone with mental illness cannot be committed for an unspecified period of time. The "standard of proof" as it pertains to involuntary civil commitment was fleshed out fully in *Addington v. Texas* (1979). In this case, the U.S. Supreme Court, understanding that the criminal standard of proof of "beyond a reasonable doubt" was impractical given the difficulty with precision in psychiatric medicine, opted for the language of "clear and convincing evidence" to satisfy due process (*Addington v. Texas* 1979).

The movement away from "imminent risk" toward a probability or likelihood in many states speaks to the need to identify those in need of help before they become dangerous in the moment. "Imminent risk" does not lend itself to societal needs of predicting risk and addressing it beforehand. Returning to Cho, there were a plethora of events that strongly suggested Cho's likelihood for potential violence. However, the "imminent risk" language of involuntary civil commitment only allowed the court to address his state at the time. Balancing this is the language of "least restrictive means," and there has been much controversy over the balancing of the rights of the mentally ill (or not) patient and the safety of society. A standardized risk assessment tool, given in the context of a psychiatric evaluation, can ensure that dangerousness as part of civil commitment is being evaluated without bias. Rather than opinions being offered to the court, data from a risk assessment tool may be better suited in the context of a civil commitment.

Summary

The expectations for evaluations within the forensic setting are unique and very different from those in the general clinical arena. Many individuals working in this area require specific training to make reliable forensic assessments. Many have only been studied within the scope of correctional/forensic settings, and results may not be verifiable or relatable to a standard inpatient setting. A clear understanding of what is being asked, the relevant legal standards, and the body of relating case law are paramount in being able to conduct an appropriate forensic evaluation. Lastly, we as a profession are expected—by our patients, their families, our peers, society at large, and the justice system—to be able to conduct meaningful and accurate assessments of risk of aggression. While many clinicians on the frontlines of medicine feel that clinical, unstructured interviews yield the best assessment of risk, the research consistently shows that structured risk assessments have more validity than unstructured assessments.

Key Clinical Points

- Structured assessments are better than unstructured.
- Even the best structured assessments are limited, and fidelity to the original design and use is required.
- The legal and forensic management of aggression is modulated by the type (impulsive/affective, predatory/psychopathic, psychotic) and severity of the violence.
- When conducting legal assessments, the examiner should be clear about the questions to be addressed; this will in turn guide the structured assessments to be used and the extent of the clinical assessment to be pursued.

References

Addington v Texas, 441 U.S. 418, 1979

Belfrage H, Fransson R, Strand S: Prediction of violence using the HCR-20: a prospective study in two maximum-security correctional institutions. J Forensic Psychiatry 11(1):167–175, 2000

Bourget D, el-Guebaly N, Atkinson MJ: Assessing and managing violent patients. CPA Bull 34:25–27, 2002

Calhoun MC: Scientific evidence in court: Daubert or Frye, 15 years later. Legal Backgrounder 23(37):1–4, 2008

Daffern M, Mayer MM, Martin T: Environmental contributors to aggression in two forensic hospitals. Int J Forensic Ment Health 3:105–114, 2004

Daubert v Merrell Dow Pharmaceuticals, Inc 509 U.S. 579, 1993

Elbogen E, Calkins CM, Scalora M, et al: Perceived relevance of factors for violence risk assessment: a survey of clinicians. Int J Forensic Ment Health 1:37–47, 2002

Grove WM, Meehl PE: Comparative efficiency of informal (subjective, impressionistic) and formal (mechanical, algorithmic) prediction procedures: the clinical–statistical controversy, 2. Psychology, Public Policy, and Law 2(2):293–323, 1996

Hanson RK, Thornton D: Improving risk assessments for sex offenders: a comparison of three actuarial scales. Law Hum Behav 24(1):119–136, 2000 10693322

Hare RD: Manual for the Revised Psychopathy Checklist, 2nd Edition. Toronto, ON, Canada, Multi-Health Systems, 2003

Harper FV, Kime PM: The duty to control the conduct of another. Yale Law Journal 43(6):886–905, 1934

Helmus L, Hanson RK, Thornton D: Reporting Static-99 in light of new research on recidivism norms. Forum 21(1):38–45, 2009

Katz P, Kirkland FR: Violence and social structure on mental hospital wards. Psychiatry 53(3):262 277, 1990 2217651

Lake PF: Revisiting Tarasoff. Alabama Law Review 58:97–111, 1994

Large M, Nielssen O: The limitations and future of violence risk assessment. World Psychiatry 16(1):25–26, 2017 28127932

Link BG, Stueve A: Psychotic symptoms and the violent/illegal behavior of mental patients compared to community controls, in Violence and Mental Disorder: Developments in Risk Assessment. The John D and Catherine T MacArthur Foundation Series on Mental Health Development. Edited by Monahan J, Steadman HJ. Chicago, IL, University of Chicago Press, 1994, pp 137–159

Lipari v Sears, Roebuck and Co., 497 F. Supp. 185 (D. Neb. 1980)

McDermott BE, Holoyda BJ: Assessment of aggression in inpatient settings. CNS Spectr 19(5):425–431, 2014 25296966

McDermott BE, Quanbeck CD, Busse D, et al: The accuracy of risk assessment instruments in the prediction of impulsive versus predatory aggression. Behav Sci Law 26(6):759–777, 2008 19039802

Monahan J, Steadman HJ, Robbins PC, et al: An actuarial model of violence risk assessment for persons with mental disorders. Psychiatr Serv 56(7):810–815, 2005 16020812

Nederlof AF, Muris P, Hovens JE: Threat/control-override symptoms and emotional reactions to positive symptoms as correlates of aggressive behavior in psychotic patients. J Nerv Ment Dis 199(5):342–347, 2011 21543954

Nicholls TL, Ogloff JR, Douglas KS: Assessing risk for violence among male and female civil psychiatric patients: the HCR-20, PCL:SV, and VSC. Behav Sci Law 22(1):127–158, 2004 14963884

Quanbeck CD, McDermott BE, Lam J, et al: Categorization of aggressive acts committed by chronically assaultive state hospital patients. Psychiatr Serv 58(4):521–528, 2007 17412855

Quinsey VL, Harris GT, Rice ME, et al: Violent Offenders: Appraising and Managing Risk. Washington, DC, American Psychological Association, 1998

Shaw v Glickman, 45 Md., 1980

Singh JP, Grann M, Fazel S: A comparative study of violence risk assessment tools: a systematic review and metaregression analysis of 68 studies involving 25,980 participants. Clin Psychol Rev 31(3):499–513, 2011

Singh JP, Grann M, Fazel S: Authorship bias in violence risk assessment? A systematic review and meta-analysis. PLoS One 8(9):e72484, 2013 24023744

Soulier MF, Maislen A, Beck JC: Status of the psychiatric duty to protect, circa 2006. J Am Acad Psychiatry Law 38(4):457–473, 2010 21156904

Stanford MS, Mathias CW, Dougherty DM, et al: Fifty years of the Barratt Impulsiveness Scale: an update and review. Pers Ind Diff 47(5):385–395, 2009

Stompe T, Ortwein-Swoboda G, Schanda H: Schizophrenia, delusional symptoms, and violence: the threat/control override concept reexamined. Schizophr Bull 30(1):31–44, 2004 15176760

Swanson JW: Mental disorder, substance abuse, and community violence: an epidemiological approach, in Violence and Mental Disorder: Developments in Risk Assessment. The John D. and Catherine T. MacArthur Foundation Series on Mental Health and Development. Edited by Monahan J, Steadman HJ. Chicago, IL, University of Chicago Press, 1994, pp 101–136

Swogger MT, Walsh Z, Christie M, et al: Impulsive versus premeditated aggression in the prediction of violent criminal recidivism. Aggress Behav 41(4):346–352, 2015 25043811

Tarasoff v Regents of the University of California, 17 Cal. 3d 425, 551 P.2d 334, 131Cal. Rptr. 14 (Cal. 1976)

Thompson v County of Alameda, 27 Cal.3d 741, 1980

Torrey EF, Stanley J, Monahan J, et al: The MacArthur Violence Risk Assessment Study revisited: two views ten years after its initial publication. Psychiatr Serv 59(2):147–152, 2008 18245156

Webster CD, Douglas KS, Eaves D, et al: Assessing risk of violence to others, in Impulsivity: Theory, Assessment, and Treatment. Edited by Webster CD, Jackson MA. New York, Guilford, 1997a, pp 251–277

Webster C, Douglas K, Eaves D, et al: HCR-20: Assessing Risk for Violence (Version 2). Vancouver, BC, Canada, Simon Fraser University, 1997b

Index

Page numbers printed in **boldface** type refer to tables. Page numbers followed by *n* refer to note numbers.